Probability, Statistics and Modeling in Public Health

Probability, Statistics and Modeling in Public Health

Editor: Phillis Cousins

hayle medical
New York

Hayle Medical,
750 Third Avenue, 9th Floor,
New York, NY 10017, USA

Visit us on the World Wide Web at:
www.haylemedical.com

ISBN 978-1-64647-589-6 (Hardback)

Cataloging-in-publication Data

Probability, statistics and modeling in public health / edited by Phillis Cousins.
p. cm.
Includes bibliographical references and index.
ISBN 978-1-64647-589-6
1. Public health--Statistical methods. 2. Medical statistics.
3. Public health--Mathematical models. 4. Probability measures.
5. Probabilities. I. Cousins, Phillis.
RA409 .P76 2023
610.727--dc23

Contents

Preface

This book was inspired by the evolution of our times; to answer the curiosity of inquisitive minds. Many developments have occurred across the globe in the recent past which has transformed the progress in the field.

Public health is an interdisciplinary field that draws from fields such as epidemiology, biostatistics, social sciences, and management of health services. The primary aims of public health include preventing disease, prolonging life and promoting health. The objectives of public health can be achieved through organized efforts and choices made by society, public and private organizations, communities, and individuals. The study of public health also involves the role of environmental health, community health, behavioral health, health economics, public policy, mental health, health education, health politics, occupational safety, disability, oral health, and reproductive health. The pivotal role of public health is to inform, educate, and empower people about the various health-related problems and their resolutions. This can be performed by assessing current services, ascertaining the requirements of health professionals, and supporting decision making in health care. This book is compiled in such a manner, that it will provide an in-depth knowledge about public health as well as the application of probability, statistics and modeling in this field. It is appropriate for those seeking detailed information in this area of study.

This book was developed from a mere concept to drafts to chapters and finally compiled together as a complete text to benefit the readers across all nations. To ensure the quality of the content we instilled two significant steps in our procedure. The first was to appoint an editorial team that would verify the data and statistics provided in the book and also select the most appropriate and valuable contributions from the plentiful contributions we received from authors worldwide. The next step was to appoint an expert of the topic as the Editor-in-Chief, who would head the project and finally make the necessary amendments and modifications to make the text reader-friendly. I was then commissioned to examine all the material to present the topics in the most comprehensible and productive format.

I would like to take this opportunity to thank all the contributing authors who were supportive enough to contribute their time and knowledge to this project. I also wish to convey my regards to my family who have been extremely supportive during the entire project.

Editor

Part 1
Methodological, Conceptual and Theoretical Context

1

Multilevel Analysis of Public Health and Health Services Research: An Overview

Abstract In this chapter we describe in general terms what we mean by the equivalent terms multilevel analysis (MLA) or multilevel modelling. We place MLA in the context of public health and health services research. Most of our readers will be working in this field, and this book is specifically written for them. As public health and health services research is an applied research, it is strongly oriented towards solving practical problems in health, healthcare and health policy. Therefore we will also discuss the relationships between research on the one hand and policy and practice on the other. We end with some conclusions on the relevance of MLA for public health and health services research.

Keywords Multilevel analysis · Public health research · Health services research · Health policy · Health system organisation · Inequalities in health

The fact that we are willing to consider 'Health in context' means that people's health depends on the context in which they live. This is a basic credo of social medicine and public health (Rosen 1993). Not only health and well-being but also health behaviour and healthcare utilisation depend partly on people's personal resources and partly on shared resources and circumstances—in other words, their context. People's personal resources can be their personal stock of health—their health capital in other words—as well as other more tangible resources. So if we talk about health, we are implicitly talking about two distinct levels: people and their context.

MLA makes it possible to handle this reality of health operating at different levels. Although MLA is a statistical method, it would be too narrow to restrict the teaching of multilevel modelling to statistical methods courses. Statistics is a tool to solve problems, so the methods should not be seen to be isolated from the problems themselves. In other words, if we want to understand MLA, we should also pay attention to the substantive fields of public health and health services research and to the origins of their research problems. Moreover, in sociology, a lot of attention has been paid to the relationships between different levels, from the micro level of individual people, via intermediate levels of families, schools and work organisations, to the macro social levels of cities or countries. Social science helps us to conceptualise these different levels and to decide which levels are relevant for certain research problems. Therefore, it is not only statistics that we will be dealing with in this book; theoretical considerations about levels and about human behaviour in context are equally important. We should add a third pillar to this book: study design and methodology. Between theory and statistics stand the study design and methodology—the way we design our research and collect data to test our theoretical ideas.

Importance of MLA for Research in Health and Care

MLA is important for research in the fields of public health and healthcare for two reasons. The first is substantive: many of the problems studied involve different levels or contexts. To analyse such problems with state-of-the-art methods, MLA is the most appropriate statistical tool. Secondly, research in the fields of public health and healthcare increasingly uses MLA. It is therefore important that even if you do not apply MLA yourself, you are able to understand research that uses MLA. Nowadays it is nearly impossible to understand, appreciate and critically appraise published articles in our field of research if you are not acquainted with MLA.

The pioneering development of MLA methodology has been in education where researchers have been interested in studies examining how pupil outcomes (such as examination scores) are related to both the characteristics of the pupils themselves and those of the schools (Aitken and Longford 1986; Snijders and Bosker 2012). The use of MLA has since been widespread in the overlapping fields of health services research, epidemiology and public health (Diez-Roux 2000; Leyland and Groenewegen 2003; Merlo et al. 2005a, b, c, 2006; Rice and Leyland 1996; Subramanian et al. 2003), assisted by the development of specialist multilevel software and the addition of multilevel capabilities to common statistical packages (de Leeuw and Kreft 2001). The educational example may be transferred to a public health context in several ways. For example, when studying outcomes in hospitalised patients, interest focuses on the roles played by both hospitals *and* patients. The individual *and* the workplace may both influence absence from work due to sickness. Regional differences in incidence of heart disease may reflect differences in the composition of populations *and* in the success of local health promotion programmes.

The Scope of Public Health and Health Services Research

The intended readership of this book consists of researchers with an interest in public health and health services research. We will now briefly discuss the scope of these two areas of research and will show that they are often related. Public health research studies the conditions in which populations can be healthy. Health at group or population level is the focal point of interest. According to the Lalonde model

Fig. 1.1 Influences on population health

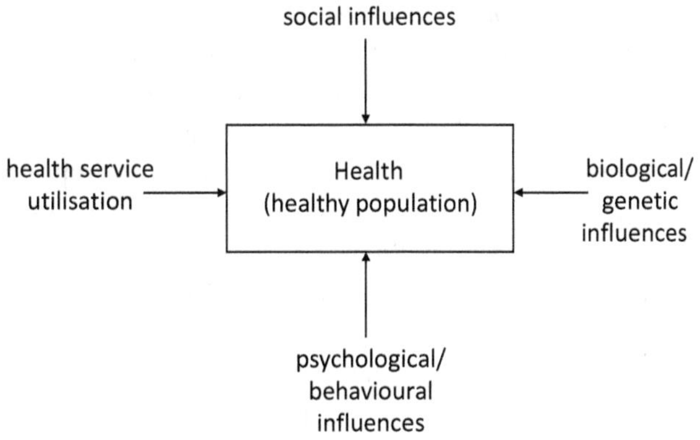

Fig. 1.2 Influences on healthcare utilisation (and health)

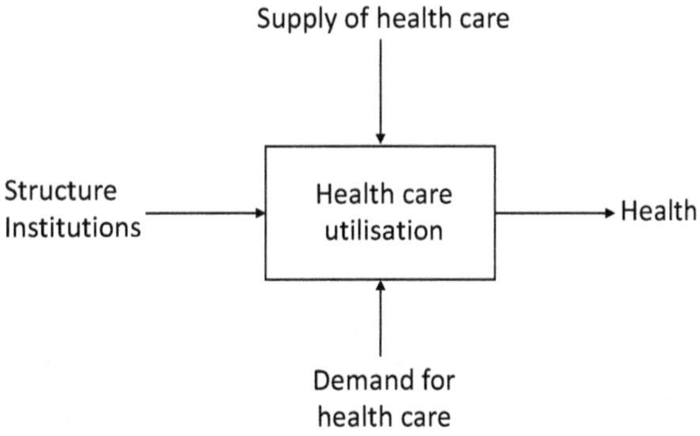

(1974), the health of the population is influenced by social, psychological, biological and healthcare determinants (see Fig. 1.1). In some form, this model has been at the root of public health policy in numerous countries. Health and health inequality at a group or population level are based on some aggregation or transformation of the health status of the people who form the group or population. The determinants of health can be both individual level and group or population level. Psychological determinants of health are typically individual characteristics. However, in the form of shared ideas and common psychological traits, they could build a collective characteristic, such as a group mentality. Biological characteristics can be individual, but they can also be shared characteristics of larger populations of genetically related individuals or those exposed to the same environmental hazard. Healthcare determinants are typically group or population-level characteristics determined by the administration or government, whether this is at the local (e.g. municipality) or national level. Social influences will also often operate through various higher (population) levels such as family, peer group or neighbourhood.

Compared to public health research, the scope of health services research places more emphasis on healthcare and healthcare utilisation than on health per se (Fig. 1.2). Health services research focuses on the relationships between demand for care and supply of care, as influenced by the structure and institutions of the healthcare system. It is a multidisciplinary field of scientific investigation that studies how social factors, financing systems, organisational structures and processes, health technologies and personal behaviours affect access to healthcare, the quality and cost of healthcare and ultimately our health and well-being. Its research domains are individuals, families, organisations, institutions, communities and populations (AcademyHealth 2005). Quality of care is an important research area, and this can be defined in relation to structures, processes and outcomes in the provision of health services (Donabedian 2003).

Healthcare utilisation is traditionally the centre of attention in health services research. It is influenced by the *demand* for healthcare. The demand for healthcare is partly based on health—people with health problems tend to use health services—but not completely. There are also social and psychological influences on healthcare utilisation. People differ individually in the way they cope with ill health, and the threshold at which they will visit a healthcare professional also differs. There are also social influences, such as family or group norms as to when to invoke the help of others. The supply of healthcare also influences healthcare utilisation. The availability of hospital facilities, for example, influences their utilisation. And the organisation of healthcare facilities also affects utilisation; supply of and demand for healthcare exert their influence within an institutional context. This is the way in which the system is organised and funded. Whether or not general practitioners (GPs) have a gatekeeping role influences the utilisation, not only of the services that GPs provide but also of specialist services. Financial accessibility, in terms of organisation in systems of insurance or other funding of healthcare, also influences utilisation. Again we can say that these influences can be individual characteristics but often they are group- or population-level characteristics. Countries differ regarding the structure of their healthcare system, regions differ in the supply and mix of services, and social groups differ in how quickly they invoke healthcare.

Figures 1.1 and 1.2 also show the relationship between public health research and health services research. In public health research, the utilisation of health services is one of the determinants of health whilst in health services research one of the influences on healthcare utilisation is ill-health, and one of the outcomes of health service utilisation is the creation of health. Both public health research that does not take healthcare into account as an input and health services research that does not take health into account as an outcome can exist.

This brief discussion of the scope of public health and health services research has drawn our attention to different influences. Researchers with different educational backgrounds can study each of these influences on their own. Public health and health services research is populated by researchers who studied medicine, health sciences, epidemiology, psychology, sociology, statistics, human geography, economics, political science, etc. (and we must still have forgotten some). This diversity is the reason why we discuss rather broad substantive and theoretical issues in the first two chapters of this book. This ensures that we have a common understanding of the kind of research we are doing before proceeding to the statistical approach.

Research and Policy

Although researchers in the health and healthcare realm come from different disciplinary backgrounds, they typically do not derive their research problems from their original disciplines. Public health and health services research derives the problems from the healthcare sector. They are applied fields of research, in the sense that researchers in these areas apply their skills to problems that have their base in the healthcare sector and in the sense that they try to produce insights that can be used to solve problems in that same sector. The issues we study are rooted in the problems that practitioners and policymakers encounter in the healthcare sector. In the standard theoretical–empirical cycle of research within a specific discipline, the problems for research are generated within the discipline and are usually based on earlier research. This refers to the right-hand side of Fig. 1.3, where the conclusions of previous research typically feed back to new research questions. However, in public health and health services research, the problems we study are very strongly influenced by the current practical and policy problems in the healthcare sector (Bensing et al. 2003). Our research is part of a broader cycle that also involves the application of our results in health policy and practice.

To get a better feeling for this extended policy and research cycle and to illustrate the importance of different levels in studying problems in policy and practice of healthcare, we will spend some time on a very broad grouping of policy problems.

Governments have a responsibility for the health of their subjects. In the Netherlands, for example this responsibility for protecting and improving population health is part of the Constitution. Governments take this responsibility by designing and implementing policies. Some of these policies are directly related to health, whereas others are intended to improve healthcare. As the history of public health shows, policies directed towards standards for housing quality and public services in areas such as waste disposal and clean water supply have been very important. Often

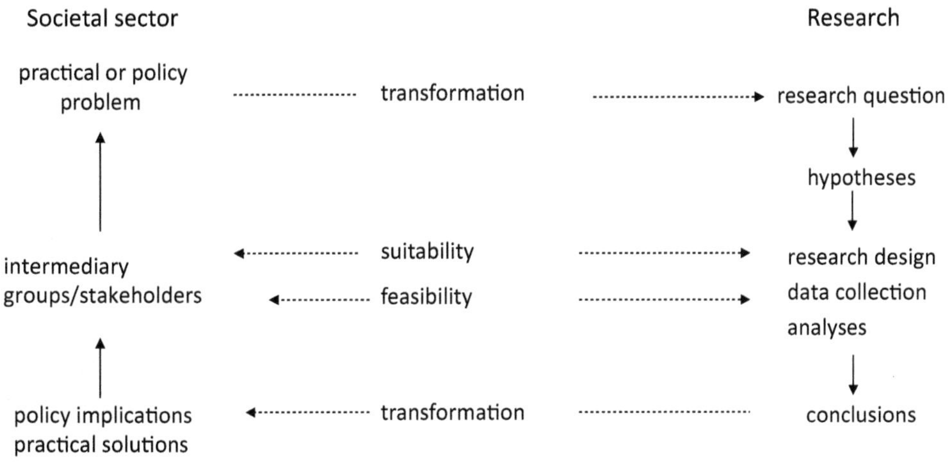

Fig. 1.3 Relationships between the societal sector of healthcare and health (services) research

these are policies that originate outside the direct jurisdiction of ministries of health. They require crosscutting policies and analysis of the health impacts of sector-specific policies (Puska 2007).

The central aim of health (care) policy is to improve population health. This aim is very general. It can be approached through policies in several important fields, and we can see these as being instrumental in reaching the overarching aim. As an example, the Dutch Ministry of Health published a document in 2009 with the title 'Societal challenges for public health and health care' (Ministry of Health 2009). According to this document, the big societal challenges were living longer in good health, anticipating changing care demands, quality of care and patient safety, dealing with limits to care and governance of the system. Here we can distinguish three instrumental aims:

- Increasing the coherence and responsiveness of the system
- Diminishing inequalities in health and in access to healthcare
- Increasing the efficiency of the system (stewardship)

We use these three aims because, basically, most social systems are concerned with problems of coherence and responsiveness, inequalities and efficiency in one way or another, and healthcare is no exception. For example, a country's educational system can be seen as trying to cope with these three basic problems: the way different types of school are tuned in to different educational needs, geographical and social inequalities in access to schooling and the efficiency of teachers and educational programmes. Therefore, we might get our inspiration to develop research in the healthcare field by looking at experiences in other sectors of society. We might also look at more general theories of how societal systems are organised or about the causes of inequalities. So we might use this insight in a horizontal way—looking at other sectors—or in a vertical way—looking at more general theories. An example of a book that does both is 'The spirit level: why more equal societies almost always do better' (Wilkinson and Pickett 2009).

Going back to healthcare, the emphasis that is placed on each of these three instrumental aims may vary over time or differ between countries (Tenbensel et al. 2012). If we look at the past few decades, we could say that in the 1970s the emphasis was on structuring the healthcare system, by strengthening primary care and by using planning as an instrument (Saltman and Von Otter 1992). In contrast, efficiency and stimulation of evidence-based healthcare were much more at the centre of policy attention during the 1990s (Sackett et al. 1996). The performance movement in healthcare is also intended to increase the efficiency of the system but performance indicators of healthcare in themselves, such as those developed by the World Health Organization (WHO) for the World Health Report 2000 (WHO 2000), try to incorporate indicators of inequality and responsiveness. Inequalities in access to healthcare are central to a model, developed in the early 1970s in the USA, called the Andersen–Newman model (Aday and Andersen 1974). This model looks at and subsequently analyses the influence of the need for healthcare; predisposing variables, such as attitudes about health and healthcare; and enabling variables, such as income or insurance status, and is still often used. Inequalities in health have featured prominently on the political agenda over the past decades from the Black report

(Department of Health and Social Security 1980) to more recent reviews of the state and extent of inequalities (Commission on Social Determinants of Health 2008; Marmot Review 2010).

These aims of health policy give us a basic classification to enable us to position our own research problems. We can think of examples of a research problem addressing one of these central aims of health policy. In doing so, we will see that again different levels are involved. The central aims can be used to introduce the relationships between macro, intermediate and micro levels, and the idea is that more than one level is usually involved when you analyse a problem. We will briefly go through each of the three instrumental aims.

Our research problem might concern the reasons why some people receive the care that they need, whilst others do not get the care that they require or are given care that they do not need. This is a well-known problem in areas such as home care where some people, who just need some help with shopping, receive help cleaning their house, or where people who need specialised nursing attendance receive home help. Some of the explanation for such discrepancies might be at the intermediate level, which could be the level of the organisation that supplies home care. Home care might not cooperate effectively with the hospitals that discharge patients with certain needs or with GPs who have a clear view of the exact nature of a person's needs. So the way the actions of different healthcare providers are tuned in to each other might influence the outcome for individual users of home care. The extent of cooperation with other service providers might vary between home care organisations. As a consequence, badly tuned care might be more prevalent among the clients of some organisations than among clients of other organisations. In other words, to some extent the outcome of whether a patient receives the appropriate care is clustered within home care organisations. The extent of cooperation between health and home care providers might vary between regions or health care systems. We then come to the macro level where health system organisation may influence cooperation at the intermediate level, for example in terms of an emphasis on planning or the market, or in the public/private mix (Fig. 1.4).

Problems of inequality might be defined in terms of health, determinants of health, access to healthcare or healthcare utilisation. In this example we consider

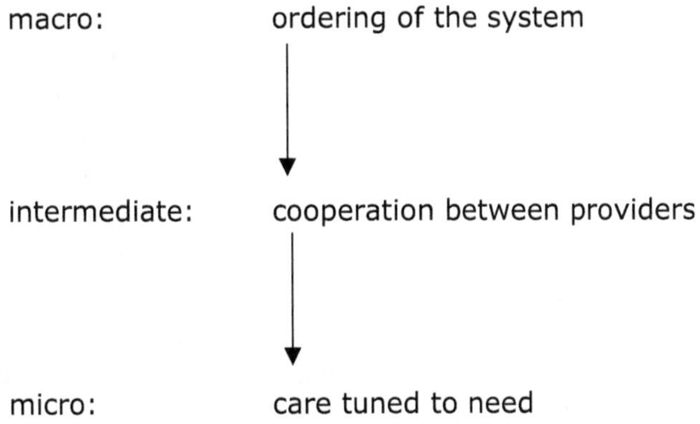

Fig. 1.4 Problems of coherence and responsiveness

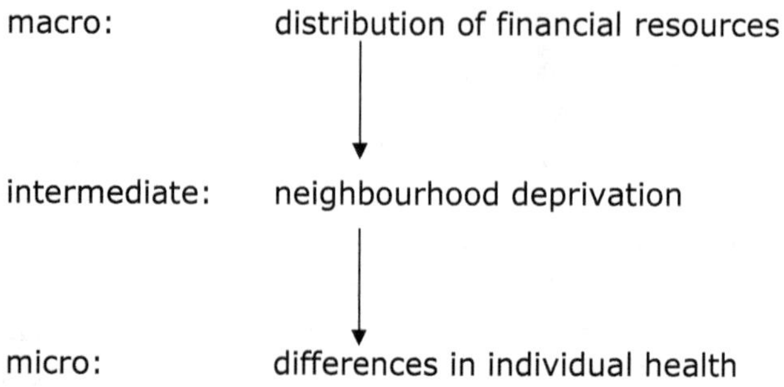

Fig. 1.5 Problems of inequality

health. We might want to explain the relationship between neighbourhood deprivation, individual socioeconomic resources and health behaviour and some measures of health. Variation in health (which is an indication of health inequalities) might be greater in some neighbourhoods and smaller in others. This might be partly related to individual people's resources (such as whether or not they are unemployed) and health behaviours (e.g. smoking). However, some of the variations might persist and indicate differences between neighbourhoods. These might be related to neighbourhood (as distinct from individual) deprivation. At the macro level, we could look at the cities where these neighbourhoods are located. We could, for example, relate the financial or social policies of different cities to neighbourhood deprivation. Again we see that we can subsume a specific research question under the umbrella of problems of inequality. And we can specify different levels that contribute to the explanation of health inequalities (Fig. 1.5).

The third example relates to problems of efficiency. As we mentioned before, one of the manifestations of a healthcare policy that is oriented to increasing the efficiency of healthcare is evidence-based medicine. We might define appropriate care at the micro level as being whether or not a patient receives care according to current guidelines. Some patients might receive appropriate care and others not. Some of the reasons for that might have to do with individual circumstances, such as the existence of a co-morbidity which can be a reason to deviate from single morbidity guidelines. Part of the explanation might be that the patient is treated by a GP who is not in favour of this particular guideline or of guidelines in general, or who is just too busy to take the time and effort to work according to the guideline. Consequently, some of the variation in whether a patient receives appropriate care is generated at this intermediate level of GPs. Groups of GPs might be organised within larger practices or primary care groups or trusts. These larger groups then form a macro context that may influence the behaviour of individual GPs by agreeing on the use of guidelines or sanctioning their non-use (Fig. 1.6).

In these examples, we have used three different levels and named the higher two intermediate and macro. It is important to realise that there is no 'law of three levels'. The number of levels in any study depends on a combination of theoretical analysis and practical considerations of data collection or availability. What is micro or macro depends on your point of view. Although the micro level is often the level of individuals, we will see in Chap. 4 that the micro level or lowest level in a multilevel analysis can also be a number of repeated observations on the same person. The

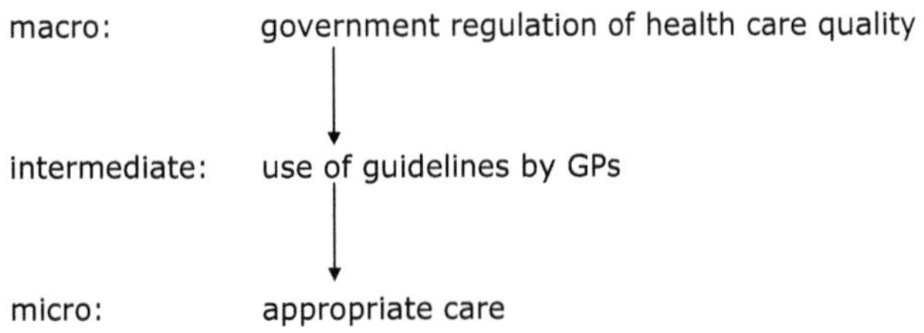

Fig. 1.6 Problems of efficiency

lowest level can also be a small area, for example when we do not have access to individual health data for reasons of data confidentiality. In such a case we might obtain small area data and analyse them within a higher level of regions or countries. The macro level is also relative. In some research problems, this level might be formed by countries, but in others by GP practices.

Conclusion

The issues we have raised in this introductory chapter relate directly to the philosophy behind the book. Firstly, we feel that it is important to try to integrate substantive issues, methodology and statistics. Secondly, these substantive issues relate to the field in which we are working and our approach: application, policy and practice oriented. Thirdly, MLA has a close correspondence with the substantive issues; health and healthcare are context dependent. And, finally, we have to learn to think in multilevel concepts: to develop hypotheses, conceptualise contexts and define levels.

References

AcademyHealth (2005). www.academyhealth.org/about/whatishsr.htm

Aday LA, Andersen R (1974) A framework for the study of access to medical care. Health Serv Res 9:208–220

Aitken M, Longford N (1986) Statistical modelling in school effectiveness studies. J R Stat Soc Ser A 149:1–43

Bensing JM, Caris-Verhallen WMCM, Dekker J, Delnoij DMJ, Groenewegen PP (2003) Doing the right thing and doing it right: toward a framework for assessing the policy relevance of health services research. Int J Technol Assess Health Care 19:604–612

Commission on Social Determinants of Health (2008) CSDH final report: closing the gap in a generation: health equity through action on the social determinants of health. World Health Organization, Geneva

de Leeuw J, Kreft IGG (2001) Software for multilevel analysis. In: Leyland AH, Goldstein H (eds) Multilevel modelling of health statistics. Wiley, Chichester, pp 187–204

Department of Health and Social Security (1980) Inequalities in health: report of a research working group. DHSS, London

Diez-Roux AV (2000) Multilevel analysis in public health research. Annu Rev Public Health 21:171–192

Donabedian A (2003) An introduction to quality assurance in health care. Oxford University Press, Oxford

Lalonde M (1974) A new perspective on the health of Canadians. Government of Canada, Ottawa

Leyland AH, Groenewegen PP (2003) Multilevel modelling and public health policy. Scand J Public Health 31:267–274

Marmot Review (2010) Fair society, healthy lives. Marmot Review, London

Merlo J, Chaix B, Yang M, Lynch J, Råstam L (2005a) A brief conceptual tutorial of multilevel analysis in social epidemiology: linking the statistical concept of clustering to the idea of contextual phenomenon. J Epidemiol Community Health 59:443–449

Merlo J, Chaix B, Yang M, Lynch J, Råstam L (2005b) A brief conceptual tutorial on multilevel analysis in social epidemiology: interpreting neighbourhood differences and the effect of neighbourhood characteristics on individual health. J Epidemiol Community Health 59:1022–1029

Merlo J, Yang M, Chaix B, Lynch J, Råstam L (2005c) A brief conceptual tutorial on multilevel analysis in social epidemiology: investigating contextual phenomena in different groups of people. J Epidemiol Community Health 59:729–736

Merlo J, Chaix B, Ohlsson H, Beckman A, Johnell K, Hjerpe P, Råstam L, Larsen K (2006) A brief conceptual tutorial of multilevel analysis in social epidemiology: using measures of clustering in multilevel logistic regression to investigate contextual phenomena. J Epidemiol Community Health 60:290–297

Ministry of Health (2009) [Societal challenges for public health and health care]. Ministry of Health, Welfare and Sports, The Hague

Puska P (2007) Health in all policies. Eur J Pub Health 17:328

Rice N, Leyland AH (1996) Multilevel models: applications to health data. J Health Serv Res Policy 1:154–164

Rosen G (1993) A history of public health [1958]. The Johns Hopkins University Press, Baltimore

Sackett DL, Rosenberg WMC, Gray JAM, Haynes RB, Richardson WS (1996) Evidence based medicine: what it is and what it isn't. Br Med J 312:71

Saltman RB, Von Otter C (1992) Planned markets and public competition: strategic reform in Northern European health systems. Open University Press, Buckingham

Snijders TAB, Bosker RJ (2012) Multilevel analysis: an introduction to basic and advanced multilevel modeling. Sage, Los Angeles

Subramanian SV, Jones K, Duncan C (2003) Multilevel methods for public health research. In: Kawachi I, Berkman LF (eds) Neighborhoods and health. Oxford University Press, New York

Tenbensel T, Eagle S, Ashton T (2012) Comparing health policy agendas across eleven high income countries: islands of difference in a sea of similarity. Health Policy 106:29–36

WHO (2000) World health report 2000. World Health Organisation, Geneva

Wilkinson RG, Pickett KE (2009) The spirit level: why more equal societies almost always do better. Allen Lane, London

2

Relationship between Macro and Micro Level

Abstract With multilevel analysis, we can model the relationship between the context in which people live or act and an outcome at the individual level. In this chapter we discuss the relationship between the context or macro level and the individual or micro level. Sociologists have developed ways of analysing these relationships that may help our understanding of MLA. At the micro level, it is important to have a theory of human behaviour that takes context into account. But what contexts are relevant? That depends on the research question, and the phenomenon we are studying.

Keywords Multilevel analysis · Social production function theory · Health behaviour · Healthcare providers · Social context · League tables

Multilevel analysis enables us to analyse individual-level outcomes in relation to independent variables at the same level and independent variables at a higher level. This higher level is what we usually call the context or the macro level. In this chapter we give a theoretical analysis of the relationships between individual- or micro-level outcomes and contexts. However, the relationship between macro and micro levels has two dimensions. Not only does the context, such as the availability of health services in an area, influence behaviour (e.g. health service utilisation), there is also an influence the other way around: from micro to macro level. Continuing this example, the health service utilisation of many individuals will result in a high level of healthcare expenditure in an area. Often we are interested in both directions. MLA is especially suited for analysis in one direction, from macro to micro level, and less so the other way around. However, when we are analysing 'league tables' of hospital performance at the end of this chapter, we can use MLA to arrive at estimates of hospital effects, taking differences in the composition of the patient populations (case-mix differences) into account.

We start this chapter examining the relationship between macro-level context and individual, micro-level outcomes. The other dimension, from micro level to macro level, will be addressed at the end of this chapter. At that stage we will also briefly introduce league tables. In between we discuss theories about behaviour (the micro level) and the relevance of different contexts.

Relationships Between the Macro and Micro Levels

Social context influences what people do, their behaviour and interactions, and what people do leads to certain outcomes in which we are interested such as their health or the decision to consult a healthcare provider. These outcomes are the results of decisions people make. To clarify this statement, people usually do not choose to be unhealthy, but this outcome is partly the consequence of their behavioural choices and partly the outcome of circumstances that influence either their choices or the outcomes directly. We will discuss three heuristic models of the relationships between macro and micro levels that maybe helpful in conceptualising your own research (Raub et al. 2011). Heuristic means that these models are not conceived as descriptions of reality, but as a means of helping you to understand phenomena, to conceptualise your own research, and arrive at hypotheses (Groenewegen 1997).

The first heuristic approach brings the relationship between two phenomena at the macro level to centre stage. For example, consider the relationship between mean income level and income inequality on the one hand and the standardised mortality rate of states on the other hand. The explanation of a relationship like this requires the specification of a mechanism that connects the macro contexts (mean income and income inequality) with individuals at the micro level (Hedström and Swedberg 1998). The outcome at the micro level is whether individuals of a specified age and sex die. The mechanism might be partly behavioural, such as health damaging habits, partly social, such as comparison to other people, and partly biological, such as the effect of exposure to dangerous substances. Based on the individual deaths at the micro level and additional information about the populations involved, standardised mortality ratios can be calculated. Figure 2.1 shows the basic scheme as developed by (Coleman 1986, 1990).

Van Beek et al. (2013) applied Coleman's diagram to establish and explain a relationship between social networks of staff in nursing home wards (A) and treatment of residents by ward staff (D). The explanation runs via organisational identification (B) and motivation (C) of nursing staff. Figure 2.2 illustrates this.

In ecological analyses, we only analyse the relationships at the macro level (the arrow from A to D). We run the danger of attributing these macro relationships to relations at the individual level (a phenomenon known as the ecological fallacy, described in Chap. 3). In behavioural research, we analyse the relationship at the micro level (the arrow from B to C). We then run the opposite risk to the ecological

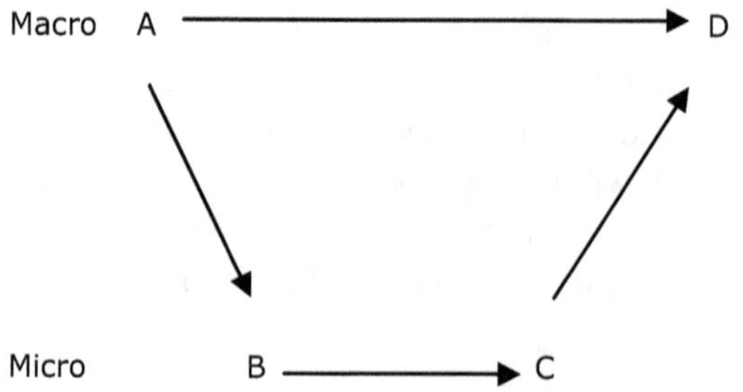

Fig. 2.1 Coleman's diagram of relations between macro and micro level

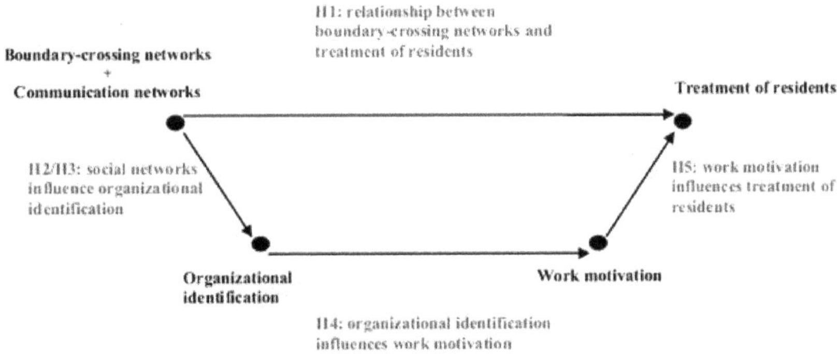

Fig. 2.2 Application of Coleman's diagram to explain the relationship between social networks of nursing staff and treatment of residents. (Reproduced with permission from Elsevier, Social Networks)

fallacy—that of the atomistic fallacy. In instances of an atomistic fallacy, the analysis is carried out at the micro (individual) level, but inference is made at the macro (group) level (Diez-Roux 1998).

Sometimes the relationship at the micro level is analysed, using information about the context as a distributed variable at the individual level. That is, every single individual in the same context is assigned the same value for a contextual variable. In this case we would run into a statistical problem. The observations on individuals that share the same context or macro variable are not independent. This violates an important assumption in standard regression analysis. Moreover, standard statistical techniques would misestimate the precision of the coefficients of the distributed variables. They would not distinguish between the (usually much smaller) number of contexts and the number of individual observations. However, when using MLA we are able to analyse macro and micro levels—the contexts and the individuals—in a statistically appropriate way. In Chap. 3 we will elaborate on this further.

Figure 2.1 shows that ecological research and behavioural research are not mutually exclusive approaches. The two complement each other, and there is a clear relationship between them; to explain an ecological relationship, you need to go into the micro-level mechanisms. MLA helps us to analyse part of the diagram: the arrows from A to B to C. In other words, MLA provides us with the tools to examine how aspects of the context in which people live (A), together with their personal characteristics and resources (B), influence some outcomes at the individual level (C).

Coleman's heuristic shows the basic structure of the explanation of macro-level relations. It is, however, more easily applied to static situations than to problems involving social change. Boudon (1979) explicitly designed a heuristic to analyse processes of social change. He distinguishes between the *Environment*, which includes the social and institutional structure, the *Interaction System*, which includes the relevant actors and the choices they make, and the *Outcomes*, which form a distribution of the choices of many actors, such as the percentage of people who choose to behave in a certain way. These elements correspond to Coleman's A, B

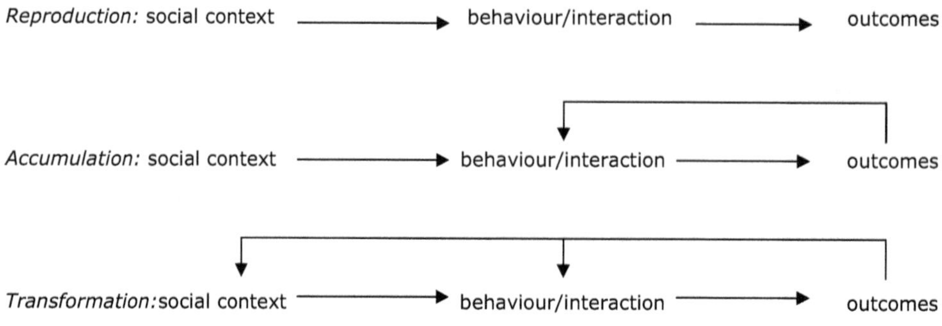

Fig. 2.3 Boudon's diagram of social change

and C, and D, respectively: 'environment' influences 'interaction system', which produces certain collective 'outcomes'. However, Boudon's next step makes the system a dynamic one. 'Outcomes' might feed back to the processes in the 'interaction system' or to the 'environment'.

Boudon distinguishes three processes of social change (see Fig. 2.3). In the first, called reproduction, there is no feedback and outcomes stay the same. In the second, there is feedback from outcomes to the interaction system, causing a process of accumulation or the gradual change of a distribution. Finally, if there is also feedback to the environment, then a process of transformation occurs.

As an example of these processes of social change, one could look at the system of care around childbirth (Schuller 1995). As outcomes we are interested in the changing distribution of the place where women give birth to their children. By the end of the nineteenth century and the beginning of the twentieth century in Western countries, most children were born at home with the assistance of a midwife. With the single exception of the Netherlands, where, at the beginning of this century, approximately 30% of children were stillborn at home, in Western countries childbirth had become a hospital affair. How did this change come about? The interaction system consists of childbearing women and their direct social relations, midwives and physicians. The environment consists of the broader healthcare and hospital system, both in the structural sense of accessibility and supply and in the institutional sense of the regulation of the professions involved, and developments in medicine and medical technology.

Until the early twentieth century, the system was in equilibrium and could be characterised as a reproduction process: there was not much choice, and nearly all women delivered their babies at home, attended by a midwife. However, with the development of the modern hospital, improved hygiene and new medical technology, the outcome of hospital deliveries in terms of the health of child and mother became as good and under some conditions better than the outcome of home deliveries. From that time on there was a choice, and physicians developed an interest in hospital obstetrics, the safety arguments appealed to expectant mothers, and midwives were not in a position to counteract.

These good and sometimes better results of hospital births fed back to the interaction system and influenced the decision-making process regarding the place of birth, especially in the case of a first child or following an earlier difficult delivery. The decrease of family size during the twentieth century resulted in a higher proportion of births being first children. Combined with the changing decision regarding place of birth, this resulted in a rapid increase of the share of hospital births—a process of accumulation. In most European countries, at some point in the 1960s, the number of home births reached such a low point that the possibility of a home delivery virtually disappeared as an alternative. Market shares became too low for self-employed community midwives, and physicians undertaking home deliveries would be scandalised within their profession. So eventually even the environment was affected, and again there was no choice whatsoever; hospital birth became not just the norm but the rule. Among Western industrialised countries, the Netherlands was the only exception to this process, probably due among other reasons to a stronger position of midwives in terms of their legal position, the reimbursement rules of public insurance and their professional education (De Vries 2005).

Generally, in this heuristic the interaction system is the micro-level process. The environment is the macro-level and determines the range of options available to the actors within the interaction system, and the outcome is the macro-level result of interaction. Again, using MLA we can statistically analyse the relationships between the environment, the micro-level conditions of the actors that influence the choices of pregnant women, and the choice of women to have a home or hospital birth as the dependent variable. The macro-level outcomes (the percentage of home deliveries) and the feedback steps are best explored using approaches beyond the scope of this book, such as complex systems theory (Diez-Roux 2011) and specific techniques, e.g. structural equation modelling (Bentler and Stein 1992).

The third heuristic that we will briefly discuss relates to the transformation of individual behaviour to macro-level outcomes. Often these outcomes are the unintended consequences of individual behaviour. Students flock to studies that educate them for occupational fields with high-income potential due to current shortages, only to find out that so many did the same that the shortage turns into over-supply and decreasing wages.

Unintended consequences are part and parcel of processes of social change. For example, as we have seen, decreasing family size has the unintended consequence of speeding up the accumulation process of the share of hospital deliveries. Such unintended consequences of behaviour are of primary interest to many social scientists (Boudon 1982; Popper 1963; Wippler 1981). If, as a first approximation, human behaviour is seen as being goal-directed, the question arises as to why people do not always achieve their goals. Part of the answer is in the transformation from micro to macro level. Two important sources of unintended consequences are the interdependencies of individual behaviour and incorrect anticipation of the reactions of others. An example of interdependencies leading to unintended consequences can be found in what has been called fee inflation. This occurs when there is a macro budget for specialist care, for example, and when individual specialists are paid on a fee-for-service basis. If they bill for too many services, the budget is exceeded and fees are adapted downwards. If individual physicians want to maintain their income, then they have to increase the number of services they undertake, and, since all other physicians are doing the same, the unintended consequence is that they all have to work harder to achieve the same income (Delnoij 1994).

Health policy struggles with unintended consequences due to the incorrect anticipation of the reactions of policy subjects. One example is of the reaction of health insurers within the field of healthcare to the announcement of the basic ideas for health system reform in the Netherlands in the second half of the 1980s. The aim of the intended reforms was to improve the performance of the system by introducing market elements and competition in healthcare. Health insurance organisations anticipated this policy by undertaking a huge chain of mergers. This in its turn made it very difficult to realise the original aims of the policy when competition was actually introduced because of the reduced number of competitors (Groenewegen 1994).

We have briefly discussed three heuristics that connect the micro and macro levels. Macro-level structures and institutions influence individual behaviour and the interaction between individuals, and individual behaviours form macro-level outcomes, both intended and unintended. In the following sections, we will first discuss some aspects of behavioural theory at the micro level. Following this we will discuss the transformations from macro to micro level and vice versa.

Micro Level: Behaviour of Patients and Providers

An important element in the analysis of macro-level phenomena is a behavioural theory at the micro level. The point of departure is that people act in a goal-directed manner and are sensitive to incentives. They act rationally in a restricted sense, set against the background of their knowledge and ideas about goals and their means to reach them (Boudon 1979). The extent to which people achieve their goals will be determined by the constraints imposed upon them as well as by the resources at their disposal. In as far as constraints and resources are structurally or institutionally determined, they are the way to bridge the gap between the macro and micro levels (Wippler and Lindenberg 1987).

If we apply the theory of goal-oriented behaviour as part of the explanation, we need to know the background against which people weigh up their alternatives—in other words, what their goals are. A systematic approach to this is given in social production function theory (Lindenberg 1996). The assumption here is that people have a limited number of ultimate goals, namely physical and social well-being. The theory proposes that people produce their physical and social well-being through their activities and use of resources (Fig. 2.4).

How and through which activities people achieve their ultimate goals depend on individual circumstances and resources and on macro-level social, structural and institutional conditions. This theory has been successfully applied to explain the loss of quality of life among the elderly (Gerritsen 2004; Ormel et al. 1997). It was also the basis of the empirical material we use in the tutorial on multilevel logistic regression in Chap. 12.

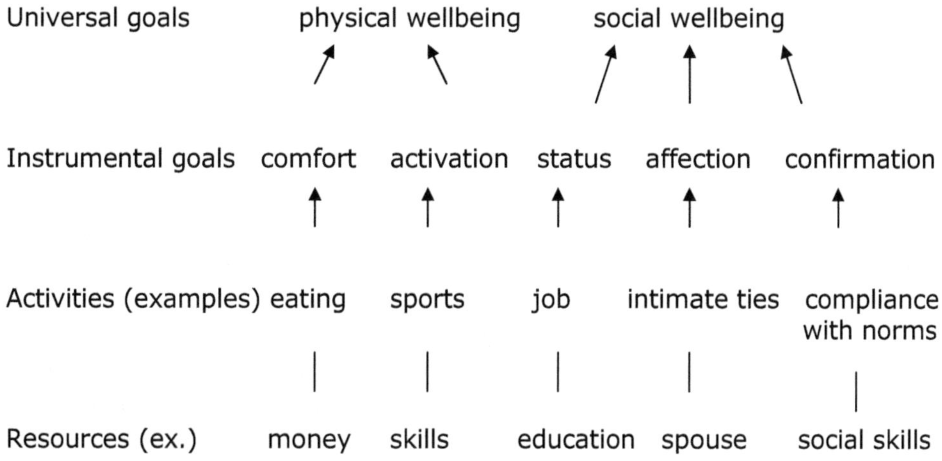

Fig. 2.4 Outline of the social production function theory. (Adapted from Ormel et al. (1997))

The Behaviour of Healthcare Providers

We assume that healthcare providers strive to achieve the same general goals of physical and social well-being as everyone else. An important instrumental goal for producing social well-being specific to health workers is the promotion of the health of their patients or clients. The importance of this goal is firmly established through a long period of socialisation in medical school and internships and during postgraduate specialisation. The patient's health is usually the first and dominant element in determining the physician's definition of a decision situation. This also underlines the mutual dependence of health workers' and patients' goals.

The fact that health workers also have other instrumental goals makes it understandable that they are not necessarily perfect agents for their patients (Domenighetti et al. 1993; Mooney and Ryan 1993). Their actions towards the improvement of their patients' health have consequences for their other goals; they take time, generate income, and obtain approval or disapproval from colleagues. Structural conditions, at the system level, for example, might influence the ability to achieve an optimal mix of income and leisure time. Fee-for-service payment makes it attractive to perform more services, because that increases income, as was hypothesised by Westert (1992). Physicians that work in single-handed practices depend more on their patients to gain social approval, whilst those in group practices have a greater dependency on their colleagues to achieve the same goal (Freidson 1970, 1975).

The Behaviour of Patients

Models of patients' behaviour have been elaborated mainly from a social psychological point of view. A common model is the Health Belief Model (Janz and Becker

1984) based on attitude theory. A more sociologically oriented model is the so-called Andersen–Newman model (Andersen and Newman 1973; Andersen 1995) that evaluates healthcare utilisation from three groups of influences: predisposing variables (attitudes, patterned by age and gender); enabling variables (or constraints), such as insurance status or the availability of health services; and needs variables, such as the experience of symptoms of ill health. These models lack a theory of preferences, such as social production function theory. They either take the goals of patients for granted (as in the Anderson–Newman model) or just ask people for their preferences (as in the Health Belief Model). Within health economics, the Grossman model (Grossman 1972; Van Doorslaer 1987) assumes that healthcare utilisation is one of several instrumental goals that people use to create health. The basic idea is that people invest in maintaining their 'stock of health capital' by their lifestyle, preventive actions and use of healthcare. Apart from maintaining or regaining health, people also have other instrumental goals such as reducing anxiety or uncertainty (Ben Sira 1986) or have quick or slow solutions to their problems (depending on sickness benefits, for example).

Patient–Provider Interaction

Utilisation of health services, the meeting point of supply and demand, is determined in the interaction between healthcare providers and patients—usually the consultation. A typical feature of this interaction is its asymmetry. Firstly, asymmetry exists in the importance of the consultation. For a particular patient, there is only one problem and that is his or her problem, whilst for the health worker there are many patients with many problems (Gillon 1988). Secondly, there is asymmetry in information. Providers have information that patients do not have, and the former use that information to reach a diagnosis or to advise therapy. Finally, healthcare providers sometimes govern access to scarce resources, such as drugs that are only available on prescription or sickness certificates that entitle the patients to certain benefits (Stone 1979).

Given these asymmetries, one would hypothesise that the expectations of health workers and providers would often diverge from those of patients (Persoon 1975). In addition, both parties have instrumental goals other than regaining or maintaining health. In situations in which expectations diverge, patients have different alternative courses of action, for example:

- To negotiate or enter into conflict with the health worker: the alternative of the knowledgeable patient
- To find another healthcare provider: the alternative of 'doctor shopping' or consulting complementary healers
- To act as if they accept the situation, but neglect the advice dispensed: the alternative of non-compliance.

Both the occurrence of diverging expectations and the alternatives that are subsequently chosen depend on constraints and resources.

From Macro to Micro Level

The gap between macro and micro levels is bridged by assumptions about structural and institutional constraints that influence the way people can realise their goals. These constraints are located at different levels. Basically, the organisation of the phenomenon under study determines what the relevant levels are and where they are located. In the case of health services research, three levels might be relevant: the level of the healthcare system, the level of the practice or organisation (hospital) in which providers work or the social context of the patient and the level of the actual consultation between provider and patient. The upper half of Fig. 2.5 shows these levels.

The structure and institutions of the healthcare system influence both healthcare providers and patients. The result of the interaction between patient and provider, in

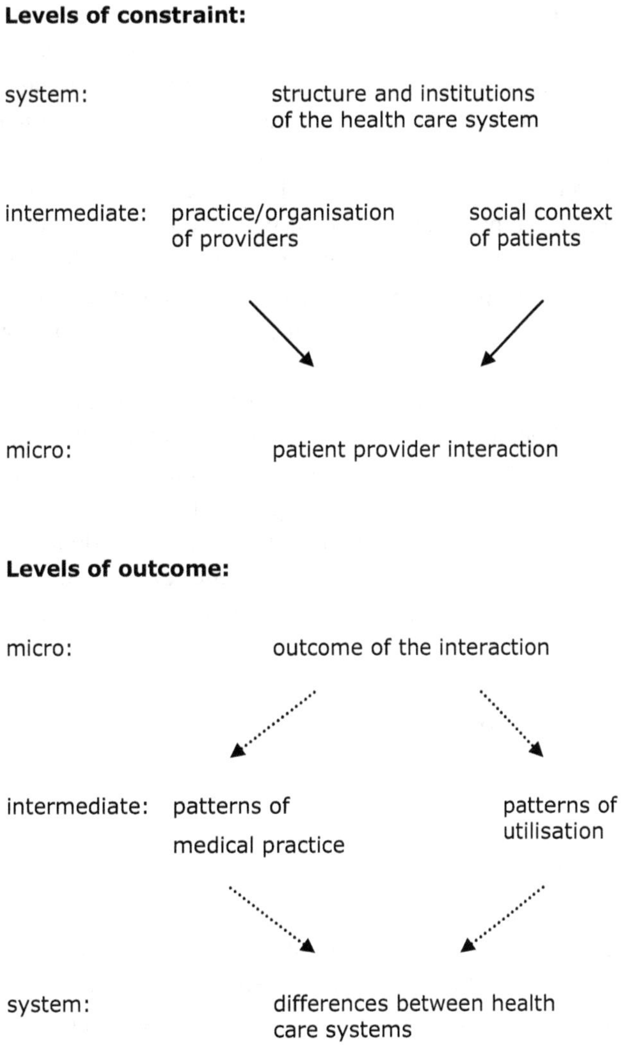

Fig. 2.5 Context at different levels and outcomes at different levels

terms of alternative modes of action distinguished above, is influenced at the system level by the extent to which consultations are embedded in an existing patient–provider relationship. This is notably the case when patients are on the list of a specific healthcare provider. In such circumstances, what happens in the current consultation may be influenced both by the common past of the patient and the provider and by the expectation of a common future. Moreover, in some systems, it is more difficult to change your doctor than in others (Thomas et al. 1995). If providers are paid on a fee-for-service basis, patients and providers are usually not institutionally tied to each other or, if they are, then this tends to be only for a restricted time period. In such a case, one would expect patients to negotiate when expectations diverge. If providers are paid on a capitation basis, patients and providers are tied to each other and usually there are administrative barriers to changing your doctor. The reaction to diverging expectations in this case is more likely to be non-compliance. If providers are in salaried service, patients are usually tied to a group of providers but not to an individual doctor. In this case, we would expect to find a higher incidence of doctor shopping.

The second, intermediate level at which constraints operate is at the level of the practice or organisation of the provider and the social context of the patient. Doctors in single-handed practices are more dependent on their patients to gain social approval, whilst doctors who work in larger practices depend more on each other to gain this good (Freidson 1970). As a consequence, the former might be more willing to negotiate with their patients. From the viewpoint of patients, the tendency to negotiate might be influenced by their ability to communicate their goals to healthcare providers, which is probably related to their educational level, and by the need to communicate their goals (such as the time or money costs of the proposed treatment), which may be related to their economic position (Westert et al. 1991).

Finally, there are constraints at the level of the consultation. The more urgent that a healthcare problem is, the less important any alternative goals of the patient will be and the greater the inclination of patients will be to follow professional advice. If the health problem is less urgent, goals will coincide to a lesser extent. If, in such a case, the freedom of the doctor to make an individual decision has been reduced as a consequence of professional guidelines or protocols, patients might be more inclined to go doctor shopping, for example by seeking a second opinion.

What Contexts Are Relevant?

Contexts are important because they define the action space of individuals and the alternatives they have. Many problems in health and healthcare are related to people's behaviour. People behave within the social and institutional context of their community or workplace, for example. These contexts influence the resources and the range of options (opportunities and constraints) that actors have.

The question 'Which contexts are relevant?' is answered by analysing the research problem and asking: 'What kind of opportunities and constraints determine people's behaviour, and across which units are these opportunities and constraints patterned?' This abstract notion can be illustrated with an example as follows.

If you are trying to explain neighbourhood differences in health, different contexts might be relevant, each related to a different mechanism. And each of these contexts has different requirements regarding the kind of geographical unit you would prefer to use.

1. People live in social units, and these offer opportunities and constraints that influence their health and health behaviour. Neighbourhoods differ in terms of how close the relationships between people are within those neighbourhoods and the availability of support networks. Social integration and social support are known to influence people's health. A relevant context would comprise small-scale, socially homogeneous units. The relevance of small homogeneous areas has been discussed from a theoretical and methodological point of view in criminology by Oberwittler and Wikström (2009) in their chapter 'Why small is better'.
2. People also live in administrative and planning areas which are used to plan and organise healthcare facilities, including community health centres and hospitals, and to organise public health activities, such as the delivery of smoking cessation services or vaccination campaigns. Here the opportunities and constraints are more institutional. A relevant context would be administrative areas.
3. People's health is also influenced by exposure to the physical environment. Areas differ in exposure to factors including noise and air pollution. When analysing such physical influences, sometimes very small units are used, especially in urban areas.

Different constraints related to several higher levels could influence health at the same time, either separately or jointly. Different levels may work in conjunction; for example, municipalities may have certain policies, and the effectiveness of these policies may depend on the characteristics of neighbourhoods (such as deprivation, remoteness or rurality) within these municipalities.

In conclusion, examples of higher level units relevant in public health and health services research are administrative areas, such as municipalities; social units, such as groups of neighbours or peers; service areas of healthcare institutions, such as hospitals; places of work, such as schools or different departments of a large enterprise; and exposure areas to physical agents.

Ideally, the choice of higher level units should not depend on what routinely collected administrative data are available but on a substantive analysis of the research problem. However, for practical reasons, one often has to compromise and use data based on administrative units, even though the preference might be for data based on small areas with different levels of exposure. In such suboptimal cases, it is important, when interpreting results, to be aware that the units of interest may not coincide exactly with those that have been analysed.

From Micro to Macro Level

Usually the aim of health services research is not to explain the individual choices made by healthcare providers or patients. From the viewpoint of the providers, the main focus is on patterns of medical practice rather than the individual choice of a therapy. In the same way, from the patient's viewpoint, the main interest is in patterns of healthcare utilisation. The behaviour of individual providers and patients, therefore, has to be transformed to higher levels (see the lower half of Fig. 2.5). Just as we distinguished different levels at which constraints operate, we can also distinguish different levels of results: from the results of the interaction of provider and patient in particular consultations to intermediate-level results in terms of practice patterns and utilisation patterns, to differences between health systems at a system level.

The transformation of micro level to macro level can have a number of different forms. We can distinguish four such forms.

- Aggregation: in this case, individual behaviour is transformed through the application of a mathematical function. An example is the rate of Caesarean sections in a region, which is the count of the individual decisions by gynaecologists to perform a section divided by the total number of births in certain time period.
- Partial definition (or definition by convention): when the incidence of an individual outcome reaches a certain level, a collective outcome is supposed to exist by definition. An example is the existence of an epidemic. One might use the partial definition that if a certain percentage of the population at risk is infected, it is called an epidemic.
- The application of institutional rules: in this case the transformation is not made through a more or less arbitrary definition, but is based on an institutional rule. An example is the process of creating consensus statements or protocols for medical treatment. In a process like this, implicitly or explicitly, a majority rule is used as a necessary step in transforming individual expert opinion into a consensus document.
- Game theory and simulation: the analogy of a game can be used to predict the collective outcomes of joint individual actions. Game theory can, for example, be applied to the analysis of fee inflation. When formal, mathematical solutions cannot be reached, simulation can be used to transform individual effects to collective outcomes.

The Use of "League Tables"

In the wake of the performance indicator movement, governments increasingly want to monitor the success of public and semi-public organisations, such as hospitals. Moreover, knowledgeable healthcare consumers want information on which to base their choice of healthcare provider. League tables order organisations from high to low performing on a given criterion. The English NHS, for example, publishes league tables for GP practices, based on the Quality and Outcomes Framework, on its website.

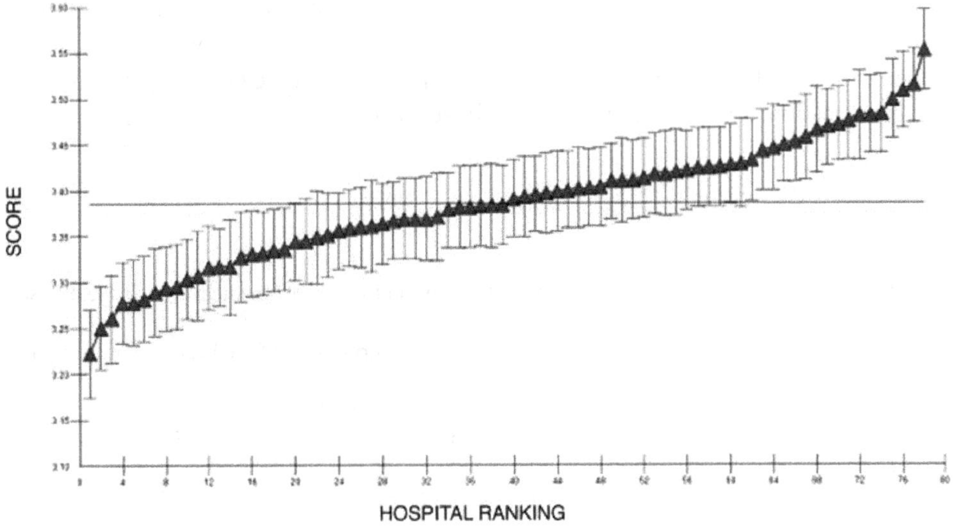

Fig. 2.6 Hospital performance scores (and confidence intervals) on the patients' experience of their room and stay (78 hospitals; 22,000 patients). (Source: Sixma et al. (2009))

Such performance indicators are usually aggregated from individual outcomes. Examples include patient deaths, complications, and readmissions within a given time period, and patient satisfaction. A big problem with league tables is how we can make a fair comparison between organisations that may have very different patient populations. Specialised hospitals differ from general hospitals in the composition of the patient population in terms of severity of conditions, and this in turn might affect outcomes that are used to construct league tables (Jacobson et al. 2003; Leyland and Boddy 1998). MLA can be used to adjust the differences in outcomes between organisations for case-mix differences. Importantly, however, it also ensures that adjustments are made based on the assumption that there may be an institutional effect (Goldstein and Spiegelhalter 1996).

Organisations also differ in size and, as a consequence, the confidence intervals for estimates of the average outcomes differ. With MLA we can estimate these confidence intervals. A further discussion of this and related issues will follow in Chaps. 5 and 8. Figure 2.6 gives an example from a comparison of 78 hospitals in the Netherlands. The measured effect shown here relates to people's experience of how clean sanitary facilities were.

Conclusion

In this chapter we have put health and healthcare in a micro to macro context. This provides the readers with heuristic tools to analyse their own research problems. Characteristics of macro-level contexts define people's action space and thus influence their behaviour. The outcome of people's individual behaviour aggregates to collective outcomes, and these in turn might influence future behaviour. Different heuristics and models of (health) behaviour may be helpful when defining your own research and when developing hypotheses. The individual research problem determines which contexts are relevant. We come back to this in the next chapter when we ask the question: 'What is a level in multilevel research?'

References

Andersen RM (1995) Revisiting the behavioral model and access to medical care. J Health Soc Behav 36:1–10

Andersen R, Newman JF (1973) Societal and individual determinants of medical care utilization in the United States. Milbank Mem Fund Q 81:95–123

Ben Sira Z (1986) Stress, disease and primary medical care. Avebury, Aldershot

Bentler PA, Stein JA (1992) Structural equation models in medical research. Stat Methods Med Res 1:159–181

Boudon R (1979) The logic of social action. Routledge, London

Boudon R (1982) The unintended consequences of social action. Macmillan Press, London

Coleman JS (1986) Social theory, social research and a theory of action. Am J Sociol 91:1309–1335

Coleman JS (1990) Foundations of social theory. Belknap Press of Harvard University Press, Cambridge

De Vries R (2005) A pleasing birth: midwives and maternity care in the Netherlands. Amsterdam University Press, Amsterdam

Delnoij DMJ (1994) Physician payment systems and cost control. Nederlands Instituut voor Onderzoek van de Gezondheidszorg (NIVEL), Utrecht

Diez-Roux AV (1998) Bringing context back into epidemiology: variables and fallacies in multilevel analysis. Am J Public Health 88:216–222

Diez-Roux AV (2011) Complex systems thinking and current impasses in health disparities research. Am J Public Health 101:1627–1634

Domenighetti G, Casabianca A, Gutzwiller F, Martinoli S (1993) Revisiting the most informed consumer of surgical services: the physician-patient. Int J Technol Assess Health Care 9:505–513

Freidson E (1970) Profession of medicine: a study in the sociology of applied knowledge. Harper & Row, New York

Freidson E (1975) Doctoring together: a study of professional social control. Elsevier, Amsterdam

Gerritsen DL (2004) Quality of life and its measurement in nursing homes. PhD thesis, Free University, Amsterdam

Gillon R (1988) Ethics, economics and general practice. In: Mooney G, McGuire A (eds) Medical ethics and economics in health care. Oxford University Press, Oxford

Goldstein H, Spiegelhalter DJ (1996) League tables and their limitations: statistical issues in comparisons of institutional performance. J R Stat Soc Ser A 159:385–443

Groenewegen PP (1994) The shadow of the future: institutional change in health care. Health Aff 13:137–148

Groenewegen PP (1997) Dealing with micro–macro relations: a heuristic approach with examples from health services research. In: Westert GP, Verhoeff RN (eds) Places and people: multilevel modelling in geographical research. Nederlandse Geografische Studies, Utrecht

Grossman M (1972) On the concept of health capital and the demand for health. J Polit Econ 80:223–255

Hedström P, Swedberg R (1998) Social mechanisms: an analytical approach to social theory. Cambridge University Press, Cambridge

Jacobson B, Mindell J, McKee M (2003) Hospital mortality league tables. Question what they tell you—and how useful they are. Br Med J 326:777–778

Janz NK, Becker MH (1984) The health belief model: a decade later. Health Educ Q 1:1–47

Leyland AH, Boddy FA (1998) League tables and acute myocardial infarction. Lancet 351:555–558
Lindenberg S (1996) Continuities in the theory of social production functions. In: Ganzeboom H, Lindenberg S (eds) Verklarende sociologie: opstellen voor Reinhard Wippler. Thesis Publishers, Amsterdam
Mooney G, Ryan M (1993) Agency in health care: getting beyond first principles. J Health Econ 12:125–135
Oberwittler D, Wikström P-OH (2009) Why small is better: advancing the study of the role of behavioral contexts in crime causation. In: Weisburd D, Bernasco W, Bruinsma GJN (eds) Putting crime in its place: units of analysis in geographic criminology. Springer, New York
Ormel J, Lindenberg S, Steverink N, Vonkorff M (1997) Quality of life and social production functions: a framework for understanding health effects. Soc Sci Med 45:1051–1063
Persoon J (1975) [Changes in the general practitioner—patient relationship]. Dekker & Van de Vegt, Nijmegen
Popper KR (1963) Prediction and prophecy in the social sciences. In: Conjectures and refutations: the growth of scientific knowledge. Routledge & Kegan Paul, London
Raub W, Buskens V, Van Assen MALM (2011) Introduction: micro-macro links and microfoundations in sociology. J Math Sociol 35:1–25
Schuller R (1995) [Parallel modernisation in midwifery: explanation of differences in birth culture in Western societies in the 20th century]. MA thesis, Faculty of Spatial Sciences, Utrecht
Sixma H, Spreeuwenberg P, Zuidgeest M, Rademakers J (2009) [Consumer quality index hospital stay]. NIVEL, Utrecht
Stone DA (1979) Diagnosis and the dole: the function of illness in American distributive policies. J Health Polit Policy Law 4:507–521
Thomas K, Nicholl J, Coleman P (1995) Assessing the outcome of making it easier for patients to change general practitioner: practice characteristics associated with patient movements. Br J Gen Pract 45:581–586
van Beek APA, Wagner C, Frijters DHM, Ribbe MW, Groenewegen PP (2013) The ties that bind? Social networks of nursing staff and staff's behaviour towards residents with dementia. Soc Networks 35:347–356
Van Doorslaer EKA (1987) Health, knowledge and the demand for medical care. PhD thesis, Maastricht University, Maastricht
Westert GP (1992) Variation in use of hospital care. Van Gorcum, Assen
Westert GP, Groenewegen PP, Lindenberg S (1991) [The influence of hospitalized patients on their length of stay]. Tijdschrift voor Sociale Gezondheidszorg 69:184–194
Wippler R (1981) [The explanation of unintended consequences of action]. In: Mathes J (ed) Lebenswelt und Soziale Probleme. Campus, Frankfurt am Main
Wippler R, Lindenberg S (1987) Collective phenomena and rational choice. In: Alexander JC, Giesen B, Münch R, Smelser NJ (eds) The micro-macro link. University of California Press, Berkeley

3

An Integrated Study of Multilevel Modeling

Abstract In this chapter, we will introduce the basic methodological background to multilevel modelling in verbal form. The underlying graphs and algebra are not covered until Chap. 5. There are two principal reasons for the increasing popularity of multilevel analysis. Firstly, it is more efficient and uses more of the available information than the alternative approaches of distributing contextual information to all individual observations or of aggregating all individual observations to the contextual level. Secondly, multilevel analysis enables the testing of more interesting hypotheses, especially those referring specifically to variation in outcomes or concerning the interactions between characteristics of the context and of individuals. This chapter also covers the idea of what constitutes a level in multilevel research.

Keywords Multilevel analysis · Random intercepts · Fixed effects · Random slopes · Cross-level interaction · Multilevel hypotheses

In public health, we are often interested in discovering what factors are associated with certain outcomes or what the strength of the relationship is between a variable and an outcome. Such relationships are commonly explored using regression analysis, but standard regression analysis makes certain assumptions that are untenable. Most pertinent among these is the assumption that the outcomes are independent of each other for all of the individuals in our study. We have seen from the previous chapter that the behaviour of individuals often cannot be isolated from the macro context in which they operate: the neighbourhood in which people live or the practice in which physicians work, for example. The influence of the context means that outcomes are unlikely to be independent, violating the assumption on which the standard regression model is based. Our solution is to use MLA to take the different levels into account in our analysis.

Methodological Background

We use multilevel modelling when we are analysing data that are drawn from a number of different levels and when our outcome is measured at the lowest level. Such a situation arises, for example, when we analyse the self-rated health of individuals, and we want to relate this both to individual characteristics, such as age and social class, and to contextual characteristics, such as the population density of the neighbourhood. If we had only one observation for each neighbourhood—that is, if we had sampled and interviewed just one person in each neighbourhood—and sufficient observations in total, then we would just conduct an ordinary single-level regression analysis. Our observations would be independent of each other; although there may be an influence of the neighbourhood context, our observation of this would differ for each individual in our sample as though it were an individual characteristic. Alternatively, if our entire sample were taken from the same neighbourhood, then we would again be able to treat the observations as though they were independent; although there may be a contextual effect, the identical effect would apply to everyone in our sample.

However, the above sampling designs of one person per neighbourhood or of a sample from a single neighbourhood are unusual ones; more commonly, we will have a number of individuals living in each of a number of neighbourhoods. If the place in which people live influences their health, then the observations are no longer independent. Two individuals living in the same neighbourhood have a common context influencing their self-rated health; as a result, some contribution to self-rated health is common for all individuals living in the same neighbourhood that is not shared by those from other neighbourhoods. The ways in which the environmental contexts in which individuals live or work may influence or constrain behaviour were explored in Chap. 2; an example might be that health behaviours are shared within social networks meaning that there is a common influence on self-rated health.

The average level of self-rated health in any particular neighbourhood may be higher or lower than the average for all neighbourhoods, all other factors being equal. Then within that neighbourhood, some individuals will have self-rated health above the neighbourhood average and some below average. So the overall difference between an individual's self-rated health and the population average will be partly attributable to the differences between neighbourhoods and partly due to the differences between individuals within neighbourhoods. When we look at the differences between individuals in our sample, we use the variance as a summary measure of the total variation. The first important feature enabled by multilevel analysis is the ability to split up or partition this variation into that part which is attributable to the neighbourhood and that which is attributable to the individual. The neighbourhood part of the variation consists of the variation of the average self-rated health of each neighbourhood around the overall average. In multilevel analysis, the neighbourhood averages are assumed to be sampled from a distribution of all neighbourhood averages; this is similar to a random effects analysis of variance

(Gelman and Hill 2007). In regression terms we can think of the neighbourhood average as a regression intercept since this then generalises to the introduction of independent or explanatory variables; the fact that these neighbourhood intercepts are assumed to be drawn from a statistical distribution of all possible intercepts gives rise to the term *random intercepts* model.

Earlier we considered two studies in which we would not need MLA. In the first we sampled one person from each of a number of neighbourhoods. In such a situation, we have no variability within neighbourhoods; the average score in each neighbourhood cannot be distinguished from the score of the single person sampled. In the second example, we took our entire sample from a single neighbourhood; this time there is no variability between neighbourhoods, as the population (sample) mean is equal to the mean observed in that neighbourhood. Neither design enables us to distinguish between the levels of individual and area, and so neither is a true multilevel design.

As discussed earlier, the assumption that our observations are independent is violated if our data are hierarchically structured, and we believe that the context may influence the outcomes; the shared context introduces a correlation between two individuals from the same neighbourhood. This has consequences both for the estimation of regression coefficients—measures of the relationships between individual or contextual characteristics and outcomes—and for the standard errors of these estimates (our measures of precision, which determines the extent to which we find a relationship to be statistically significant). Failing to take into account the correlation between individuals within their contexts leads to the phenomenon known as *misestimated precision* (Aitken et al. 1981); ignoring the clustering of individuals within higher level units leads to an overestimation of the effective sample size and hence the tendency to find more relationships significant at a given significance level than the data can actually support.

The *random intercepts* regression model is based on the assumption that, whilst the intercept or average outcome for individuals with a given set of characteristics varies between higher level units, the relationship between the dependent and independent variables is consistent across all contexts. Returning to the example of how self-rated health varies across neighbourhoods, we might find a relationship with income such that those with higher incomes tend to enjoy better health. A linear relationship would suggest that for every unit increase in individual income, we can expect to see a fixed increase in self-rated health. The use of a *random intercepts* model would be based on the assumption that such a relationship between income and self-rated health holds in all neighbourhoods despite health on average being higher or lower in some neighbourhoods. A *random slopes* or *random coefficients* model allows us to relax this assumption and to let the relationship between self-rated health and income vary across contexts; in some neighbourhoods, the health gain associated with a fixed increase in income may be larger than in others. As with the intercepts, the slopes—the relationship between health and income in each neighbourhood—are assumed to come from a distribution of all possible slopes. Moreover, we can examine the relationship between the intercepts and slopes to see whether, for example, the health gain associated with a fixed increase in income is larger or smaller among neighbourhoods in which the average health rating is lower.

Why Use Multilevel Modelling?

We can think of a number of alternatives to multilevel analysis. The most common of these are:

- Aggregate or ecological analysis: ignore the level of the individual and restrict the analysis to the relationship between contexts
- Individual analysis: ignore the effect of context on our estimates of relationships and their associated precision
- Separate individual analyses within each higher level unit
- Individual level analysis with the inclusion of dummy variables to estimate the effect of each higher level unit

As we mentioned in Chap. 2, these alternative approaches may easily lead to inferences at the wrong level, the ecological and atomistic fallacies (Diez-Roux 1998).

Aggregate Analysis

Imagine that we are interested in examining the relationship between the time spent undertaking recreational physical exercise each week and certain individual characteristics (including age, sex, education and income) and environmental characteristics (including area deprivation and the availability of green spaces). The aggregate analysis would involve averaging the time spent exercising by individuals in each neighbourhood and regressing these means on averages of the individual variables (average age, proportion of males, average education and average income) as well as the contextual variables. Such an analysis involves considerable loss of power since the number of observations in our data set is reduced from the total number of individuals to the total number of neighbourhoods in our study. But, more importantly, the analysis may be misleading; the average income in a neighbourhood may reflect opportunities available to everybody in the area (Diez-Roux 1998) and as such may exhibit a different relationship from that seen with individual income. We return to this issue in our discussion of context and composition in Chap. 7 and provide an example of the way in which aggregated individual variables can take on a different meaning in the practical work in Chap. 13.

Individual Analysis

As we have discussed above, conducting the analysis at the individual level when the context is important, and outcomes are therefore correlated, causes problems with misestimated precision (Liang and Zeger 1993). This can be illustrated most easily for (although is not restricted to) *contextual variables*; that is, variables that have been observed, measured or created at the higher level. Whereas in the above example we have measures of education and income for every participant in the study, the contextual variables—area deprivation and the availability of green spaces—are measured at the area level. The number of observations available on each is therefore limited to the number of neighbourhoods in the study and not the number of individuals. Yet in an individual analysis, we would behave as if we had taken a measure of area deprivation for every study participant, resulting in artificially small standard errors and confidence intervals around those regression coefficients. We show the potential effect of even a small degree of clustering on sample size calculations when we consider the importance of variation at different levels in Chap. 6.

Separate Individual Analyses Within Each Higher Level Unit

If the analysis is conducted separately for every high level unit, then this is fine as far as it goes. We can overcome the effects of the clustering of individuals within contexts by making each analysis context-specific. But there are severe limitations to such an analysis. Firstly, we are unable to share relevant information across contexts. So if, for example, the gender effect—the difference between the mean time spent exercising each week for men and women—does not differ significantly between areas, then the separation of the analysis into specific blocks means that we have lost the ability to estimate a single shared regression coefficient. In general we will estimate a complete set of regression coefficients for each neighbourhood. So a regression on four independent variables—plus an average or intercept term—will be undefined without a minimum of five observations in each area. (In practice we would probably want considerably more than five observations if we were to estimate five parameters; a rough guide is to have ten observations per parameter being estimated, meaning that a more realistic minimum might be 50 observations per area.) But secondly, and more importantly, we have lost the ability to estimate contextual effects. Our contextual variables do not vary between individuals within neighbourhoods and so we are unable to estimate directly the effect that area deprivation or the availability of green space has on recreational exercise. A two-stage "slopes-as-outcomes" approach was developed to enable the combination of such separate regression coefficients, and even to permit the introduction of contextual effects to explain variation in regression parameters between context, but such an approach has several notable limitations (Raudenbush and Bryk 1986).

Individual-Level Analysis with Dummy Variables

Our final alternative to fitting a multilevel model is to fit a fixed effect—a dummy or indicator variable—for every higher level unit in our model. This is rather inefficient in that it can require a large number of dummy variables. Fitting a dummy variable to model the intercept in each neighbourhood may not stretch modern computational capability; however, if a dummy variable were required for every household in a study of individuals nested within households, then the large number of single-person households would result in a large proportion of the total available degrees of freedom being used up in a very unparsimonious model. This would effectively remove the characteristics of individuals living in single person households from our model. The equivalent of a *random slopes* model would require a further dummy variable to estimate the regression coefficient for each neighbourhood. But once again the biggest problem with this approach is the inability to estimate the relationship between a contextual variable and the individual outcome. The inclusion of $(n - 1)$ dummy variables to model the intercepts for n neighbourhoods means that there are no remaining degrees of freedom at the neighbourhood level. It is for this reason that these "*fixed effects*" models (as opposed to *random effects* or multilevel models) can only be used to adjust for the potentially confounding influences of contexts on individual-level relationships rather than to explore contextual influences per se. *Fixed effects* models may also change the interpretation of regression parameters in subtle but important ways, particularly regarding the analysis of panel (repeated measures) data (Leyland 2010).

What Is a Multilevel Model?

By now it should be clear that a multilevel model is a form of regression model that is appropriate when the data have some form of a hierarchical structure. We have also covered what a multilevel model is not, including the *fixed effects* model that uses dummy variables to remove the effects of higher level units. But how do multilevel models work? The key is in the distributional assumption made about the higher level units. Rather than estimate a mean for each higher level unit, as is necessary when using a *fixed effects* model, a multilevel model summarises the distribution of the higher level units using a population mean for all contexts and a variance. A single-level regression model already estimates the mean (or intercept), so the additional requirement of a two-level multilevel model is just one parameter—the variance—regardless of the number of higher level units. When we turn a random intercepts model into a random slopes model, rather than including an additional parameter (the dummy variable modelling the slope) for each of $(n - 1)$ neighbourhoods, we need to add just two parameters—the variance of the slopes and the covariance between the intercepts and slopes. This reduction in the number of parameters required means that multilevel models provide a more efficient approach to data analysis.

But how much information is there in a variance? Is this sufficient for our needs? Often we require estimates of the effects or residuals at higher levels in our model; an example would be for models of institutional performance or the "league tables" discussed in Chap. 2. If we are not estimating the effect of each hospital, we can still use multilevel modelling to make inferences about the performance of contexts, such as hospitals. The distributional assumption that we make about the higher level units—usually that they are normally distributed—means that the estimated effect for each unit is shrunk towards the mean for all units. The extent to which the estimated effect for a particular hospital is shrunk towards the overall mean depends on two factors: the extent of clustering in our data and how much information we have about that hospital. The extent of the clustering can be summarised in a simple fashion by the intraclass or intraunit correlation coefficient—the proportion of the total variance that is attributable to the higher level units. Returning to our earlier example, this is the proportion of the variance between individuals in the time spent exercising that is attributable to neighbourhoods. The intraclass correlation coefficient, sometimes referred to as the variance partition coefficient (Goldstein et al. 2002), is also a measure of the correlation in outcomes between two individuals in the same higher level unit, ranging between 0 (no correlation—time spent exercising is completely independent of the neighbourhood of residence) and 1 (perfect correlation—all individuals from the same neighbourhood spend exactly the same time exercising, given their individual characteristics). The estimated effect for each higher level unit is then a weighted average of what the data for that particular unit tell us and the population average; with less information about a given neighbourhood, we have little evidence that the effect is different from the average and hence the greater the shrinkage towards the mean. Small units about which we have little information are said to "borrow strength" from the rest of the sample (Ghosh et al. 1998). Of course the amount of information that we have about each unit is reflected in the (un)certainty around any estimate; confidence intervals will be smaller for neighbourhoods for which we have a lot of information. See for example Fig. 2.6 in Chap. 2.

There are numerous published examples comparing multilevel analyses with alternative methods that illustrate how different the results can be and how the results and conclusions that can be drawn from the studies are dependent on the method of analysis employed. We briefly describe three such studies below.

The first example concerns a training programme in diabetes care for GPs. When the data were analysed at the level of the individual patients, the conclusion was that the training programme had a positive influence on diabetes outcomes. However, because the training programme targeted GPs and not patients and because the patients are nested within the GPs, a multilevel analysis was also performed. In this analysis, the training programme was no longer significant (Renders et al. 2001).

Our second example concerns the impact of an indoor dichlorodiphenyltrichl oroethane (DDT) house-spraying programme, introduced at the village level, on individual malaria parasitaemia in Central Highland Madagascar (Mauny et al. 2004). As well as showing that the standard errors (and hence confidence interval s) of estimates were somewhat larger for the multilevel analysis, the authors showed how the population size of the village appeared to be strongly associated with the presence of parasites when using a conventional logistic regression model, but that this relationship was not significant when a multilevel analysis was conducted.

Finally, Moerbeek et al. (2003) considered the analysis of multicentre intervention studies based on the analysis of data collected on children clustered within classes and schools from the Television School and Family Smoking Prevention and

Cessation Project (TVSFP) (Flay et al. 1988). They showed that not only did ordinary (least squares) and *fixed effects* regression approaches tend to underestimate the standard error of the treatment effect on the post-intervention Tobacco and Health Knowledge Scale (THKS), these two approaches also provided incorrect estimates of the treatment effect.

What Is a Level?

In the first two chapters, we have given a number of examples of contexts that are relevant for people's health and for healthcare utilisation. When dealing with multilevel analysis, these contexts are called levels. We define a level as a *sample* (or a total population if the number is too small to use a sample or if all of the data are available) of contexts; moreover, we may have one or more *characteristics* (or variables) that vary between contexts.

Earlier in this chapter we introduced an example in which we focused on the time spent undertaking recreational exercise. We used information about individuals: the length of time spent exercising each week and information about individual demographic and socio-economic factors that might influence the time spent exercising. We also had information about the context in which these individuals live: the neighbourhood. Now we have two levels: individuals and neighbourhoods. The average of the time spent by individuals within each neighbourhood on recreational exercise varies between neighbourhoods, and a random intercepts model assumes that the neighbourhood means are sampled from some hypothetical distribution of all neighbourhood means. Such an exercise assumes that the higher level consists of units that can be meaningfully sampled. In this case, that would be a sample of neighbourhoods from a population of neighbourhoods. In practice we often work with *all* neighbourhoods rather than a sample; in such a situation, these can still be considered a sample for the generalisability of results. The data for each neighbourhood form a sample of data that could possibly have been collected at different times (if the sample had been drawn and interviews conducted a week earlier or a month later, the results would have differed) and allow us to make inferences about those neighbourhoods and neighbourhoods in general.

To summarise, levels comprise units that can be observed, sampled and analysed. These units have characteristics that can either be directly observed and measured, such as the availability of green spaces in a neighbourhood, or aggregated from individual characteristics, such as average income.

The distinction between a level and its characteristics is important. A characteristic, such as the degree of urbanisation of regions, is not a level. Degree of urbanisation may have a number of values; for example, it may be categorised in six classes from highly urban to sparsely populated countryside. (Some statistical software refers to these classes as levels, but these are clearly quite different from the levels that we are talking about in MLA.) We can sample regions from each of the classes of degree of urbanisation to form a stratified sample, but that does not make degree of urbanisation the level. Categories of urbanisation are not something that we would usually sample. We do, however, sample neighbourhoods or municipalities and then categorise them according to urbanisation, or we may stratify the sampling frame by urbanisation and draw a sample of neighbourhoods from each stratum to ensure that all strata are represented. Urbanisation is a variable, and neighbourhoods are units that, among other things, can be characterised by their degree of urbanisation.

In survey research urbanisation can be used at both the individual and municipality level depending on the sampling design. In health interviews among a random population sample, people are asked questions about health-related behaviour and subjective health. Characteristics of the place where people live may also be requested or recorded. The dataset comprises details about the individuals interviewed and a variable concerning the place where they live. It is possible to study the relationship between degree of urbanisation and, for example, mental health. All units are still at the individual level; there is no sampling of municipalities and the identity of the municipality of residence is not recorded just the *nature* or characteristic of the local area. Such a design might be employed to ensure confidentiality using a random dial telephone survey. Alternatively, the sample design of the same health interview survey could be two-stage such that, firstly, a number of municipalities is sampled, and, within each of the sampled municipalities, a sample of interviewees is drawn. The dataset now contains individual data and the identity of the municipality. Characteristics of the municipality can be added from other sources or constructed by aggregating individual variables. The result is a database with sampled units at two levels. (Multistage sampling designs are covered, along with other multilevel data structures, in Chap. 4.)

In survey practice, a simple random sample is often not considered for pragmatic reasons—consider the costs of conducting face-to-face interviews with people dispersed over a large area, such as a country. In such circumstances a staged sample is used. To take this data structure into account, often simple adjustments are made to the standard errors of parameter estimates. With the diffusion of MLA in health-related research, there are now tools enabling us to treat a multistage sample in an appropriate way, and it has become more common to theorise about the way context affects people's health, health-related behaviour, and health service utilisation.

As long as we only see the pragmatic reason of not having to send interviewers to a large number of different places as the rationale for using a two-stage sample design, the higher level in the data structure is just a nuisance. It is important to take the two-stage nature of the sample into account in statistical analysis, because the outcomes for individuals clustered within the same higher level sampling unit may not be independent. However, if we think of the higher level units as a context for human behaviour, they become interesting in themselves.

In intervention studies, to use another example, the intervention can be made at the individual level or at a higher level related to the provider of the intervention, such as a physician, health centre or community. If the intervention is a new drug, and patients are recruited from one site or the administration of the drug is strictly controlled and independent of where the patients get it, we again have a traditional single level analysis. One of the variables, the marker of the intervention, is whether the patients were given the new drug or a placebo. More complicated interventions often require healthcare providers to follow a protocol when treating eligible patients after randomisation. In this case the sampling design might be that physicians or centres are sampled and then patients are recruited among the eligible population that visit these physicians or centres. In such a case there might be differences in the way the intervention is administered, and it is important to take this into account. Often researchers are only interested in the effect of the intervention, in which case they tend to see the higher level as no more than a nuisance. For example, in a discussion of the advantages of MLA over single-level regression when analysing the relationship between patients' age and blood cholesterol levels, Twisk (2006) states "... the medical doctor variable was only added to the regression analysis to be corrected for, and there is no real interest in the different cholesterol values for each of the separate doctors" (p. 9).

How Many Units Do We Need at Each Level?

This question is usually more pressing for the higher level units than for the lower level units. Starting with the number of higher level units we need, we can say that it is not an easy question to answer, and there are no clear rules to follow. We will only give a number of considerations.

First of all, the number needs to be sufficient to estimate a mean and a variance. So the question is: with what number of units would we be confident that we can do that? With somewhere around ten higher level units, it would make sense to do so. With a smaller number it is perhaps better to do a single-level analysis and include dummy variables for the higher level units (a fixed effects model). The accuracy of different parameter estimates from a multilevel model, together with their standard errors, may be dependent on the sample size. Maas and Hox (2005) showed that in general estimates were unbiased in two-level linear multilevel models if there were sufficient (at least 50) higher level units. With fewer higher level units, the only estimate that was affected was the standard error of the high level variance.

Secondly, the research question can impact on the number of higher level units needed. If the research question or hypothesis is about the effect of characteristics of higher level units, such as hospitals, then we need enough hospitals to estimate the effect of the hospital characteristics or test the hypothesis. As a rule of thumb you need an additional ten higher level units for each independent variable at this level that you want to include in the analysis. So if you want to test a specific hypothesis and take into account a few confounders at the higher level, the number of higher level units needed quickly increases.

A related consideration has to with the power available to answer specific research questions (discussed further in Chap. 6). The smaller the number of higher level units, the more difficult it is to find an effect of a given size of a characteristic of the higher level units. If you do not want to be too quick to reject a hypothesis—after all, the hypothesis may be true even if you do not find a significant effect of the variable in question—then one option is to use a different threshold when testing the coefficient of a higher level variable (such as $p < 0.10$ instead of the more common $p < 0.05$).

Cost is often an important factor when making decisions about the number of higher level units to be sampled, especially when data collection for each extra higher level unit is very expensive or burdensome. Snijders (2001) shows how costs may be taken into account when calculating the sample size for a multilevel study.

A final consideration is related to the nature of the higher level units. Sometimes only a certain number of higher level units exist. There are only (currently) 28 European Union Member States, 12 provinces in the Netherlands and 14 health boards in Scotland. So if one of these units is relevant for our research, we are restricted in terms of the numbers available.

In general the number of units within each higher level unit is less of a problem. Even with small numbers of lower level units within each higher level unit, we can estimate a mean and a variance. An example where we have small numbers within higher level units is when we study individuals within households (see e.g. Cardol et al. 2005). There are some situations where it is important. An example is when we want to make league tables to inform patients about quality of care in different hospitals. In this case it is important to have enough observations in each hospital to be able to show significant differences between hospitals; our interest is in estimating the hospital effects, and there have to be enough observations in each hospital to estimate these effects reliably. Another example is when we want to construct new independent variables on the basis of individual observations. This is the case in the field of ecometrics (discussed in Chap. 8) where we might want to say something about safety in neighbourhoods on the basis of survey questions answered by individuals and use that as a neighbourhood characteristic in an analysis of the relation between neighbourhood safety and health. In this case the number of individuals is important to reach a satisfactory reliability of the construct "neighbourhood safety". However, in general, if we have a choice, it will be better to increase the number of higher level units than the numbers within the higher level units.

Hypotheses That Can Be Tested with Multilevel Analysis

As we argued in Chaps. 1 and 2, higher level units are important because they define the action space of individuals. Many problems in public health and health services research are related to people's behaviour; people behave within the social and institutional context of, for example, their community or workplace. This context influences the resources and the range of options (opportunities and constraints) that actors have (Groenewegen 1997). The question "Which levels are relevant?" is answered by analysing the research problem and asking: "What kind of opportunities and constraints determine people's behaviour, and in which units are these opportunities and constraints patterned?" The answers to these questions provide us with hypotheses, and we can now examine the kind of hypotheses that we can test using multilevel analysis.

There is a two-sided relationship between the theories that you want to test and the methodology to do so. Researchers usually do not formulate hypotheses that they are unable to test. If important hypotheses come up that cannot be tested with the standard statistical techniques available at the time, then attempts will be made to develop new techniques. As soon as new statistical techniques are disseminated, new hypotheses develop. This general observation also applies to MLA and the hypotheses that can be tested with it.

MLA makes it possible to test different kinds of hypotheses (Leyland and Groenewegen 2003):

- Hypotheses about variation.
- Hypotheses about the relationship between an outcome variable and individual-level independent variables.
- Hypotheses about the relationship between an outcome variable and higher level (contextual) independent variables.
- Hypotheses about cross-level interactions.

Hypotheses About Variation

The first step in MLA is to consider the variation in an outcome and to split this variation into that part that is attributable to differences between individuals and the part attributable to differences between their contexts. The statistical aspects of this will be introduced in Chap. 5. At present, it is sufficient to know that we can analyse how much of the total variance in our outcome variable is determined by the individual level (e.g. patients) and how much by a higher level, such as doctors or hospitals. In this manner we can get a sense as to how *important* each level is. In MLA we stop seeing variance only as a nuisance parameter that describes uncertainty, but we can also focus on the information that it represents (Merlo 2011).

We can therefore also develop hypotheses about where to expect more variation: at the individual level or at the higher level (Merlo et al. 2005). In many practical applications, the majority of the variation will be at the individual level. If we analyse treatment decisions by physicians, it is reasonable to expect there will be substantially more variability between patients than between doctors. Physicians take into account the situation of individual patients and apply their knowledge and skills according to each patient's circumstances. However, if the patient's situation does not strongly influence the physician's course of action, possibly because there is considerable disagreement between physicians as to the relative value of alternative treatments, more variability might be associated with the physicians. So receipt of treatment A rather than treatment B might be more strongly influenced by the physician consulted than by individual patient characteristics or circumstances.

There are other situations in which we might expect more variation to be at the higher level. This is for instance the case with repeated measures data (this and other data structures will be detailed in Chap. 4). When we analyse repeated measures made on the same individuals (the measures are then the lower level units and the individuals the higher level units), most of the variations will tend to be located at the higher level of the individuals themselves. Think, for example, of repeated measures of a subject's weight; there is likely to be more variability between people than between the measures made at different times on the same individual.

We might also be interested in patients treated by physicians who work together in group practices or hospitals. We now have three levels in our model: the patients, the physicians and the practices in which they work or, alternatively, the patients, hospital departments and hospitals. In this case we can develop hypotheses about the partitioning of variation between physicians and their practices or between hospital departments and the hospitals in which they are situated.

De Jong et al. (2006) considered how the hospital in which physicians worked could influence decisions regarding the length of stay of patients treated. Using data relating to patient discharges from all hospitals in New York State for different medical and surgical diagnostic-related groups (DRGs), they developed and tested a hypothesis based on variation. Believing that physicians would adapt to their local operating circumstances, they hypothesised that there would be more variation in length of stay between hospitals than between physicians working in the same hospital. The variation between individual patients, although substantially larger than the variation between physicians or between hospitals, was not of primary concern for this hypothesis.

In a more exploratory analysis, with no prior hypothesis, it is still important to analyse how variation is distributed between levels. This might provide clues as to what mechanisms could potentially explain variation (Merlo et al. 2009). The extent to which variation is distributed over different levels is also highly relevant when it comes to the development of interventions to influence a certain outcome. Think, for example, about patients' evaluation of their hospital stay. These patient evaluations may be influenced by the attending consultant, by the department where the patients were treated and by the hospital as a whole. Some aspects of the evaluation by patients may relate to the consultant level, such as the patients' judgement as to whether they had received sufficient information from their doctor, whilst other aspects, such as the quality of meals, will be related to the hospital rather than the consultant or department. The extent to which variation is distributed over different levels will give an indication as to the starting point for policies designed to improve patient satisfaction with their hospital stays (Hekkert et al. 2009). Zegers et al. (2011) analysed the occurrence of adverse events in hospitalised patients. From the partitioning of the variance between hospitals and hospital departments, they concluded that interventions to reduce adverse events should not only target hospitals as a whole, but also hospital departments.

Sundquist et al. (2011) studied how individual physical activity was related to objective measures of the built environment among a sample in Sweden. Realising the potential importance of neighbourhood as an influence on individual activity levels, given that neighbourhood is a relevant context for physical activity and that it is an environment that might be amenable to intervention, one of the stated aims of the study was to determine the proportion of the variability in moderate-to-vigorous physical activity that was attributable to neighbourhoods. Finding a rather small proportion of the total variation attributable to neighbourhoods, the authors suggested that the role of urban redevelopment in improving activity levels may be limited.

Apart from splitting the variation in an outcome between the different levels in our model, we can also develop hypotheses about differences in variation between groups. Variation across groups is usually seen by researchers as a nasty statistical problem that is best avoided as opposed to a source of hypotheses (Stinchcombe 2005). In their study on the impact of physician behaviour on patient length of stay, de Jong et al. (2006) reasoned that greater dependencies meant that there would be less variability among physicians who practiced in just one hospital (compared to those working in two or more hospitals). They therefore hypothesised that the variation between physicians (within hospitals) would decrease as the proportion of physicians practicing in just one hospital increased; that is, that there would be more variability within those hospitals in which a larger proportion of doctors worked in more than one hospital.

Ohlsson and Merlo (2007) evaluated the effect of the natural experiment of introducing a decentralised drug budget in Scania county, Sweden, using a before and after design. Believing that the increased economic responsibility given to those responsible for prescriptions would lead to efficient drug prescription, they hypothesised that not only would the prescription of recommended statins increase but also that the variation between healthcare centres and healthcare areas would decrease following budget decentralisation.

In a study of regional inequalities in mortality, Leyland (2004) found that the variance between the mortality rates of districts in Great Britain differed between the 11 regions and tended to increase over time, although the increases were not uniform. These variances were used as a measure of inequality within regions and were considered quite separately from the mean mortality rate for each region.

Although there may not be specific hypotheses concerning differences in variability between subgroups, it should be appreciated that *not* testing for differences in the variance is equivalent to assuming that the variance is the same for all subgroups but failing to test this assumption.

The emphasis on variation is a typical feature of MLA. If you are used to analysing your data at a single level with regression analysis, you probably will not consider differences in the variance between subgroups in your data. Ordinary regression analysis only predicts the means and not the distribution (Stinchcombe 2005). The coefficient of determination (R^2) is used to see how much variation is explained by a set of independent variables, but how much variation there was to begin with is usually not discussed. If you usually use analysis of variance, you might be more aware of differences in variation between groups. When you start using MLA, thinking about variation is an important first step. We return to the subject of variation in more detail in Chap. 6.

Individual-Level Hypotheses

In the case of individual-level hypotheses, a relationship is hypothesised between two variables at the same, lower, level. An example would be the relationship between the educational level of a patient and the amount of negotiating the patient initiates in a consultation with the GP. Why would we use MLA in a case like this? Basically because we know that the relationship cannot be adequately estimated without taking the structure of the data into account. We know that there are numerous other influences on what happens in a consultation, some of which are related to the individual patients and some to the GPs. In that sense the hypothesis about the relationship between educational achievement and initiating negotiations is incomplete, and we cannot simply assume that all other influences are the same (or that they only lead to random variation at the individual level).

Apart from the specific relationship between two variables at the lower level, we can also test the hypothesis that only individual characteristics are responsible for differences in outcomes between contexts such as health differences between communities. If individual characteristics related to health cluster in some communities, one might mistake this for differences produced by community characteristics or circumstances. For example, some communities may have poorer health outcomes but at the same time have older populations. MLA makes it possible to distinguish these so-called *compositional* effects from real *contextual* or area effects. This issue will be dealt with in more detail in Chap. 7. One could of course pose the question as to why people with certain characteristics should cluster together as opposed to being randomly distributed throughout areas. The identification of compositional effects therefore does not solve the problem of the importance of individual choice versus material conditions.

Context Hypotheses

In health services and public health research, as opposed to clinical research, we tend to be more interested in hypotheses relating the context to the outcome when applying MLA. We can distinguish between two kinds of contextual variables: those that are aggregated on the basis of individual characteristics at the lower level, such as the average level of education of the members of a group, and those that are only defined as characteristics of the higher level units. An example of the latter would be the number of years that a group has been in existence. This cannot be deduced from the characteristics of the individuals, but can only be observed for the group as a whole. Context hypotheses can refer to either kind of variable. The interpretation, of course, depends on the researcher's substantive theory. We will only give some possible interpretations here, to emphasise the importance of thinking in terms of possible mechanisms underlying a relationship in order to form hypotheses. We make no pretence that these are the only plausible interpretations.

Aggregated Individual-Level Characteristics

In this case, the higher level variable is constructed by aggregating an independent variable from the lower level to the higher level. (We come back to the way we can construct aggregated variables within MLA in Chap. 8.) There are numerous examples and associated interpretations. We will briefly discuss three.

The first example concerns the number diabetics in a GP's practice and how this number—obtained from counting all diabetics within the practice—might influence the regulation of individual patients. The hypothesis could be that the more diabetics there are in a practice, the greater the chances are that an individual diabetic is more poorly regulated. In this case the mechanism would be *competition*: all diabetics in a practice compete for the scarce and finite resource that is the GP's time and, in so doing, they have to divide the GP's time between them. The consequence is that, as the number of diabetics increases, each of them has less time with the GP and so all of them will be worse off.

The second example is substantively the same, but this time the hypothesis is framed the other way around: the more diabetics there are in a practice, the greater the chances are that an individual diabetic is better regulated. In this case the interpretation could be that a GP with more diabetics on their books is more attentive or more *experienced* in the treatment of diabetics and individual patients within that practice have better results as a consequence.

The aggregation of individual characteristics to a higher level may result in different kinds of variables; we could construct a count of the numbers of subjects having a certain characteristic, as in the previous two examples, the average value of a variable such as age, the proportion of subjects that have a particular attribute or trait (such as smoking), or an aspect of the distribution of a variable. The third example addresses this last possibility. There is a large (and much debated) research literature about income distribution and mortality rates. Henriksson et al. (2010) considered the effect of municipal level income inequality on the incidence of AMI in Sweden, adjusting for individual- and parish-level socio-economic characteristics. Income inequality was measured using the Gini coefficient, a statistical measure of dispersion, and the authors hypothesised that increasing municipality-level income inequality would be associated with elevated risk of AMI.

Higher Level Characteristics

In this case direct observations or measurements are made on the higher level units. These higher level characteristics can be indicators of the same processes that are implicated in the examples using aggregated variables. Competition for a GP's time could also be measured using the booking intervals in office consultations; experience in treating diabetics could be measured directly by testing the knowledge or skills of GPs involved in the study.

The number of higher level units may not be very large; as a rule there will be fewer higher level than lower level units. This may make it feasible to use observation or other more qualitative methods, such as the content analysis of documents as a means of constructing higher level characteristics. For example, if we study the effects of characteristics of urban neighbourhoods on the health behaviours of the people in these neighbourhoods, we can go out into the neighbourhoods and observe, for example, aspects of disorderliness. This is feasible with (perhaps) 20 neighbourhoods; however, it would be very costly to collect information on health behaviour through observation of (perhaps) 50 individuals in each neighbourhood. This means that MLA provides opportunities to combine quantitative and more qualitative approaches. A quantitative survey of patients at the individual level, where we usually deal with large numbers, can be combined with qualitative measures at the higher level. It may also be the case that geocoding provides a simple means to link the availability of structures derived from publicly available lists to specified areas (Macintyre et al. 2008).

The big advantage of MLA is that, if contextual information is available, MLA enables the testing of hypotheses about the relationship between contextual characteristics and individual outcomes, whilst simultaneously taking individual influences on health into account. This provides better estimates of the relationship between context and health. This means that, for example, we can analyse the effect of community wealth on population health, taking individual income into account.

Cross-Level Interactions

The fourth type of hypothesis that can be tested using MLA is that relating to cross-level interactions. These are combinations of (or interactions between) variables at different levels. It is the combination of a particular characteristic of the higher level with a particular individual level variable that is hypothesised to have a specific effect on the dependent variable of interest. Below we consider a couple of examples.

In another study of the effect of income inequality on health, Henriksson et al. (2007) hypothesised that manual workers were at higher risk of death than non-manual workers when living in areas of high-income inequality, arguing that such an effect might be supported by both psychosocial and neomaterial explanations. With data on individuals nested within the municipalities of residence, and following adjustment for both individual occupational social class and area income inequality, testing this hypothesis then equated to testing the significance of the interaction between the individual and contextual variables.

Finch et al. (2010) explored whether the relationship between health—measured using allostatic load, a measure of cumulative physiologic stress—and neighbourhood advantage or disadvantage varied according to an individual's educational status. Their hypothesis—that the relationship between context and the individual outcome would vary depending on individual characteristics—again amounted to a test of the significance of the cross-level interaction between a neighbourhood-level education index of concentration at the extremes (ICE) and individual socioeconomic status (operationalised using educational status).

The ability to analyse cross-level interactions is a major advantage of MLA that follows on from the ability to incorporate both individual and contextual independent variables in an analysis. In our thinking and theorising about health and healthcare, the relationships between context, individual characteristics and outcomes are of central importance. MLA affords the opportunity to test our ideas about these relationships.

Conclusion

In this chapter we have covered the basic concepts of multilevel modelling and have explained its potential and application in non-statistical terms. We have also covered the rationale for MLA and an explanation of what it is and how it differs from other regression approaches. We will return to the important subjects of variance and hypothesis testing at later stages in this book; for the moment it is important that you are aware that variance is not just a nuisance (the unexplained part of a model) and that, whether you are interested in formal hypothesis testing or concerned only with exploratory analysis, variances and contexts add new dimensions to research based solely on individual variables.

References

Aitken M, Anderson D, Hinde J (1981) Statistical modelling of data on teaching styles. J R Stat Soc Ser A 144:419–461

Cardol M, Groenewegen PP, de Bakker DH, Spreeuwenberg P, van Dijk L, van den Bosch W (2005) Shared help seeking behaviour within families: a retrospective cohort study. Br Med J 330:882–884

de Jong JD, Westert GP, Lagoe R, Groenewegen PP (2006) Variation in hospital length of stay: do physicians adapt their length of stay decisions to what is usual in the hospital where they work? Health Serv Res 41:374–394

Diez-Roux AV (1998) Bringing context back into epidemiology: variables and fallacies in multilevel analysis. Am J Public Health 88:216–222

Finch BK, Do DP, Heron M, Bird C, Seeman T, Lurie N (2010) Neighborhood effects on health: concentrated advantage and disadvantage. Health Place 16:1058–1060

Flay BR, Brannon BR, Johnson CA, Hansen WB, Ulene AL, Whitney-Saltiel DA, Gleason LR, Sussman S, Gavin MD, Glowacz KM, Sobol DF, Spiegel DC (1988) The television school and family smoking prevention and cessation project. I. Theoretical basis and program development. Prev Med 17:585–607

Gelman A, Hill J (2007) Data analysis using regression and multilevel/hierarchical models. Cambridge University Press, Cambridge

Ghosh M, Natarajan K, Stroud TWF, Carlin BP (1998) Generalized linear models for small-area estimation. J Am Stat Assoc 93:273–282
Goldstein H, Browne W, Rasbash J (2002) Partitioning variation in multilevel models. Underst Stat 1:223–231
Groenewegen PP (1997) Dealing with micro–macro relations: a heuristic approach with examples from health services research. In: Westert GP, Verhoeff RN (eds) Places and people: multilevel modelling in geographical research. Nederlandse Geografische Studies, Utrecht
Hekkert KD, Cihangir S, Kleefstra SM, Van den Berg B, Kool RB (2009) Patient satisfaction revisited: a multilevel analysis. Soc Sci Med 69:68–75
Henriksson G, Allebeck P, Ringbäck Weitoft G, Thelle D (2007) Are manual workers at higher risk of death than non-manual employees when living in Swedish municipalities with higher income inequality? Eur J Pub Health 17:139–144
Henriksson G, Ringbäck Weitoft G, Allebeck P (2010) Associations between income inequality at municipality level and health depend on context—a multilevel analysis on myocardial infarction in Sweden. Soc Sci Med 71:1141–1149
Leyland AH (2004) Increasing inequalities in premature mortality in Great Britain. J Epidemiol Community Health 58:296–302
Leyland AH (2010) No quick fix: understanding the difference between fixed and random effect models. J Epidemiol Community Health 64:1027–1028
Leyland AH, Groenewegen PP (2003) Multilevel modelling and public health policy. Scand J Public Health 31:267–274
Liang K-Y, Zeger S (1993) Regression analysis for correlated data. Annu Rev Public Health 14:43–68
Maas CJM, Hox JJ (2005) Sufficient sample sizes for multilevel modeling. Methodology 1:86–92
Macintyre S, Macdonald L, Ellaway A (2008) Do poorer people have poorer access to local resources and facilities? The distribution of local resources by area deprivation in Glasgow, Scotland. Soc Sci Med 67:900–914
Mauny F, Viel JF, Handschumacher P, Sellin B (2004) Multilevel modelling and malaria: a new method for an old disease. Int J Epidemiol 33:1337–1344
Merlo J (2011) Contextual influences on the individual life course: building a research framework for social epidemiology. Psychosoc Interv 20:109–118
Merlo J, Chaix B, Yang M, Lynch J, Råstam L (2005) A brief conceptual tutorial of multilevel analysis in social epidemiology: linking the statistical concept of clustering to the idea of contextual phenomenon. J Epidemiol Community Health 59:443–449
Merlo J, Ohlsson H, Lynch KF, Chaix B, Subramanian SV (2009) Individual and collective bodies: using measures of variance and association in contextual epidemiology. J Epidemiol Community Health 63:1043–1048
Moerbeek M, van Breukelen GJP, Berger MPF (2003) A comparison between traditional methods and multilevel regression for the analysis of multicenter intervention studies. J Clin Epidemiol 56:341–350
Ohlsson H, Merlo J (2007) Understanding the effects of a decentralized budget on physicians' compliance with guidelines for statin prescription—a multilevel methodological approach. BMC Health Serv Res 7:68
Raudenbush S, Bryk AS (1986) A hierarchical model for studying school effects. Sociol Educ 59:1–17
Renders CM, Valk GD, Franse LV, Schellevis FG, van Eijk JT, Van der Wal G (2001) Long-term effectiveness of a quality improvement program for patients with type 2 diabetes in general practice. Diabetes Care 24:1365–1370
Snijders TAB (2001) Sampling. In: Leyland AH, Goldstein H (eds) Multilevel modelling of health statistics. Wiley, Chichester
Stinchcombe AL (2005) The logic of social research. University of Chicago Press, Chicago

Sundquist K, Eriksson U, Kawakami N, Skog L, Ohlsson H, Arvidsson D (2011) Neighborhood walkability, physical activity, and walking behavior: the Swedish Neighborhood and Physical Activity (SNAP) study. Soc Sci Med 72:1266–1273
Twisk JWR (2006) Applied multilevel analysis. Cambridge University Press, Cambridge
Zegers M, De Bruijne MC, Spreeuwenberg P, Wagner C, Van der Wal G, Groenewegen PP (2011) Variation in rates of adverse events between hospitals and hospital departments. Int J Qual Health Care 23:126–133

4

Diverse Data Structures for Multilevel Modeling

Abstract This chapter covers different data structures for which multilevel modelling is appropriate, giving examples of each. The first such structure is the strict hierarchy, which may be the structure that first comes to mind when you think about multilevel models: patients who are treated in hospitals or individuals living in certain areas. Then there are multistage sampling designs and the evaluations of community interventions, in which it is the study design that imposes the hierarchical structure on the data. There are studies that collect data over time, either through repeated cross-sections or through repeated measures on an individual. This introduces another hierarchy to the data. Such models can be expanded to include multiple responses: more than one measure on each individual. These can be analysed simultaneously and considered as being nested within individuals. Then there are structures which are not strictly hierarchical. Firstly, the cross-classified model, in which there is an overlap between different classifications meaning that units at one level are not nested neatly within units at another level. Secondly, the multiple membership model in which an individual at one level can be a member of a number of different units at a higher level. Thirdly, the correlated cross-classified model, used when cross-classifications are repeated over time. Finally, this chapter briefly covers some further structures that can be modelled as multilevel structures. The idea of including these further structures is to make the reader aware of the range of models that could potentially be fitted to data rather than to cover them in detail.

Keywords Multilevel analysis · Hierarchy · Community interventions · Time dependent data · Multiple responses · Cross-classified models · Multiple membership models

In Chap. 3, we considered why levels were important and what might constitute a level in your data. We now expand on these ideas as we show a wide range of data structures that can be considered to be hierarchical and for which MLA is therefore the appropriate form of analysis. We draw largely on the model classifications used by Duncan et al. (1996) and Subramanian et al. (2003).

Strict Hierarchies: The Basic Model

We start off with the strict hierarchies. A lot of the theory and practice of multilevel modelling was developed in educational research in which the aim was to determine whether the shared environment of the school that pupils attended contributed to educational attainment, after adjusting for differences between schools in pupil characteristics (Aitken and Longford 1986; Goldstein 1986). From there it is not a big leap to consider a design of, for example, patients nested within hospitals (Fig. 4.1). The hierarchies have a pyramid structure with patients at the lower level (level one) nested within hospitals at the higher level (level two). The lowest level—the patient level in this example—is the level at which the outcome is measured. The reason for considering a multilevel model for these data is because the outcome for an individual patient may be influenced by the hospital that they attend or, in general, the shared context means that the patient outcomes may well be correlated, violating the standard regression assumption of independence. So whilst there is variability between patient outcomes, some of this variability may be due to differences between hospitals. The ability to partition variation into that attributable to different levels is an important feature of multilevel models. It is easy to think of examples of these basic models, whether they be patients in hospitals, survey respondents in residential neighbourhoods or GPs nested within practices.

We might have a three-level model in which the individuals at level one are the persons for whom we have measured a response (Fig. 4.2). These individuals are clustered within households at level two and then within neighbourhoods at level three. The idea of all of these strict hierarchies is that we have many units at one level nested within fewer units at the next level. Of course, the real world is not restricted to two or three levels and nor need our multilevel models be; the inclusion of relevant contexts may increase the number of levels that we need to consider. For example, in a study of diagnostic practice style in Alberta, Canada, Yiannakoulis et al. (2009) used a model including not only the individual physicians, for whom the outcome of diagnostic style was recorded, and the facilities in which they worked but also the municipality and census division—a strict hierarchy of four levels. And when

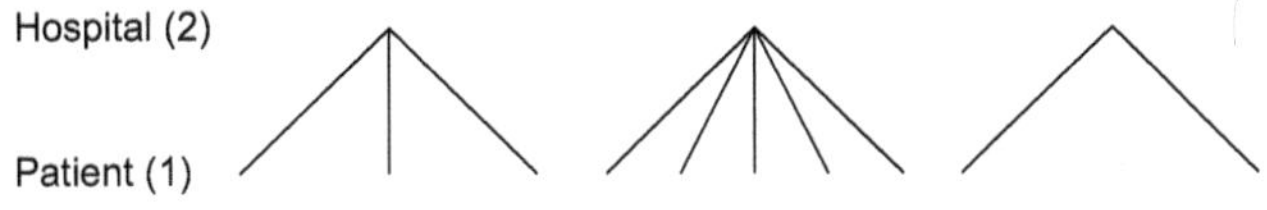

Fig. 4.1 Basic two-level model

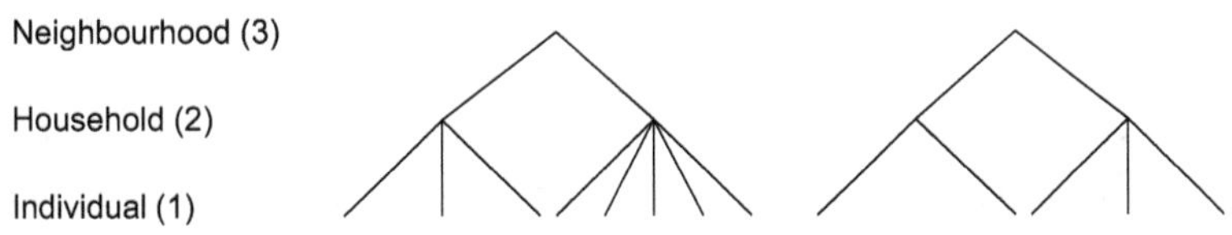

Fig. 4.2 Basic three-level model

exploring the consumption of tobacco in India, Subramanian et al. (2004) included household, local areas, districts and states as relevant contexts for the survey respondents in a five-level model.

It is important to note two features of these basic designs. Firstly, we do not need to have a balanced design. Our sample does not need to have the same number of patients in every hospital, or the same number of individuals in every household, or the same number of households in every neighbourhood. Secondly, the examples that we have discussed have the person as the lowest level, whether this is a patient, survey respondent or physician. Although this is a common occurrence, and there have been instances in previous chapters where we have referred to the individual and level one as though the two were synonymous, this need not necessarily be the case. For example, in a study of the variation in the use of drug-eluting stents (DESs) in the treatment of coronary heart disease in Scotland, Austin et al. (2008) took into account the fact that patients may have more than one lesion treated during a procedure by using lesions as the lowest level (the level at which the outcome, DES use, is measured) with these in turn nested within patients, operators and hospitals. The use of a multilevel model in this instance took into account the possible clustering of DES use within patients. And in periodontology, in a study of factors influencing the closure of pockets observed at different sites around teeth, Tomasi et al. (2007) used a hierarchy of sites within teeth within patients, patients forming the highest level in this analysis.

It may also be the case that data are not available at the individual level but rather are aggregated to an administrative area level. Such data restriction may reflect issues surrounding data confidentiality, whereby agencies are unwilling to release potentially identifiable individual data, or may just represent the constraints of official data systems. Cavalini and Ponce de Leon (2008) undertook an ecological analysis of the association between various socio-economic, political and healthcare indicators and differing morbidity and mortality outcomes in Brazil. With no data on individuals they used the levels of municipality, region and state; the outcomes were all measured at municipality level. No matter whether the data we have refer to individuals, aggregations of individuals or are collected within individuals, the lowest level is always the level at which the outcome is measured.

Multistage Sampling Designs

For a multistage sampling design, the hierarchy is imposed during data collection. The structure of the survey dictates the hierarchical design and straight away this implies that MLA is necessary. If the survey design is a simple random sample, individuals are selected from a sampling frame (for example, from a population register or hospital discharge register). In a two-stage sample high level sampling units are first selected, perhaps towns or municipalities, and then within each high level unit a sample of individuals is drawn. Individuals are nested within the higher-level sampling units, and this nesting must be taken into account because of the potential for contextual influences on any outcomes. The data hierarchy will appear similar to those seen in Figs. 4.1 and 4.2. An example of such a design is the health interview survey in Belgium, as described by Demarest et al. (2013).

The primary reason for using multistage sampling is usually related to cost. It may be considerably cheaper to send interviewers to conduct several interviews within selected municipalities than conducting single interviews across a number of municipalities. Statistical methods were developed to permit the analysis of data collected from multistage samples; relatively simple sandwich estimators can be used which correct the standard error of the estimates to take the clustered sample design into account (Froot 1989). As described in Chap. 3, one effect of a multilevel data structure is to reduce the effective sample size which will in turn increase standard errors and confidence intervals. We return to the impact of clustering on power calculations in Chap. 6. The use of techniques such as sandwich estimators assumes that the hierarchical data structure is a nuisance—something for which we must make allowances but in which we have no substantive interest. But this is an over-simplification and is rarely the case; social epidemiology as a discipline is built on such substantive interests as the reasons for variations in health between areas. This is where we can start to explore the role of composition—who lives in the areas—and the context, or what it is about the areas themselves that lead to differences in outcomes between areas. These issues are explored further in Chap. 7.

Evaluating Community Interventions and Cluster Randomised Trials

There are a number of reasons for conducting an intervention at the community level; that is, when the community (as opposed to the individual) is the unit of allocation or randomisation. These include the impossibility or impracticality of introducing the intervention at an individual level (for example, in the case of water fluoridation), the desire to avoid contamination between intervention and control subjects, or as a cheaper and non-stigmatising means of targeting higher risk groups (Leyland 2010). In health services research, a cluster randomised approach may be the only appropriate means of evaluating certain interventions such as those relating to organisational change (Campbell and Grimshaw 1998). But whatever the rationale underlying the design of the study, if the intervention is at the group level and outcomes are measured at the individual level, then the data are hierarchical and must be analysed using MLA (Koepsell et al. 1992). Sample size or power calculations for cluster randomised trials differ from those for standard trials and are covered in Chap. 6.

Designs Including Time

We can think of two different types of designs including time: repeated cross-sections and repeated measures or panel data (Duncan et al. 1996; Subramanian et al. 2003). A repeated cross-sectional design might be used as a means of assessing hospital performance and how that changes over time. In such a case the hospitals form the highest level, and within each hospital every year data are collected relating to patient outcomes as a measure of that hospital's performance. The ambition is to use these data to learn how each hospital performs in comparison to its peers and how the performance of each hospital is changing over time. Since the outcomes are at the patient level, the patient forms the lowest level in the hierarchy. Figure 4.3 shows the nesting of patients within years, and years within hospitals, in a three-level model. Dee (2001) used a repeated cross-sectional design to investigate the impact of (economic) cyclical state-level income effects on individual alcohol consumption through the study of repeated cross-sectional surveys of individuals nested within states of the USA. As with previous models we have no requirement for a perfectly balanced data set and so there is no need for our samples to include the same number of patients every year. Moreover, we can include hospitals for which we do not have data in every year. This will come as a relief to those familiar with the changing patterns of health provision and the idea that hospitals may close or open during a period of data collection.

The repeated measures or panel design is similar to the repeated cross-sectional design except that the same individuals are observed on different occasions. This means that the outcome is not measured at the level of the individual but at the level of the measurement occasion nested within the individual. The outcome still refers to the individual but may differ from one moment in time to another. Figure 4.4 illustrates a study in which outcomes on individuals are assessed on an annual basis and, in this example, the individuals themselves are clustered within neighbourhoods. This means that we can analyse longitudinal data in a multilevel

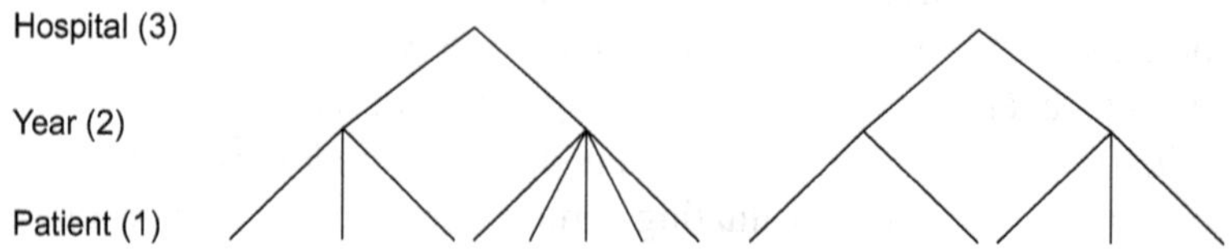

Fig. 4.3 Repeated cross-sectional design

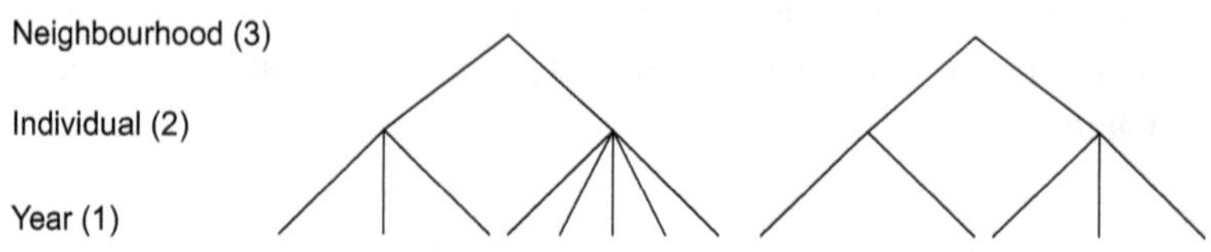

Fig. 4.4 Repeated measures or panel design

framework by taking into account the fact that measurement occasions are nested within individuals. In addition to any correlations that may exist between individuals within their contexts (hospitals, neighbourhoods, etc.), this design allows for the correlation between observations made on the same individual.

Haynes et al. (2008) looked at the risk of accidents in pre-school children using data from a longitudinal study, with measurement occasions nested within children and children nested within neighbourhoods. It is not necessary for individuals to be clustered within higher-level units; MLA can still be used to analyse repeated measures with individuals forming the higher level. Such a two-level model for changes in body mass index was used by Lipps and Moreau-Gruet (2010). Repeated measures do not have to be made on individuals; Kroneman and Siegers (2004) considered how reductions in the number of available hospital beds affected different measures of bed use using repeated measures on countries, with the outcomes (bed occupancy, average length of stay and admission rates) being observed in different years for each country. The example used in the first computing practical (Chap. 11) is based on the analysis of repeated measures of mortality rates made at the area level.

As with the previous models, it is not necessary to have information on every individual on every occasion; if we are able to make certain assumptions about missingness (that the data are *missing completely at random* or *missing at random*), then we can include individuals with incomplete data in the analysis. More detail about the different types of missing data and appropriate methods for their analysis can be found elsewhere (Carpenter et al. 2006; Little and Rubin 2002; Sterne et al. 2009).

When analysing repeated measures data, it is usually the case that we find more variation between individuals than within individuals (between measurement occasions) and so, unlike the basic models considered above, a larger proportion of the total variation may be at higher levels. This is easy to understand if you consider, for example, a study with repeated measures of people's weight; there is likely to be much less variability in individual weight from one measurement occasion to another than there is between the weights of individuals in the population. Such is the nature of individual heterogeneity.

Multiple Responses

There are strong similarities between repeated measures and multiple response designs. In the former we measure the same item on individuals at a number of different measurement occasions; in the latter we measure a number of different items on individuals, often at the same measurement occasion. This can therefore be seen as a multilevel model—we have the different responses nested within each individual—and there may be a further level such as the neighbourhood of residence as illustrated in Fig. 4.5. The multiple responses may, for example, be drawn from a questionnaire focusing on health-related behaviours; a number of individuals may be surveyed about alcohol and tobacco consumption, diet and exercise. These behaviours may be correlated within individuals; high alcohol consumption may be

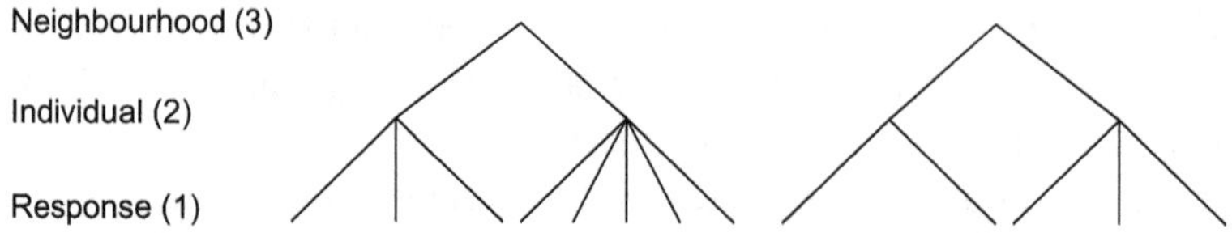

Fig. 4.5 Multiple responses

associated with poor diet, for example. This correlation may remain after adjustment for individual characteristics, particularly if an important characteristic associated with more than one behaviour is omitted or poorly recorded in the survey. But we also have the possibility of modelling and examining these correlations at higher levels. If alcohol consumption and diet both show variation between areas, is the nature of the relationship the same? That is, are those areas associated with above (below) average alcohol consumption also associated with poorer (better) diets?

Once again we can work with an unbalanced data set and so if some individuals have not responded to all questions, and provided that we can make the usual assumptions about the data being missing at random, we can include all the data that we have and do not have to consider the deletion of cases or responses. An example of a multiple response model includes a joint analysis of self-rated health and happiness on individuals nested within communities (Subramanian et al. 2005). In addition to showing the different effects of various socio-demographic variables on the two outcomes, the authors demonstrated a modest positive correlation at the individual level and a stronger positive correlation at area level, interpreting this as meaning that communities that were unhealthy were also likely to be unhappy.

It is possible to combine the analysis of different response types in a multilevel multiple response model; for example, we could include a continuous response such as blood pressure alongside a dichotomous response such as smoking status. The fact that there is no requirement for the data to be balanced or complete means that we can have structurally missing values: data which may or may not be collected depending on the response to another question. Duncan et al. (1996) looked at smoking behaviour among individuals living in areas (electoral wards) in England, considering two aspects of smoking: smoking status (whether an individual currently smoked or not) and the number of cigarettes smoked per day. For those who do not smoke the number of cigarettes smoked per day must be zero and can be ignored, removing a large peak in the (bimodal) distribution. Smoking status is therefore treated as a dichotomous outcome and the number of cigarettes smoked per day (among those who smoke) as a continuous measure. In addition to noting differences in the factors related to smoking status and cigarette consumption, the authors found a positive correlation between the two at the area level suggesting that cigarette consumption tends to be higher for individuals who live in areas in which people are more likely to smoke. A similar example is given in a study of the use of tranquillizers (benzodiazepines) in neighbourhoods in a Dutch city (Groenewegen et al. 1999). In this case the dichotomous outcome was whether or not people received a prescription and the dose of the drug, if given a prescription, was treated as a continuous response. Once again the model permitted not only the analysis of factors associated with both prescription and dose but also the analysis of the relationship between these outcomes at the area level.

Any data showing an excessive number of observations at zero are amenable to these types of mixed response models. Tooze et al. (2002) considered a range of factors associated with medical expenditure based on a sample of individuals nested within households. They interpreted the strong positive correlation between the occurrence of healthcare expenditure (dichotomous) and the intensity of expenditure (continuous) as indicating that, after adjusting for any differences in covariates, households that were more likely to seek medical care were also likely to have greater healthcare expenditure.

Non-hierarchical Structures

The data structures that we have considered up to this point are all strict hierarchies; that is, a number of units at one level are nested within one and only one unit at the level above. The reality is that healthcare systems or the social contexts affecting individuals are often more complex than this, and if we have data that reflects this complexity then this leads to hierarchies that do not have such a neat structure. Below we discuss three types of non-hierarchical structures that can be fitted using MLA: *cross-classified models*, *multiple membership models* and *correlated cross-classified models*.

Cross-Classified Models

A cross-classified model is one in which units at one level are simultaneously nested within two separate, non-nested hierarchies (Goldstein 1994). For example, we may want to examine how the outcome for an individual patient varies according both to the hospital the patient attended and to the general practitioner (GP) that referred the patient to hospital. Figure 4.6 shows how the hierarchy may appear for such a model. Although all patients are referred by one and only one GP, and each attends one and only one hospital, there is no strict nesting of GPs within hospitals; certain GPs may refer different patients to different hospitals. Similarly, hospitals are not nested within GPs since hospitals receive referrals from several different GPs. We say in

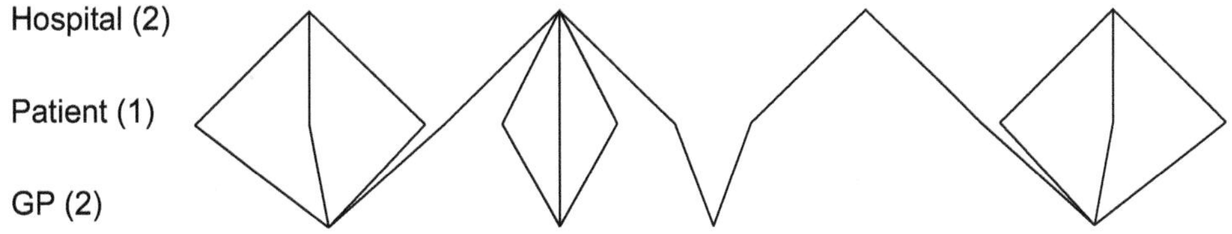

Fig. 4.6 Cross-classified model

such a case that patients are nested within a cross-classification of GPs and hospitals (Browne et al. 2001; Rasbash and Browne 2001). The way in which the computational aspects of fitting cross-classified models are handled varies according to the software used for analysis; some of the statistical packages used to fit multilevel models treat cross-classified models no differently from strict hierarchies, whilst other packages may require a distinct specification for this class of model. Readers are advised to check the reference manuals of their chosen software for further details.

As with the strictly hierarchical multilevel models, cross-classified models may be used to reflect the observed hierarchy (in which case the levels themselves may not be of substantive interest) or they may be used to explore variation and determine the relative importance of different contexts. This distinction relates to the range of hypotheses that can be tested using MLA discussed in Chap. 3. Downing et al. (2007) explored the association between deaths and hospital admissions for a range of conditions and scores assigned to GP practices through the UK's Quality and Outcomes Framework (QOF). Their data comprised patients nested within a cross-classification of GPs and residential areas, with covariates available on both contexts. Urquia et al. (2009) considered the relative impacts of neighbourhood of residence and country of origin on the birthweight of children born to recent immigrants in Ontario, Canada, following adjustment for a variety of individual factors, and concluded that the country of origin made a much larger contribution to the variation in outcomes. Virtanen et al. (2010) separated the effects of teachers' neighbourhood of residence and the neighbourhood in which the school was located on the sickness absences of teachers and found significant relationships with both (in terms of a contextual variable—mean neighbourhood income—and the variances at the two levels).

Multiple Membership Model

The second type of non-hierarchical structure used in MLA is the multiple membership model (Hill and Goldstein 1998). This model is appropriate when units at one level may belong to (or *be members of*) more than one unit at a higher level. For example, consider a patient who receives a course of treatment such as chemotherapy over a period of time. Certain patients may receive their treatment at more than one hospital as shown in Fig. 4.7. If the outcome for each patient is survival at 12 months, then we may be interested in determining whether patient survival varies between hospitals. For those patients who were treated in more than one hospital, we

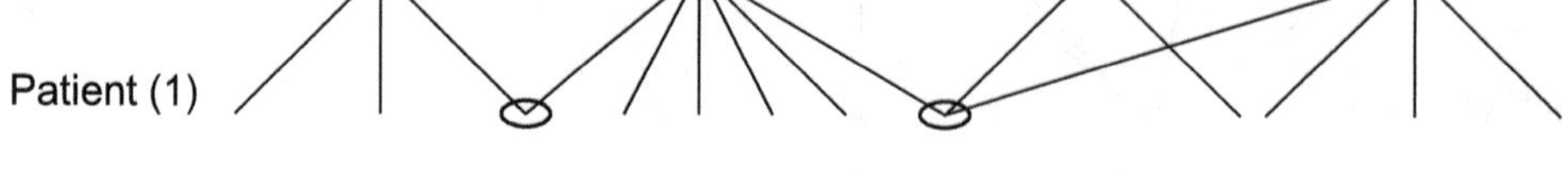

Fig. 4.7 Multiple membership model

must make assumptions about the relative contributions of different hospitals to the patients' care. This comes down to assigning a weight attributed to each hospital with the weights summing to one for each individual (so the weights are, in fact, proportions). If we know the proportion of time that a patient spent in each hospital, then these proportions may make suitable weights; otherwise, it may be sufficient to give equal weight to each hospital attended (so weights of 0.5 if a patient was seen in two hospitals, 0.33 if seen in three hospitals, etc.). The impact of different weighting schemes on the results can be examined as a form of sensitivity analysis.

Ryan et al. (2006) examined the influence of caseworkers on two child welfare outcomes: the length of stay in foster care and the probability of family reunification. Most youths in the study from Illinois were assigned more than one caseworker; multiple membership models allowed the authors to account for the complex data structure when testing hypotheses about the association of certain key caseworker characteristics on the child outcomes. Another use for a multiple membership model is to account for changes in geographical boundaries over the course of time; Leyland (2004) assigned weights based on resident populations to take account of changes in the number and boundaries of areas following administrative restructuring. Falster et al. (2018) used a multiple membership model to analyse the between-hospital variation in patient admission for preventable hospitalisations. Although the hospital of admission was known for those patients who were admitted to hospital, the population who were not admitted to any hospital were assigned to multiple hospitals based on observed admission patterns.

Correlated Cross-Classified Model

The correlated cross-classified model should be used for the analysis of repeated classifications (Leyland and Næss 2009). Such data structures are typically encountered when contextual information at regular intervals is linked to an outcome measured at the end of the study, although they may also be appropriate when different aspects of the same context are being measured such as place of residence and place of work. Figure 4.8 provides a simple example of individuals living in four areas at two different time points. The difference between this model and the cross-classified model (Fig. 4.6) is that instead of independent contexts such as GP and

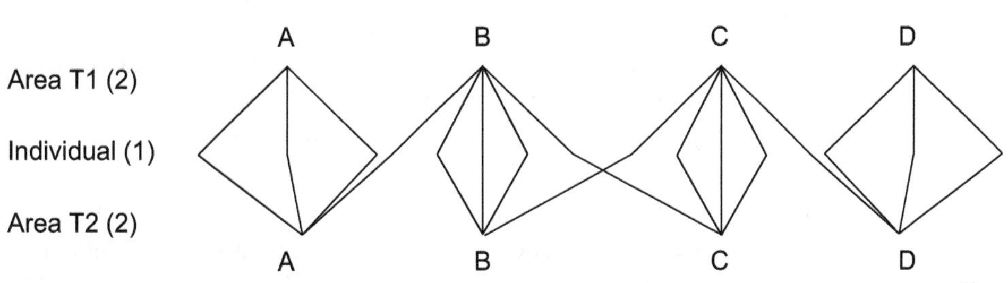

Fig. 4.8 Correlated cross-classified model

hospital, the areas are the same at each time (denoted areas A, B, C, and D). One of the assumptions underlying MLA is that the contexts are independent, whether these are the GPs and hospitals in Fig. 4.6 or the neighbourhood and households in Fig. 4.2. Standard multilevel models, including the cross-classified model, therefore assume no correlation between contexts. The multiple membership model described above is appropriate when individuals move between contexts but the contexts (e.g. areas) are the same at different points in time. The correlated cross-classified model comes somewhere between the cross-classified and multiple membership models, recognising that contexts may not be identical (due, for example, to the way neighbourhoods may change over time) but at the same time that the contexts are not completely independent of each other (the poorest area at one time point is unlikely to become the richest area at another time).

The cross-classified, multiple membership and correlated cross-classified models are described and the implications of the different assumptions underlying each are analysed from the perspective of life course epidemiology by Næss and Leyland (2010).

An example of the use of a correlated cross-classified multilevel model is based on analysis of the Oslo Mortality Study (Leyland and Næss 2009). Area of residence was known for inhabitants of Oslo at the time of the 1960, 1970, 1980 and 1990 Censuses and individuals were followed up in the mortality register until 1998. The models were used to determine the relative contribution of residence at different stages of the life course—based on known residence at the Censuses—on subsequent mortality for different birth cohorts.

Other Multilevel Models

There is a broad range of data types that can be analysed using MLA and of models that can be constructed in a multilevel framework. Some of these are dependent on the availability of specialist software, whilst others may be implemented in most packages that can be used for multilevel modelling. In this section, we briefly describe some of these models.

We have said little about the response types that can be analysed using MLA, but most of the examples presented in this chapter have assumed continuous outcomes to be normally distributed or have used logistic regression for dichotomous outcomes. Multilevel Poisson or negative binomial regression models may be used when the data take the form of counts, either because individual data are aggregated to an area level in studies of disease incidence or prevalence (Cavalini and Ponce de Leon 2008) or when the data represent counts made on individuals, such as the number of carious, extracted or filled teeth (Levin et al. 2010) or the frequency of contact with GPs (Cardol et al. 2005). Multilevel Poisson regression is also appropriate for modelling incidence or prevalence on individual data as a means of adjusting for exposure or person time at risk (Martikainen et al. 2003). Multilevel logistic regression can easily be extended to multilevel multinomial regression if the responses form unordered categories, such as place of birth being categorised as home, private hospital or public hospital in a study of maternity care provision in Ghana (Amoako Johnson and Padmadas 2009), or ordered categories, such as a measure of self-rated health (Oshio and Kobayashi 2009). Note, however, that in the presence of five or more ordered categories it may be appropriate to analyse the data as though the response was continuous and normally distributed (Mansyur et al. 2008).

Several different models have been developed for the analysis of multilevel data when the outcome of interest is the time to an event or a survival time. The simplest of these is the accelerated lifetime or log duration model, which centres on modelling the logarithm of the survival time. Such a model has been used to assess area-based inequalities in a 30-year follow-up of a large Swedish cohort (Yang et al. 2009). An alternative approach is to fit multilevel Cox proportional hazard models; these have been used, for example, to examine contextual influences on the hazard of mortality (Chaix et al. 2007). Such models have the advantage of providing answers even if a large proportion of the data are censored and of enabling the inclusion of time-varying covariates (Goldstein 2003). For example, Sear et al. (2000) examined the effect of maternal grandmothers on the survival of children in rural Gambia; the presence of the grandmother is clearly an effect which may change during a child's life. Multilevel Cox regression models require data expansion that can quickly render a dataset large and unwieldy; an alternative approach is therefore to use multilevel Weibull survival models, as employed by Chaix et al. (2008) to examine the impact of individual perception of safety and neighbourhood cohesion on mortality from acute myocardial infarction.

A multilevel repeated measures model takes into account the fact that observations made on the same individual are likely to be correlated. A *time series* model can take this one stage further by modelling the correlation between observations as a function of time such that the correlation between two measures made on the same person close together in time will be higher than the correlation between two measures made a long time apart. There are a number of different ways in which this correlation can be included (Goldstein et al. 1994). An example of the application of such methods is for the analysis of smoking cessation data in which adjustment was made for the serial dependence of observations on individuals' smoking status (Wang et al. 2006).

A similar principle applies to multilevel spatial models as to the multilevel time series models. It is possible to take geography into account to some extent by using a series of areas of increasing size. This relates to the so-called 'modifiable areal unit problem' or MAUP (Openshaw 1984). Geographical units are to some extent artificial and changing from one geographical division to another might influence the results of a study. MLA facilitates a meaningful analysis of this problem (Groenewegen et al. 1999; Jones 1993; Merlo 2011). Some of the difference between small areas (such as neighbourhoods) may be attributable to differences between larger areas such as municipalities, and the differences between municipalities may in part be due to differences between larger areas such as counties or regions. Including these different geographies in a single multilevel model ensures that there is a correlation between neighbourhoods in the same municipality and between municipalities in the same county. But this ignores the detail in the geography; the exact geographical positioning of neighbourhoods within a municipality or of municipalities within a county is not taken into account. A spatial multilevel model allows for a greater degree of correlation between areas that are geographically close than between areas that are geographically distant. A simple means of fitting such spatial dependencies is to use a *multiple membership model* (see above) in which, in addition to heterogeneous area effects, areas are modelled as multiple members of the set of their neighbours. Bartolomeo et al. (2010) used such a model to investigate the geographical patterning of hospitalisations for lung cancer and chronic obstructive pulmonary disease. Spatial modelling will also provide geographically smoothed estimates, overcoming some of the problems associated with small areas and rare outcomes leading to volatile rates and allowing the identification of clusters of disease. The methodology underlying such modelling may be complex and is described in detail elsewhere (Best et al. 2005; Lawson et al. 2003; Leyland and Davies 2005). Næss et al. (2007) used a spatial multilevel model to separate the effect of air pollution from that of social deprivation, both measured at the neighbourhood level, on individual mortality following adjustment for individual socio-economic status.

Other data which lend themselves to multilevel analysis include meta-analysis, for example a meta-analysis of the results of several clinical trials. The idea of meta-analysis is to combine information from separate studies. A fixed effects approach to meta-analysis is based on the assumption that there is a single 'true' effect which is observed with error in each study. The random effects or multilevel approach to meta-analysis assumes that there is heterogeneity between studies in the effect size. Published information on the original trials will often be extremely limited; for example, a randomised controlled trial may report the numbers of deaths and total number of patients in the treatment and control wings of a trial. In such circumstances, and if the original data cannot be made available, it is important to take into account the precision of the estimate of the effect size by giving more weight to larger studies. It is also possible to combine summary outcomes from trials with complete data on individuals from those trials for which full individual data are available or to combine trial data with observational data. Examples of multilevel meta-analyses include a study of the effectiveness of interventions to promote advance directives (such as living wills and durable power of attorney for healthcare) among the elderly (Bravo et al. 2008) and a quantification of the effects of education on self-reported health (Furnée et al. 2008).

Multilevel models have been extended to include factor analysis, latent class analysis and structural equation models. These expand upon their single-level counterparts to take into account the clustering of individuals within higher-level units. For example, Franzini et al. (2005) used multilevel structural equation models to investigate whether latent variables such as collective efficacy (comprising social cohesion, trust and helpfulness) or neighbourhood disorder (comprising physical and social disorder) mediated the relationship between neighbourhood impoverishment and self-rated health after adjusting for individual characteristics. Curry et al. (2008)

used multilevel path analysis to determine whether objectively measured neighbourhood crime rates impacted directly on individual depression or whether the impact was indirect, being mediated by subjective perceptions of neighbourhood problems. And Vermunt (2007) identified three classes of doctors and two classes of hospital on the basis of their prescribing behaviour when treating children with acute respiratory tract infection; responses for individual children were coded as indicating appropriate use, abuse of a single antibiotic or abuse of multiple antibiotics.

Multilevel latent variable analysis will be considered more extensively in Chap. 8. The reason for this is that this approach is increasingly used to construct characteristics of higher-level units on the basis of individual responses to a series of scale items. These scale items try to measure a latent variable at the higher level. For example, items about neighbourhood disorder, collected from residents in a survey, can collectively be used to indicate disorder at the neighbourhood level. This approach is also known as *ecometrics*.

Pseudo-levels

In Chap. 3, we considered what constitutes a level. In particular, we made a distinction between a level—comprising units which could be sampled—and the characteristics of a level. Although this is true in the strictest sense, it is sometimes useful to introduce characteristics as a *pseudo-level* at any level apart from the highest level in the hierarchy. This is particularly important if we want to test hypotheses about (or just to explore) variation between subgroups, as was discussed in Chap. 3. For example, suppose we have health data on a number of individuals attending different hospitals, and one focus of our interest is whether the variance in our outcome differs between men and women. Although the individual's sex is a characteristic of the individual and not a level, we can include sex as a pseudo-level in our model so that patients are nested within sex within hospitals, and then condition on the mean difference between men and women. (*Conditioning on the mean* means that we include a dummy variable to take account of the mean difference in health between men and women. This dummy variable is then a characteristic of the pseudo-level rather than the individual level since it applies to all individuals within that group.) Figure 4.9 shows how the inclusion of this pseudo-level changes the structure of our dataset. The groups at the pseudo-level are often referred to as *cells*, and sometimes individual responses are aggregated over these

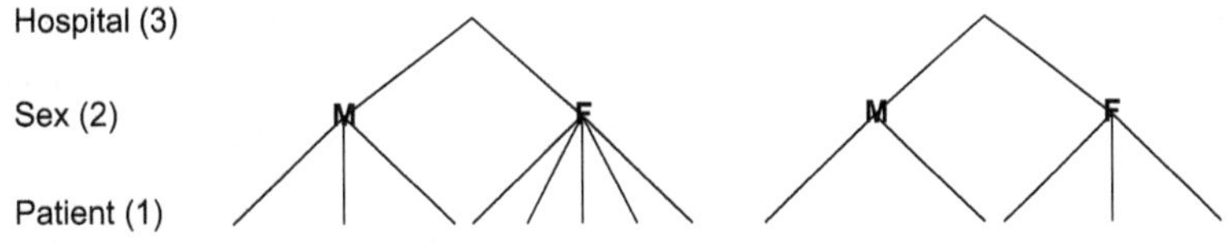

Fig. 4.9 Model with pseudo-levels

cells which then form the lowest level. For example, Judge et al. (2009) examined the rates of joint replacement in England using a hierarchy of cells defined by 5-year age group and sex (at level 1) nested within small areas (at level 2) and districts (at level 3). For each cell they had a count of the number of procedures undertaken and included an offset to adjust for differences in the population at risk in each cell whilst controlling for age and sex. And Turrell et al. (2007) investigated associations between area deprivation and mortality using cells defined by a combination of age, sex and individual occupational social class nested within a hierarchy of areas.

Incomplete Hierarchies

In general, we know to which unit at each higher level a lower-level unit belongs and so we have complete information on the hierarchy. There are two notable exceptions when this will not be the case. The first exception concerns multiple responses; the hierarchies may differ for different responses. This may be because the responses are actually measured at different levels. Goldstein gives an example of a multiple response model combining longitudinal measures (during childhood) of height and bone age with a measure of adult height (Goldstein 2003). Whilst the repeated measures during childhood are clustered within the individual, the one adult measurement is effectively at the level of individual rather than measurement occasion. The hierarchy may vary according to the number in each cluster. Dundas et al. (2014) give an example of individual children nested within sibling groups living in small areas; sibling group was omitted as a level for the 71% of children who had no siblings in the study. Alternatively, the *structured missingness* detailed under the earlier section on multiple response models may lead to differing hierarchies; Leyland and Boddy (1998) describe a model of mortality following acute myocardial infarction in which they consider the influences of both area of residence and hospital attended. Their data include both sudden deaths (death before reaching hospital) and deaths in hospital or within 30 days of discharge from hospital. These two responses (sudden death and death in or shortly after discharge from hospital) were nested within patients. The sudden deaths are clearly not affected by hospital attended; indeed, for such deaths there is no hospital attended. The second exception is when the higher-level membership is unknown. In such a situation, it is possible to use a multiple membership model with different probabilities of membership attached to the higher-level units (Hill and Goldstein 1998). Each higher-level unit (e.g. hospital) could be given equal weight or weight proportional to the total number of patients seen by that hospital in the absence of any knowledge as to group membership. However, it may be that more detailed information is available and that the precise membership of higher-level units is only partially missing; for example, it may be that a patient living in a given area is most likely to attend one of a number of local facilities.

A slightly different situation may arise when two levels are indistinguishable. Figure 4.2 illustrates a hierarchy that includes individuals nested within households.

In general, there will not be many individuals per household and many households may only contain one person. To an extent this does not matter; as long as there is at least one household comprising two or more people, then we can start to describe variation within households as well as between households. (In practice, the more households in the study in which there are at least two people, the more precise our estimate of the variance within households will be.) And clearly excluding single person households from our analysis is likely to introduce considerable bias into our sample. But our sample design may have included just one person in each household. In such a case, although it is correct to think of individuals as being nested within households, we are unable to distinguish between the individual and household levels. Not really a missing hierarchy, we are forced in practice to work with a joint individual/household level.

Conclusion

This chapter has introduced the reader to a variety of structures that can be thought of as multilevel or hierarchical. In addition to the strict hierarchies that perhaps constitute the common understanding of a multilevel model, we have discussed the appropriateness of multilevel modelling for designs including time, multiple responses and non-hierarchical structures. Furthermore, we have covered the concept of a pseudo-level and circumstances in which the unit of membership at a particular level may be missing.

When working out the data structure in your own research, it is important to bear in mind what has been said in Chaps. 2 and 3. The first step would be to analyse your research problem and specify which levels would be relevant to include from a theoretical perspective. You might end up working with data that are readily available, and the structure of these data might differ from what you would have wanted based on an analysis of your research problem. Of particular importance is whether you are missing information about a level in your data that seems to be important from a theoretical point of view. If this is the case, then your statistical model may be misspecified as a consequence. An example of this, which is discussed in more detail in Chap. 7, is the situation where you consider a health outcome of people living in neighbourhoods but omit the fact that your subjects are also clustered in families or households. This would lead to an overestimation of individual level or neighbourhood variation or both; see, for example, Sacker et al. (2006).

Some data structures may be quite complex, especially since the structures that have been discussed in this chapter can be combined. The more complicated the data structures are, the more difficult they will be to analyse and interpret. For readers who are keen to work with more complex data structures, we offer two pieces of advice. Firstly, we suggest that you simplify the data structure into a less complex, simple hierarchical structure and analyse the data in this manner before proceeding. In Chap. 9, we discuss ways of simplifying data structures as part of the modelling process. Our second piece of advice in the event of more complex data structures is to consult a colleague with experience in running and interpreting the analysis or to read some of the more technical multilevel modelling texts to gain further understanding of such analyses (for example, De Leeuw and Meijer 2008; Gelman and Hill 2007; Goldstein 2010; Snijders and Bosker 2012).

References

Aitken M, Longford N (1986) Statistical modelling in school effectiveness studies. J R Stat Soc Ser A 149:1–43

Amoako Johnson F, Padmadas SS (2009) On the spatial inequalities of institutional versus home births in Ghana: a multilevel analysis. J Community Health 34:64–72

Austin D, Oldroyd KG, McConnachie A, Slack R, Eteiba H, Flapan AD, Jennings KP, Northcote RJ, Pell ACH, Starkey IR, Pell JP (2008) Hospital and operator variations in drug-eluting stent use: a multi-level analysis of 5967 consecutive patients in Scotland. J Public Health 30:186–193

Bartolomeo N, Trerotoli P, Serio G (2010) Lung cancer and COPD rates in Apulia: a multilevel multimember model for smoothing disease mapping. Int J Health Geogr 9:15

Best N, Richardson S, Thomson A (2005) A comparison of Bayesian spatial models for disease mapping. Stat Methods Med Res 14:35–59

Bravo G, Dubois M-F, Wagneur B (2008) Assessing the effectiveness of interventions to promote advance directives among older adults: a systematic review and multi-level analysis. Soc Sci Med 67:1122–1132

Browne WJ, Goldstein H, Rasbash J (2001) Multiple membership multiple classification models. Stat Model 1:103–124

Campbell MK, Grimshaw JM (1998) Cluster randomised trials: time for improvement. Br Med J 317:1171–1172

Cardol M, Groenewegen PP, de Bakker DH, Spreeuwenberg P, van Dijk L, van den Bosch W (2005) Shared help seeking behaviour within families: a retrospective cohort study. Br Med J 330:882–884

Carpenter JR, Kenward MG, Vansteelandt S (2006) A comparison of multiple imputation and inverse probability weighting for analyses with missing data. J R Stat Soc Ser A 169:571–584

Cavalini LT, Ponce de Leon ACM (2008) Morbidity and mortality in Brazilian municipalities: a multilevel study of the association between socioeconomic and healthcare indicators. Int J Epidemiol 37:775–785

Chaix B, Rosvall M, Merlo J (2007) Assessment of the magnitude of geographical variations and socioeconomic contextual effects on ischaemic heart disease mortality: a multilevel survival analysis of a large Swedish cohort. J Epidemiol Community Health 61:349–355

Chaix B, Lindström M, Rosvall M, Merlo J (2008) Neighbourhood social interactions and risk of acute myocardial infarction. J Epidemiol Community Health 62:62–68

Curry A, Latkin C, Davey-Rothwell M (2008) Pathways to depression: the impact of neighborhood violent crime on inner-city residents in Baltimore, Maryland, USA. Soc Sci Med 67:23–30

De Leeuw J, Meijer E (eds) (2008) Handbook of multilevel analysis. Springer, New York

Dee TS (2001) Alcohol abuse and economic conditions: evidence from repeated cross-sections of individual-level data. Health Econ 10:257–270

Demarest S, Van der Heyden J, Charafeddine R, Drieskens S, Gisle L, Tafforeau J (2013) Methodological basics and evolution of the Belgian health interview survey 1997–2008. Arch Public Health 71:24

Downing A, Rudge G, Cheng Y, Tu Y-K, Keen J, Gilthorpe MS (2007) Do the UK government's new Quality and Outcomes Framework (QOF) scores adequately measure primary care performance? A cross-sectional survey of routine healthcare data. BMC Health Serv Res 7:166

Duncan C, Jones K, Moon G (1996) Health-related behaviour in context: a multilevel modelling approach. Soc Sci Med 42:817–830

Dundas R, Leyland AH, Macintyre S (2014) Early-life school, neighborhood, and family influences on adult health: a multilevel cross-classified analysis of the Aberdeen Children of the 1950s Study. Am J Epidemiol 180:197–207

Falster MO, Jorm LR, Leyland AH (2018) Using weighted hospital service area networks to explore variation in preventable hospitalization. Health Serv Res 53(Suppl 1):3148–3169

Franzini L, Caughy M, Spears W, Esquer MEF (2005) Neighbourhood economic conditions, social processes, and self-rated health in low-income neighborhoods in Texas: a multilevel latent variables model. Soc Sci Med 61:1135–1150

Froot KA (1989) Consistent covariance matrix estimation with cross-sectional dependence and heteroskedasticity in financial data. J Financ Quant Anal 24:333–355

Furnée CA, Groot W, Maassen van den Brink H (2008) The health effects of education: a meta-analysis. Eur J Pub Health 18:417–421

Gelman A, Hill J (2007) Data analysis using regression and multilevel/hierarchical models. Cambridge University Press, Cambridge

Goldstein H (1986) Multilevel mixed linear model analysis using iterative generalized least squares. Biometrika 73:43–56

Goldstein H (1994) Multilevel cross-classified models. Sociol Methods Res 22:364–375

Goldstein H (2003) Multilevel statistical models, 3rd edn. Arnold, London

Goldstein H (2010) Multilevel statistical models, 4th edn. Wiley, Chichester

Goldstein H, Healy MJR, Rasbash J (1994) Multilevel time series models with applications to repeated measures data. Stat Med 13:1643–1655

Groenewegen PP, Leufkens HG, Spreeuwenberg P, Worm W (1999) Neighbourhood characteristics and use of benzodiazepines in The Netherlands. Soc Sci Med 48:1701–1711

Haynes R, Jones AP, Reading R, Daras K, Emond A (2008) Neighbourhood variations in child accidents and related child and maternal characteristics: does area definition make a difference? Health Place 14:693–701

Hill PW, Goldstein H (1998) Multilevel modeling of educational data with cross-classification and missing identification for units. J Educ Behav Stat 23:117–128

Jones K (1993) 'Everywhere is nowhere': multilevel perspectives on the importance of place. The University of Portsmouth Inaugural Lectures, Portsmouth

Judge A, Welton NJ, Sandhu J, Ben-Shlomo Y (2009) Geographical variation in the provision of elective primary hip and knee replacement: the role of socio-demographic, hospital and distance variables. J Public Health 31:413–422

Koepsell TD, Wagner EH, Cheadle AC, Patrick DL, Martin DC, Diehr PH, Perrin EB (1992) Selected methodological issues in evaluating community-based health promotion and disease prevention programs. Annu Rev Public Health 13:31–57

Kroneman M, Siegers JJ (2004) The effect of hospital bed reduction on the use of beds: a comparative study of 10 European countries. Soc Sci Med 59:1731–1740

Lawson AB, Browne WJ, Vidal Rodeiro CL (2003) Disease mapping with WinBUGS and MLwiN. Wiley, Chichester

Levin KA, Davies CA, Douglas GVA, Pitts NB (2010) Urban-rural differences in dental caries of 5-year old children in Scotland. Soc Sci Med 71:2020–2027

Leyland AH (2004) Increasing inequalities in premature mortality in Great Britain. J Epidemiol Community Health 58:296–302

Leyland AH (2010) Methodological challenges in the evaluation of community interventions. Eur J Pub Health 20:242–243

Leyland AH, Boddy FA (1998) League tables and acute myocardial infarction. Lancet 351:555–558

Leyland AH, Davies CA (2005) Empirical Bayes methods for disease mapping. Stat Methods Med Res 14:17–34

Leyland AH, Næss Ø (2009) The effect of area of residence over the life course on subsequent mortality. J R Stat Soc Ser A 172:555–578

Lipps O, Moreau-Gruet F (2010) Change of individual BMI in Switzerland and the USA: a multilevel model for growth. Int J Public Health 55:299–306

Little RJ, Rubin DB (2002) Statistical analysis with missing data, 2nd edn. Wiley, New York

Mansyur C, Amick BC, Harrist RB, Franzini L (2008) Social capital, income inequality, and self-rated health in 45 countries. Soc Sci Med 66:43–56

Martikainen P, Kauppinen TM, Valkonen T (2003) Effects of the characteristics of neighbourhoods and the characteristics of people on cause specific mortality: a register based follow up study of 252 000 men. J Epidemiol Community Health 57:210–217

Merlo J (2011) Contextual influences on the individual life course: building a research framework for social epidemiology. Psychosoc Interv 20:109–118

Næss Ø, Leyland AH (2010) Analysing the effect of area of residence over the life course in multilevel epidemiology. Scand J Public Health 38:119–126

Næss Ø, Piro FN, Nafstad P, Davey Smith G, Leyland AH (2007) Air pollution, social deprivation, and mortality. A multilevel cohort study. Epidemiology 18:686–694

Openshaw S (1984) The modifiable areal unit problem. Geo Books, 38, Norwich

Oshio T, Kobayashi M (2009) Income inequality, area-level poverty, perceived aversion to inequality, and self-rated health in Japan. Soc Sci Med 69:317–326

Rasbash J, Browne W (2001) Modelling non-hierarchical structures. In: Leyland AH, Goldstein H (eds) Multilevel modelling of health statistics. Wiley, Chichester

Ryan JP, Garnier P, Zyphur M, Zhai F (2006) Investigating the effects of caseworker characteristics in child welfare. Child Youth Serv Rev 28:993–1006

Sacker A, Wiggins RD, Bartley M (2006) Time and place: putting individual health into context. A multilevel analysis of the British household panel survey, 1991-2001. Health Place 12:279–290

Sear R, Mace R, McGregor IA (2000) Maternal grandmothers improve nutritional status and survival of children in rural Gambia. Proc R Soc B 267:1641–1647

Snijders TAB, Bosker RJ (2012) Multilevel analysis: an introduction to basic and advanced multilevel modeling. Sage, Los Angeles

Sterne JAC, White IR, Carlin JB, Spratt M, Royston P, Kenward MG, Wood AM, Carpenter JR (2009) Multiple imputation for missing data in epidemiological and clinical research: potential and pitfalls. Br Med J 338:b2393

Subramanian SV, Jones K, Duncan C (2003) Multilevel methods for public health research. In: Kawachi I, Berkman LF (eds) Neighborhoods and health. Oxford University Press, New York

Subramanian SV, Nandy S, Kelly M, Gordon D, Davey Smith G (2004) Patterns and distribution of tobacco consumption in India: cross sectional multilevel evidence from the 1998-9 national family health study. Br Med J 328:801–806

Subramanian SV, Kim D, Kawachi I (2005) Covariation in the socioeconomic determinants of self rated health and happiness: a multivariate multilevel analysis of individuals and communities in the USA. J Epidemiol Community Health 59:664–669

Tomasi C, Leyland AH, Wennström JL (2007) Factors influencing the outcome of non-surgical periodontal treatment: a multilevel approach. J Clin Periodontol 34:682–690

Tooze JA, Grunwald GK, Jones RH (2002) Analysis of repeated measures data with clumping at zero. Stat Methods Med Res 11:341–355

Turrell G, Kavanagh A, Draper G, Subramanian SV (2007) Do places affect the probability of death in Australia? A multilevel study of area-level disadvantage, individual-level socioeconomic position and all-cause mortality, 1998-2000. J Epidemiol Community Health 61:13–19

Urquia ML, Frank JW, Glazier RH, Moineddin R, Matheson FI, Gagnon AJ (2009) Neighborhood context and infant birthweight among recent immigrant mothers: a multilevel analysis. Am J Public Health 99:285–293

Vermunt JK (2007) Latent class and finite mixture models for multilevel data sets. Stat Methods Med Res 17:33–51

Virtanen M, Kivimäki M, Pentti J, Oksanen T, Ahola K, Linna A, Kouvonen A, Salo P, Vahtera J (2010) School neighborhood disadvantage as a predictor of long-term sick leave among teachers: prospective cohort study. Am J Epidemiol 171:785–792

Wang K, Lee AH, Hamilton G, Yau KKW (2006) Multilevel logistic regression modelling with correlated random effects: application to the Smoking Cessation for Youth study. Stat Med 25:3864–3876
Yang M, Eldridge S, Merlo J (2009) Multilevel survival analysis of health inequalities in life expectancy. Int J Equity Health 8:31
Yiannakoulis N, Hill MD, Svenson LW (2009) Geographic hierarchies of diagnostic practice style in cerebrovascular disease. Soc Sci Med 68:1985–1992

Part 2
Statistical Context

5

Statistical Principles of MLA

Abstract Although we have introduced the conceptual basis for multilevel analysis in earlier chapters, it remains a statistical method; this chapter introduces the statistical principles of MLA. This is done primarily through algebraic notation, and the equations are linked to graphs where appropriate to help with the interpretation. We build up the chapter from a single-level regression analysis to a random intercept model and finally to a random slope model. We introduce the idea of intraclass correlation and provide visual examples of typical patterns of covariance between the intercept and slope residuals. We look at simple extensions to a third level and the use of complex variance functions to account for heteroscedasticity, and finally we draw comparisons between fixed effects and random effects models.

Keywords Multilevel analysis · Single-level regression · Random intercept model · Random slope model · Intraclass correlation · Variance · Covariance

Multilevel analysis is, as we have discussed, a form of regression analysis that is appropriate when the assumption of independence of observations that underlies ordinary regression models does not hold. The reason for this assumption being violated is the influence of the context; Chap. 4 has introduced a variety of contexts that may be important for our analyses and which may extend beyond 'typical' contexts such as neighbourhood, hospital or school to include, for example the individual (for repeated measures or multiple responses) or time (for repeated cross-sections).

We start this chapter with the basic, single-level, linear regression model and show how we can change this into a multilevel model by adding the context. As the chapter progresses, we cover a range of multilevel models and introduce some of the commonly encountered ideas and terminology such as the intraclass correlation coefficient and random slopes. Where possible we link these ideas to graphs as an aid to interpretation.

The chapter works through the random intercept and random slope models based on the example introduced in Chap. 3 concerning an investigation of the relationship between the time spent on exercise each week and certain individual and contextual characteristics. In this example, we have data that were collected in a health interview survey. The respondents' addresses were geo-coded, and in this manner, the respondents were allocated to neighbourhoods in the study area. We provide the algebraic notation of the regression equations and introduce the basic terminology cumulatively as we progress. For reference, this terminology is summarised in Box 5.3 at the end of this chapter.

Ordinary Least Squares (Single-Level) Regression

Using a single-level regression model, we would regress the dependent variable, the time spent exercising each week, on one or more independent variables ignoring the neighbourhood in which people live, and how this may affect our outcome. Consider a regression including only the respondent's age; the regression equation is

$$y_i = \beta_0 + \beta_1 x_{1i} + e_{0i} \tag{5.1}$$

In this equation, y_i is the dependent variable. Note that for the single-level regression model, we do not pay any attention to the area of residence of each individual and, as such, the dependent variable is uniquely identified by the subscript i. β_0 is used to denote the intercept—the number of minutes spent exercising by the reference group: respondents for whom all independent variables take the value 0. (The value 0 may not always be the best choice; in terms of respondent's age, for example we would not be interested in the time spent exercising by respondents who are 0 years old. To overcome this problem, we may choose to centre some of the independent variables such as age, so that the intercept takes on a more meaningful value, such as the time spent exercising by a respondent of average age. See Chap. 11 for an example of this in practice.) x_{1i} is the independent variable, in this case the age of respondent i. β_1 indicates the average change in time spent exercising per week associated with a 1 year increase in age. e_{0i} is the residual or error term.

This equation is illustrated graphically in Fig. 5.1. The time spent exercising tends to decrease with increasing age; the extent to which there is a decrease is determined by the slope β_1. The error term e_{0i} is the vertical distance between the regression line and each observation; in other words, it is the difference between the time that we would expect individual i to spend on exercise given their age, $\beta_0 + \beta_1 x_{1i}$, and the time that they actually spent on exercise, y_i.

Equation (5.1) is accompanied by an important assumption about the residuals e_{0i} namely that they are identically and independently distributed and can be characterised by a normal distribution with mean 0 and variance σ^2_{e0}.

$$e_{0i} \sim N\left(0, \sigma^2_{e0}\right) \tag{5.2}$$

In this equation, N indicates that the residuals are assumed to follow a normal distribution with zero mean and variance σ^2_{e0}.

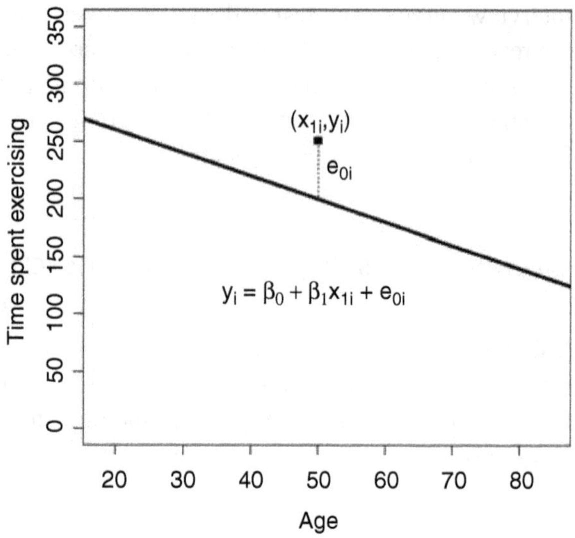

Fig. 5.1 Ordinary least square regression

As we described in Chap. 3, this error distribution is often seen as being nothing more than a nuisance; it is, after all, the part which cannot be explained by our model. But the assumption that the residuals are independent of each other is the one that we are in danger of violating if there is a level missing from our model—neighbourhood in this example. This leads us to the random intercept model.

Random Intercept Model

In a random intercept regression model, we include an effect for each area that impacts on all individuals in that area equally, regardless of their age.

$$y_{ij} = \beta_0 + \beta_1 x_{1ij} + u_{0j} + e_{0ij} \tag{5.3}$$

In this equation, the new terms introduced to Eq. (5.3) over and above those in Eq. (5.1) are as follows. y_{ij} is our dependent or response variable: the outcome for individual i living in neighbourhood j, the number of minutes per week spent exercising. Our survey respondents are numbered from $i = 1, \ldots, N$ and each lives in one neighbourhood $j = 1, \ldots, J$. There are n_j respondents in neighbourhood j so $N = \sum_{j=1}^{J} n_j$. x_{pij} are the independent or explanatory variables, again measured on individual i in neighbourhood j. The subscript p is used simply to distinguish between the different variables; for example x_{1ij} might be the individual's age in years and x_{2ij} a dummy variable indicating the subject's sex (1 = male, 0 = female). x_{pj} are also independent variables, but these are measured at the contextual or neighbourhood level; that is, they take the same value for all individuals living in neighbourhood j. These variables may be directly observed or measured at the neighbourhood level; for example, x_{3j} may be the proportion of the surface area of neighbourhood j that is characterised as being 'green space'. Alternatively, the contextual variables may represent an aggregation of individual measures; x_{4j} may be the average age of the respondents in neighbourhood j.

β_p is the regression coefficient associated with x_{pij} or x_{pj}. So β_1 would indicate the average change in time spent exercising per week associated with a 1-year increase in age and β_2 would show the average effect of being male on the time spent exercising (relative to that for the baseline category, female, for which $x_{2ij} = 0$). u_{0j} is the estimated effect or residual for area j. This is the difference that we expect to see in the time spent exercising for an individual in neighbourhood j compared to an individual in the average neighbourhood, after taking into account those (individual or neighbourhood) characteristics that have been included in the model. The 0 in the subscript denotes that this is a *random intercept* residual, a departure from the overall intercept β_0 applying equally to everyone in neighbourhood j regardless of individual characteristics. e_{0ij} is the individual-level residual or error term for individual i in neighbourhood j.

Figure 5.2 illustrates this equation graphically. As in Fig. 5.1, the time spent exercising for someone living in an average area is shown as the heavy line, and this relationship is determined by just the person's age x_{1ij}. The part of Eq. (5.3) involving the β coefficients, $\beta_0 + \beta_1 x_{1ij}$, is called the *fixed part* of the model because the coefficients are the same for everybody; the residuals at the different levels, $u_{0j} + e_{0ij}$, are collectively termed the *random part* of the model as these values depend on the individual and neighbourhood. The additional effect for inhabitants of area j, u_{0j}, applies to all inhabitants of the area regardless of age; people in the area illustrated in Fig. 5.2 tend to do more exercise than average. The time we would expect individual i to spend on exercise now depends on their area of residence and

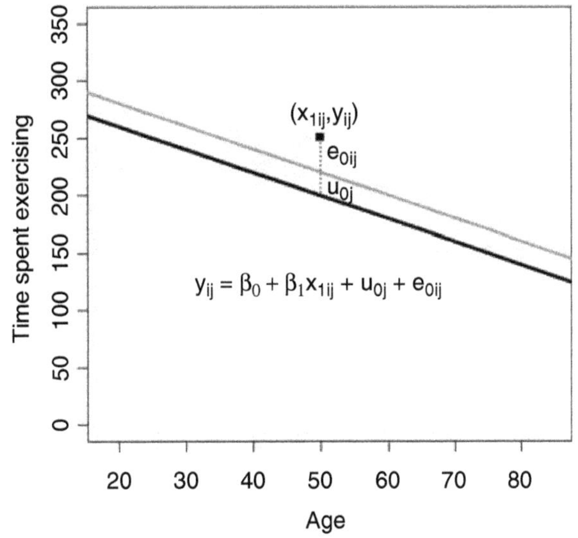

Fig. 5.2 Random intercept model

is given by $\beta_0 + \beta_1 x_{1ij} + u_{0j}$; this is shown in Fig. 5.2 as the grey line. The vertical distance between the two lines, u_{0j}, is constant (i.e., it does not depend on age).

In Fig. 5.2 we can see that the vertical distance from the observed time that person i in area j spends on exercise, y_{ij}, and the average time that someone of this age would spend on exercise, $\beta_0 + \beta_1 x_{1ij}$, is now broken down into a part that is due to the difference between area j and the average, u_{0j}, and a part that is due to the difference between individual i and the average for area j, e_{0ij}. Both the components have their associated distributions and variances:

$$\begin{aligned} u_{0j} &\sim N\left(0, \sigma_{u0}^2\right) \\ e_{0ij} &\sim N\left(0, \sigma_{e0}^2\right) \end{aligned} \tag{5.4}$$

In this equation, σ_{u0}^2 is the variance of the neighbourhood-level intercept residuals u_{0j}.

In Eq. (5.3) the fixed part of the model $\beta_0 + \beta_1 x_{1ij}$ does not vary given a person's age x_{1ij}. The total unexplained variation in the outcome (adjusted for age) is therefore equal to the variance of $u_{0j} + e_{0ij}$ or $\sigma_{u0}^2 + \sigma_{e0}^2$; that is, some of the variation in time spent exercising is due to differences between neighbourhoods and some is due to the differences between individuals within neighbourhoods. Figure 5.2 shows how the time spent exercising varies with age on average across all areas (black line) and also in area j (grey line). Figure 5.3a shows the relationship for all areas in our sample; each area is shown as a separate line. The variability between areas is then the extent to which these lines are dispersed around the average; if the lines are close together, then there is little variation between neighbourhoods and σ_{u0}^2 is small.

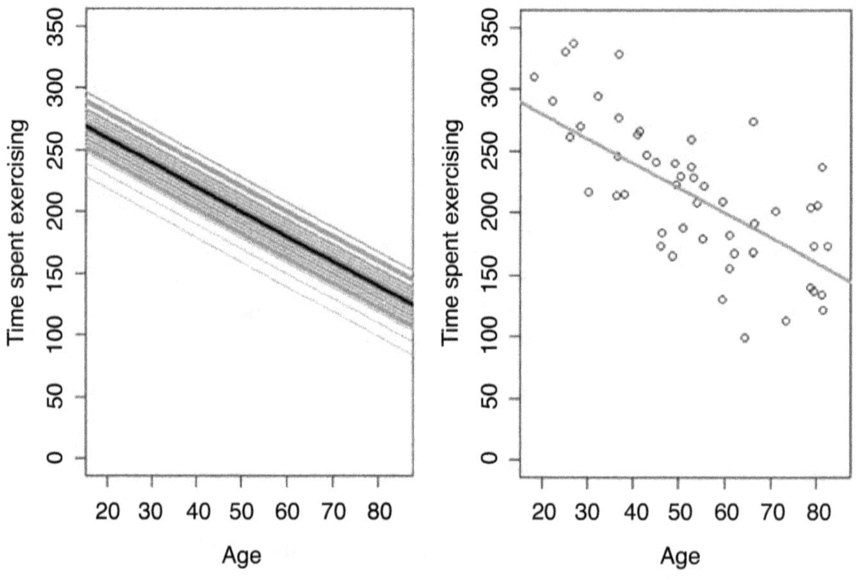

Fig. 5.3 Random intercept model showing (**a**) variation between neighbourhoods and (**b**) variation between individuals within a single neighbourhood

Figure 5.3b shows the variability of the observations made on respondents living in area j; these tend to be higher than average (given the individuals' ages) since the area mean is clearly higher than the population mean shown in Fig. 5.3a. However, there is some variability in the tendency to exercise. Some people spend more time exercising than the average for that age in the area whilst others spend less than average—indeed, some spend less than the population average as there is considerable scattering around the average for area j. The variability between individuals within areas is then the extent to which the observations are scattered around the average for each area; if the observations are close to the line, then there is little variation within neighbourhoods and σ_{e0}^2 is small.

The proportion of the total variance that is due to differences between neighbourhoods is the intraclass correlation coefficient ρ_{I}:

$$\rho_{\mathrm{I}} = \frac{\sigma_{u0}^2}{\sigma_{u0}^2 + \sigma_{e0}^2} \tag{5.5}$$

ρ_{I} is a measure of the similarity between two people from the same neighbourhood and will take a value between 0 and 1 inclusive. If there were no variation between the area effects then all of the u_{0j} would be equal (to zero) and σ_{u0}^2 would be zero meaning that $\rho_{\mathrm{I}} = 0$. If there were no variation within neighbourhoods (following adjustment for age), then the time spent exercising would be determined exactly by age and neighbourhood alone. In this case, σ_{e0}^2 would be 0 and so we can see from Eq. (5.5) that $\rho_{\mathrm{I}} = 1$; the exercise times of individuals from the same area would be perfectly correlated. The size of ρ_{I} varies between studies and is very important for power calculations; we return to a discussion of this in Chap. 6. Typically we might expect somewhere around 2–5% of the total variation to arise due to differences between contexts although there are notable exceptions in public health and health services research when this proportion might be higher. Clustering within families or households tends to be quite strong giving large intraclass correlation coefficients; Cardol et al. (2005) found that 18% of the variance in the frequency of medical contacts was attributable to the family, and Sacker et al. (2006) found 13–21% of the variation in poor general health and 20–34% of the variation in limiting illness was attributable to differences between households. For studies in which the data comprise repeated measures on individuals a large proportion of the variability is often at the individual level (which is not the lowest level in a repeated measures design—see Chap. 4). For example, Lipps and Moreau-Gruet (2010) found that over 90% of the total variance in body mass index was at the individual (as opposed to measurement occasion) level in a repeated measures analysis.

The model described by Eqs. (5.3) and (5.4) is the basic random intercept or variance components model. These terms are used interchangeably which might be confusing when reading studies that report multilevel analysis. There is, however, a glossary of the terminology used in MLA (Diez-Roux 2002) which is useful to have at hand when reading papers that use this technique. As with the single-level regression model, there are certain implicit assumptions regarding the residuals.

As well as assuming that the residuals at each level are independently and identically distributed, the model is built on the assumption that the neighbourhood residuals u_{0j} are independent of the individual level residuals e_{0ij} and that they are uncorrelated with all of the independent variables (in this case x_{1ij}). In a multilevel model described by Eqs. (5.3) and (5.4), it is possible that there will be a correlation between the independent variable x_{1ij} and the neighbourhood residuals u_{0j}. This can be avoided by including the group (contextual) mean $x_{2j} = \sum_i x_{1ij}$, so that Eq. (5.3) becomes

$$y_{ij} = \beta_0 + \beta_1 x_{1ij} + \beta_2 x_{2j} + u_{0j} + e_{0ij} \tag{5.6}$$

Random Slope Model

From Fig. 5.3a you will note that whilst the intercept—the point at which the lines cross the vertical axis—varies between neighbourhoods, the slope is the same in all areas. The lines are parallel, indicating that a fixed increase in age is associated with the same average decline in time spent exercising in all areas. A random slope model allows the relationship between the independent and dependent variables to differ between contexts; we enable this by including an area effect for the slope (the relationship between time spent on exercise and age) in addition to the area effect for the intercept.

$$y_{ij} = \beta_0 + \beta_1 x_{1ij} + u_{0j} + u_{1j} x_{1ij} + e_{0ij} \tag{5.7}$$

The new term in this equation is u_{1j}. This is the slope residual for neighbourhood j that is associated with the independent variable x_{1ij}. Just as u_{0j} denotes a departure from the overall intercept β_0, u_{1j} indicates the extent of a departure from the overall slope β_1 in a *random slope* model. In general, there may be a residual u_{pj} associated with any of the independent variables x_{pij} or x_{pj}. However, not every slope will be random and so there will not be slope residuals for every regression coefficient.

The fixed part of this model is, as before, $\beta_0 + \beta_1 x_{1ij}$, and this is shown as the black line in Fig. 5.4. The random part is now given by $u_{0j} + u_{1j} x_{1ij} + e_{0ij}$ which clearly depends on the individual's age x_{1ij}. The grey line in Fig. 5.4 is determined by the fixed part together with both area effects (the intercept residual u_{0j} and the slope residual u_{1j}), i.e. $\beta_0 + \beta_1 x_{1ij} + u_{0j} + u_{1j} x_{1ij}$. For the selected area, there is still a tendency to exercise more than average; the light line in Fig. 5.4 is consistently above the heavy line. But unlike the random intercept model in Fig. 5.2, the distance between the two lines in Fig. 5.4 varies according to the person's age; the increased mean time spent exercising in area j is greater at younger ages than at older ages. This means that the relationship between time spent exercising and age differs between areas. On average, a 1-year increase in age is associated with a change of

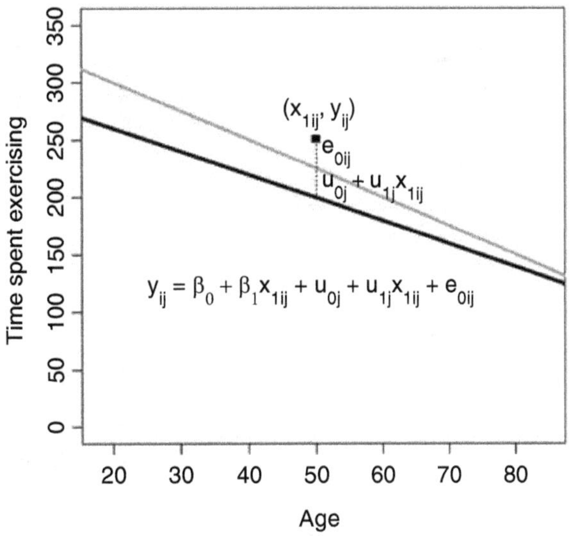

Fig. 5.4 Random slope model

β_1 in the time spent exercising, but in area j, each additional year is associated with a difference of $\beta_1 + u_{1j}$ minutes.

Just as the intercept residuals u_{0j} have an associated variance (σ^2_{u0}), the slope residuals u_{1j} also have a variance (σ^2_{u1}). What is new, however, is the introduction of a covariance (σ_{u01}) between the intercept residual and the slope residual for each area.

$$\begin{bmatrix} u_{0j} \\ u_{1j} \end{bmatrix} \sim N\left(\begin{bmatrix} 0 \\ 0 \end{bmatrix}, \begin{bmatrix} \sigma^2_{u0} & \sigma_{u01} \\ \sigma_{u01} & \sigma^2_{u1} \end{bmatrix}\right) \qquad (5.8)$$
$$e_{0ij} \sim N\left(0, \sigma^2_{e0}\right)$$

The covariance is a measure of the extent to which two variables change in the same direction. We can use the covariance between u_{0j} and u_{1j}, along with the two variances, to calculate the correlation between the two:

$$\rho_{u01} = \frac{\sigma_{u01}}{\sqrt{\sigma^2_{u0}\sigma^2_{u1}}} \qquad (5.9)$$

The unexplained variance in Eq. (5.7) is now

$$\text{var}\left(u_{0j} + u_{1j}x_{1ij} + e_{0ij}\right) = \sigma^2_{u0} + x^2_{1ij}\sigma^2_{u1} + 2x_{1ij}\sigma_{u01} + \sigma^2_{e0} \qquad (5.10)$$

The term involving the covariance σ_{u01} takes into account the fact that the intercept and slope residuals, u_{0j} and u_{1j}, are not independent of each other. The covariance matrix in Eq. (5.8)—the variances σ^2_{u0} and σ^2_{u1} and the covariance σ_{u01}—conveys a variety of information about the different relationships between time spent exercising and age for the neighbourhoods in our study. Figure 5.5 shows how

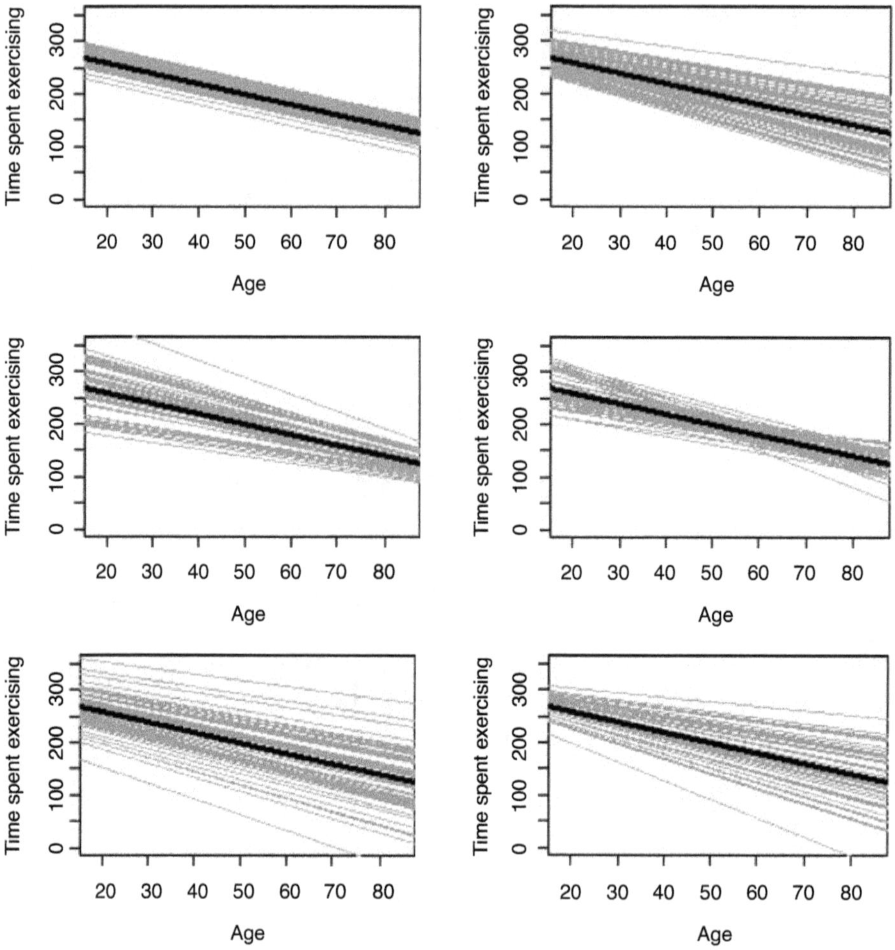

Fig. 5.5 Random slope model with differing covariance matrices showing (**a**) small (or zero) slope variance; (**b**) moderate intercept and slope variance, positive covariance; (**c**) moderate intercept and slope variance, negative covariance; (**d**) moderate intercept and slope variance, small (or zero) covariance; (**e**) large intercept variance, moderate slope variance, positive covariance; and (**f**) moderate intercept variance, large slope variance, positive covariance

various patterns in the covariance matrix can be translated into different graphs illustrating these relationships. The fixed part of the model $\beta_0 + \beta_1 x_{1ij}$ is the same in each graph, and so the black line—denoting the relationship in the average area—does not change. Firstly, Fig. 5.5a shows that if the variance of the slope is very small or zero then we are back to a random intercept model. The lines for the neighbourhoods are parallel to each other since the relationship between exercise and age does not vary between contexts. Figure 5.5b illustrates a moderate slope variance and a positive covariance between the intercept and slope residuals for each area. In general, areas with a large (small) intercept residual u_{0j} will tend to have a large (small) slope residual u_{1j}, meaning that areas with intercepts higher than average will tend to have slopes that are more positive (or less negative) than average. If the inhabitants of an area tend to do more exercise than average this will usually be the case at all ages, but this benefit is most pronounced at older ages. This leads to the general pattern of lower variability between areas at younger ages and increased variability at older ages. Equation (5.10) shows how the unexplained variance will increase with age if the covariance σ_{u01} is positive. In Fig. 5.5c the covariance between the intercept and slope is negative, meaning that areas with higher intercepts tend to have lower (or more negative) slopes. This leads to a pattern of increased variability between neighbourhoods at young ages and decreased variability at older ages. Figure 5.5d illustrates a case in which the covariance between the intercept and slope residuals is very small or zero (centred around age 50 years: see Box 5.1); in such a case, there is no relationship between the two. Unlike Fig. 5.5b, c, the knowledge that the mean time spent exercising at age 50 years in one particular area is higher than average does not impart any further information about whether the slope will be flatter or steeper than average. The lines for the neighbourhoods cross quite randomly. In Fig. 5.5e, we can see the impact of increasing the intercept variance for the model seen in Fig. 5.5b, and Fig. 5.5f demonstrates the effect of increasing the slope variance again from that seen in Fig. 5.5b. The former tends to increase the average effect or distance from the heavy line (the average area) whilst the latter tends to increase the difference between areas in the strength of the relationship between exercise and age.

The interpretation of the covariance given above is a slight simplification since this actually depends on the centring of the independent variable. This means that the size, and even the sign, of the covariance can change if the independent variable is centred around a different value although neither the data nor the pattern of convergence or divergence of areas will change. See Box 5.1 for an explanation.

Box 5.1 The Effect of Centring on the Covariance

In the equations in this chapter, x_{1ij} is the age of individual i in neighbourhood j, taking values dependent on the sample. In Eq. (5.1), β_0 is the intercept and denotes the time spent on exercise for an individual for whom all covariates are equal to zero; in other words, this is the mean time spent on exercise by a person who is 0 years old. Since this is almost certainly outside the range of our data, we can choose to centre age around another value as an aid to interpretation. To centre around age 50 years, we would replace x_{1ij} by $x^*_{1ij} = x_{1ij} - 50$, so that the random slope model in Eq. (5.7) becomes

$$y_{ij} = \beta^*_0 + \beta_1 x^*_{1ij} + u^*_{0j} + u_{1j} x^*_{1ij} + e_{0ij}$$

The new intercept, β^*_0, now indicates the mean time spent on exercise by a 50-year old. The estimate of the slope, β_1, has not changed and nor have the slope residuals u_{1j}. The u^*_{0j} are the random intercept residuals which now represent area effects for 50-year olds (as opposed to the u_{0j} which were the

(continued)

Box 5.1 (continued)
area effects for those aged 0 years). You can see from the random slope model in Fig. 5.4 that magnitude of the area effect, or the distance from the grey (area-specific) line to the black (population) line, differs by age. So changing the intercept in a random slope model also alters the area-specific intercept residual.

Since the intercept residuals change if we change the intercept, their variance also changes and so does the covariance between the intercept and slope. For a centred model, the level 2 variances and covariances given in Eq. (5.8) become

$$\begin{bmatrix} u_{0j}^* \\ u_{1j} \end{bmatrix} \sim N\left(\begin{bmatrix} 0 \\ 0 \end{bmatrix}, \begin{bmatrix} \sigma_{u0}^{*2} & \sigma_{u01}^* \\ \sigma_{u01}^* & \sigma_{u1}^2 \end{bmatrix}\right)$$

It is straightforward to show that in this example $\sigma_{u0}^{*2} = \sigma_{u0}^2 + 100\sigma_{u01} + 2500\sigma_{u1}^2$ and $\sigma_{u01}^* = \sigma_{u01} + 50\sigma_{u1}^2$. The implication of this is that the centring of a variable with a random coefficient will change the covariance and therefore the correlation between the intercept and slope residuals.

The interpretation of random slopes will vary according to the substantive nature of the research but always depends on the nature of the covariance. Damman et al. (2011) give a series of examples of random slope models examining the relationship between healthcare experiences and patient characteristics in a sample of patients drawn from 32 family practices in the Netherlands. They showed a negative covariance between the practice-level intercept and the residual for the patient's age, indicating less variability between practices for older patients; similarly variation decreased with increasing patient health status. Although the relationship between educational level and patient experiences could be seen to vary across practices, there was no correlation between the average experience and the slope across educational level. Finally, a positive correlation between the practice-level intercept and the residual for the patient's ethnicity suggested greater variation in experiences between practices for migrant patients than for those from a Dutch background.

Three-Level Model

The two-level random intercept model described by Eqs. (5.3) and (5.4) can easily be extended to include a third level. Assume that the J neighbourhoods are themselves nested within K towns, and we believe it plausible that people's exercise habits may differ between towns as well as between neighbourhoods within towns. The time spent exercising by individual i living in neighbourhood j of town k, y_{ijk}, then includes an effect or residual for town k, v_{0k}, and is given by

$$y_{ijk} = \beta_0 + \beta_1 x_{1ijk} + v_{0k} + u_{0jk} + e_{0ijk} \tag{5.11}$$

The residuals at the three levels are assumed to be independently normally distributed:

$$\begin{aligned} v_{0k} &\sim N\left(0, \sigma_{v0}^2\right) \\ u_{0jk} &\sim N\left(0, \sigma_{u0}^2\right) \\ e_{0ijk} &\sim N\left(0, \sigma_{e0}^2\right) \end{aligned} \tag{5.12}$$

It is now possible to allow the coefficient of age to vary across towns instead of (or as well as) neighbourhoods by introducing a slope residual v_{1k} in the same manner as we did for the neighbourhood level above.

Heteroscedasticity

In linear multilevel models, as with single-level models, we can allow for heteroscedasticity (also known as complex level 1 variation). The two-level random intercept model described by Eqs. (5.3) and (5.4) makes the assumption that the level 1 variance σ_{e0}^2 is constant and independent of the person's age x_{1ij}. It may be that this assumption is too simplistic and inappropriate, and instead of the observations being randomly distributed around the line for each area as in Fig. 5.3b, we find that there is more variability in the amount of exercise undertaken by older respondents. Such a scenario is illustrated in Fig. 5.6.

Heteroscedasticity of this kind can be accommodated by including a further residual term at level 1, e_{1ij}, in a manner analogous to the inclusion of a random

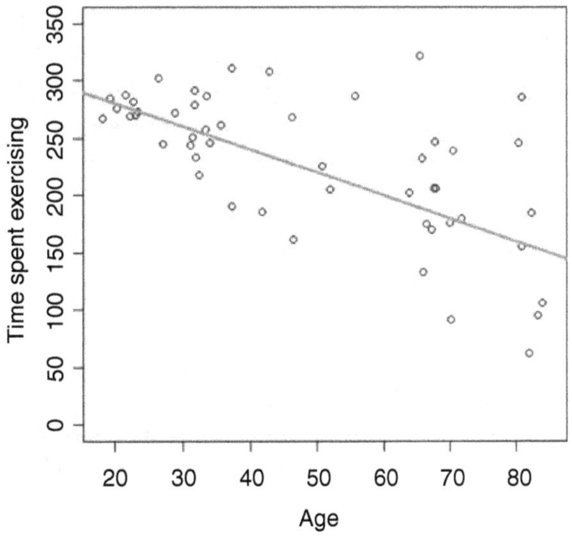

Fig. 5.6 Random intercept model showing variation between individuals within neighbourhoods, with the variance dependent on the respondent's age

slope at level 2: it is only the interpretation that is different. Equations (5.3) and (5.4) now become:

$$y_{ij} = \beta_0 + \beta_1 x_{1ij} + u_{0j} + e_{0ij} + e_{1ij} x_{1ij} \tag{5.12}$$

and

$$\begin{gathered} u_{0j} \sim N(0, \sigma_{u0}^2) \\ \begin{bmatrix} e_{0ij} \\ e_{1ij} \end{bmatrix} \sim N\left(\begin{bmatrix} 0 \\ 0 \end{bmatrix}, \begin{bmatrix} \sigma_{e0}^2 & \sigma_{e01} \\ \sigma_{e01} & \sigma_{e1}^2 \end{bmatrix} \right) \end{gathered} \tag{5.13}$$

The unexplained variation in the outcome is now given by the variance of the random part u_{0j} + e_{0ij} + $e_{1ij}x_{1ij}$ which is given by $\sigma_{u0}^2 + \sigma_{e0}^2 + 2x_{1ij}\sigma_{e01} + x_{1ij}^2\sigma_{e1}^2$. Although the variance between areas is constant, the variance between individuals within areas differs according to the individual's age.

In a single-level regression model, ignoring heteroscedasticity in the data will result in unbiased parameter estimates, but the standard errors associated with these estimates may be incorrect meaning that tests of significance may be misleading. In a multilevel regression model, the failure to model heteroscedasticity that is present in the data may result in the erroneous detection of a random slope (Snijders and Berkhof 2008).

Fixed Effects Model

We introduced the fixed effects model as an alternative to MLA in Chap. 3 and show its algebraic representation here to highlight the differences between the multilevel and fixed effects approaches. Since the fixed effects model introduces a series of $J - 1$ dummy variables to model the effect of the neighbourhoods it is an extension of the single level models described by Eqs. (5.1) and (5.2). We let x_{pi} take the value 1 if individual i lives in neighbourhood p, $p = 2, \ldots, J$, and 0 otherwise. Equation (5.1) then becomes

$$y_i = \beta_0 + \beta_1 x_{1i} + \sum_{p=2}^{J} \beta_p x_{pi} + e_{0i} \tag{5.14}$$

The parameters associated with the dummy variables, β_p, now denote the difference between the mean time spent exercising in neighbourhood p compared to neighbourhood 1 (the baseline). There is only one term in the random part of Eq. (5.14)—e_{0i}—as no assumptions are made about the distribution of the area effects β_p.

When we introduced the fixed effects model in Chap. 3, we mentioned that such models may change the interpretation of the (fixed part) regression parameters. This is because under the fixed effects model, the higher level units are regarded as nuisance parameters and all associated contextual effects are removed from the analysis. However, as described in Chap. 2 when considering the transformation from micro-level to macro-level, the contextual variables available to us include the mean of the characteristics measured at the individual level. The fixed effects model effectively centres all our level 1 independent variables around their mean, so Eq. (5.14) is more appropriately written as

$$y_{ij} = \beta_0 + \beta_1 \left(x_{1ij} - \overline{x}_{1j}\right) + \sum_{p=2}^{J} \beta_p x_{pij} + e_{0ij} \tag{5.15}$$

where $\overline{x}_{1j}$ is the average of the x_{1ij} for neighbourhood j. Whilst the parameter estimate β_1 in the multilevel models indicates the association between the time spent exercising and the individual's age, in the fixed effects model β_1 represents the association between the time spent exercising and the extent to which an individual's age differs from the average age of respondents in their neighbourhood. These two effects, and their interpretations, are not necessarily the same (Leyland 2010).

We have tried to ensure that we are internally consistent in terms of the algebraic notation that we use in this book. However, some papers use alternative notations; we describe a common alternative in Box 5.2.

Box 5.2 Alternative Notation Used in MLA

To a large extent the alternative notation used is a substitution of one letter or symbol for another which is trivial if confusing. However, multilevel models are sometimes broken down into separate equations representing distinct parts of the model. This box details the equivalence of the notation that we use in this book to that used by Diez-Roux (2002). We can expand the random slope model given by Eqs. (5.7) and (5.8) to include a contextual variable x_{2j} and the cross-level interaction between the individual and contextual variables $x_{1ij}x_{2j}$:

$$y_{ij} = \beta_0 + \beta_1 x_{1ij} + \beta_2 x_{2j} + \beta_3 x_{1ij} x_{2j} + u_{0j} + u_{1j} x_{1ij} + e_{0ij}$$

The equivalent notation

$$Y_{ij} = \gamma_{00} + \gamma_{10} I_{ij} + \gamma_{01} G_j + \gamma_{11} I_{ij} G_j + U_{0j} + U_{1j} I_{ij} + \varepsilon_{ij}$$

represents a substitution of γ_{00} for β_0, γ_{10} for β_1 and I_{ij} for x_{1ij} etc. and is also sometimes written as

(continued)

Box 5.2 (continued)

$$Y_{ij} = b_{0j} + b_{1j}I_{ij} + \varepsilon_{ij}$$

where

$$b_{0j} = \gamma_{00} + \gamma_{01}G_j + U_{0j}$$
$$b_{1j} = \gamma_{10} + \gamma_{11}G_j + U_{1j}$$

Rankings and Institutional Performance

The higher level residuals in multilevel models are also termed effects because, in the simple case of a random intercept model, the residuals represent the estimated effect of a higher level unit on all of the individuals (level 1 units) contained in that higher level unit. If the levels in a model include an institution such as a care home, school or hospital, then we might like to provide some comparison of institutions to identify those that are performing well or poorly in comparison to their peers—a "league table" of performance. Although the use of performance indicators requires careful consideration and should not be adopted universally (Smith 1995), it is clear that if they are to be used, then their construction should be methodologically sound and that necessitates the use of MLA (Goldstein and Spiegelhalter 1996; Marshall and Spiegelhalter 2001).

In a random intercepts model such as that identified by Eqs. (5.3) and (5.4), the level 2 residual u_{0j} is our estimate of the effect of institution j. As mentioned in Chap. 3, the estimates of the u_{0j} are shrunk towards zero, the mean for all hospitals. The extent of this shrinkage is dependent on the number of observations that we have for any given hospital. The u_{0j} are not known with certainty, hence the need to estimate them. They can typically be plotted together with a measure of uncertainty such as 95% confidence intervals as shown in Fig. 5.7, previously shown as Fig. 2.5; the smaller the confidence interval, the more certain we are about the estimate. Hospital effects in this example comprise the hospital residual u_{0j} added to the mean score for all hospitals, and these are plotted in rank order from the hospital with the lowest mean score (following adjustment for the patient's age, sex, education and physical and mental health) on the left to that with the highest score on the right. Typically there is substantial overlap between the estimates for different hospitals as is the case in Fig. 5.7, meaning that despite having a higher mean score, it is difficult to say with any certainty that one particular hospital is better than a hospital a few positions lower in the rankings.

The production of a measure of institutional performance following adjustment for patient characteristics using a random intercept model can be illustrated by Fig. 5.5a. Although the outcome varies according to the individual's age, the

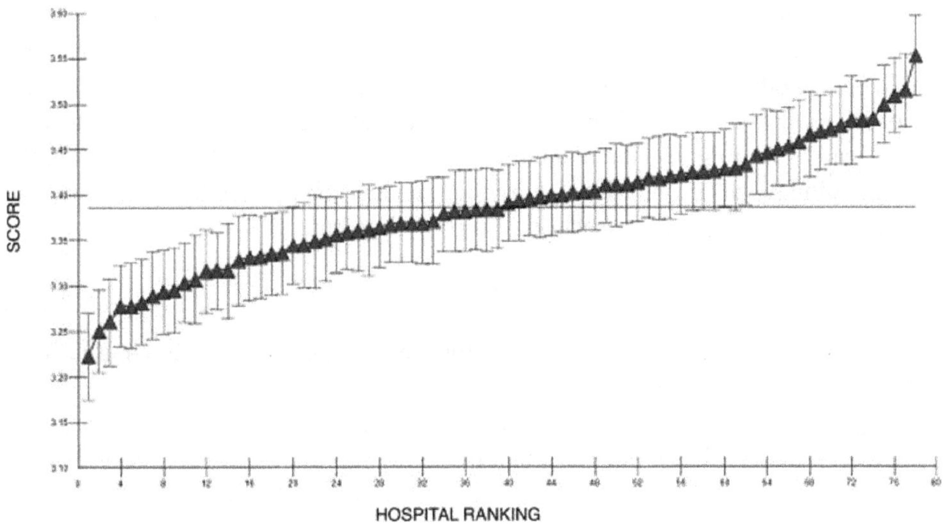

Fig. 5.7 Hospital performance scores (and confidence intervals) for patients' experience of their room and stay (78 hospitals; 22,000 patients). (Source: Sixma et al. 2009)

hospital effect—the distance between the line for any particular hospital and the fixed part of the model (the black line)—is the same for all ages. As a consequence the ranking of the hospitals—the ordering of the lines from lowest to highest—is the same at all ages. With a random slope model, this becomes more complicated; Fig. 5.5d illustrates how the lines in a random slope model may cross each other meaning that the ranking of hospitals will differ according to the patients' age. In the random slopes model defined by Eqs. (5.7) and (5.8), the random part of the model is given by $u_{0j} + u_{1j}x_{1ij}$; this is the composite residual and clearly varies according to the age of the individual x_{1ij}. So in a random slope model, it is unlikely that a single league table would capture all of the differences in rankings, but effects can be estimated (together with confidence intervals) and rankings produced for any given age.

The use of 95% confidence intervals around the residuals in plots such as Fig. 5.7 enables the reader to gauge whether the estimate for any particular unit differs significantly from the effect for the average level 2 unit. Depending on the intended use of such a plot, it may make more sense to adjust the confidence intervals so as to enable comparisons between pairs or sets of units; Goldstein and Healy (1995) describe the mechanics of making such an adjustment.

Conclusion

This chapter has introduced the algebraic notation for the models that are detailed in the rest of the book. The notation system is flexible in that it can readily be extended to include some of the more complex models that were described in Chap. 4. There are three reasons for needing to understand the algebraic representation of multilevel models. Firstly, it provides a concise means to describe your work in a manner that would enable others to replicate your models. Secondly, it facilitates an understanding of the models used by other researchers when reading literature relevant to your own research. And finally, the algebraic elements introduced in this chapter are the basic building blocks of multilevel regression models constructed using MLwiN, the software used in the practical section of this book (Chaps. 11–13).

Box 5.3 Basic Terminology

This box summarizes the terminology for the various algebraic terms used in the models in this chapter.

y_{ij} is the dependent variable: the outcome for individual i living in neighbourhood j. Individuals are numbered from $i = 1, \ldots, N$ and each lives in one neighbourhood $j = 1, \ldots, J$. There are n_j individuals from neighbourhood j so $N = \sum_{j=1}^{J} n_j$.

x_{pij} are the independent variables, measured on individual i in neighbourhood j. The subscript p is used to distinguish between the variables.

x_{pj} are independent variables, measured at the neighbourhood level; this variable takes the same value for all individuals living in neighbourhood j.

β_0 is used to denote the intercept.

β_p is the regression coefficient associated with x_{pij} or x_{pj}.

u_{0j} is the estimated effect or residual for area j. This is the difference in the outcome for an individual in neighbourhood j compared to an individual in the average neighbourhood, after taking into account those characteristics that have been included in the model. The 0 in the subscript denotes that this is a *random intercept* residual, a departure from the overall intercept β_0 applying equally to everyone in neighbourhood j regardless of individual characteristics.

u_{pj} is the slope residual for neighbourhood j that is associated with the independent variable x_{pij} or x_{pj}. Just as u_{0j} denotes a departure from the overall intercept β_0, u_{pj} indicates the extent of a departure from the overall slope in a *random slope* model.

e_{0ij} is the individual-level residual or error term for individual i in neighbourhood j.

σ_{u0}^2 is the variance of the neighbourhood-level intercept residuals u_{0j}.

σ_{up}^2 is the variance of the neighbourhood-level slope residuals u_{pj}.

σ_{u0p} is the covariance between the neighbourhood-level intercept residuals u_{0j} and slope residuals u_{pj}.

σ_{e0}^2 is the variance of the individual-level errors e_{0ij}.

ρ_I is the intraclass correlation coefficient or the proportion of the total variation in the outcome that is attributable to differences between areas.

References

Cardol M, Groenewegen PP, de Bakker DH, Spreeuwenberg P, van Dijk L, van den Bosch W (2005) Shared help seeking behaviour within families: a retrospective cohort study. Br Med J 330:882–884

Damman OC, de Boer D, Hendriks M, Meuwissen LE, Rademakers J, Delnoij DMJ, Groenewegen PP (2011) Differences between family practices in the associations of patient characteristics with health care experiences. Med Care Res Rev 68:725–739

Diez-Roux AV (2002) A glossary for multilevel analysis. J Epidemiol Community Health 56:588–594

Goldstein H, Healy M (1995) The graphical presentation of a collection of means. J R Stat Soc Ser A 158:175–177

Goldstein H, Spiegelhalter DJ (1996) League tables and their limitations: statistical issues in comparisons of institutional performance. J R Stat Soc Ser A 159:385–443

Leyland AH (2010) No quick fix: understanding the difference between fixed and random effect models. J Epidemiol Community Health 64:1027–1028

Lipps O, Moreau-Gruet F (2010) Change of individual BMI in Switzerland and the USA: a multilevel model for growth. Int J Public Health 55:299–306

Marshall EC, Spiegelhalter DJ (2001) Institutional performance. In: Leyland AH, Goldstein H (eds) Multilevel modelling of health statistics. Wiley, Chichester

Sacker A, Wiggins RD, Bartley M (2006) Time and place: putting individual health into context. A multilevel analysis of the British household panel survey, 1991-2001. Health Place 12:279–290

Sixma H, Spreeuwenberg P, Zuidgeest M, Rademakers J (2009) [Consumer quality index hospital stay]. NIVEL, Utrecht

Smith P (1995) On the unintended consequences of publishing performance data in the public sector. Int J Public Adm 18:277–310

Snijders TAB, Berkhof J (2008) Diagnostic checks for multilevel models. In: De Leeuw J, Meijer E (eds) Handbook of multilevel analysis. Springer, New York

6

Multilevel Analysis and Apportioning Variation

Abstract The starting point of multilevel analysis is to separate the variance in an outcome into the parts that are associated with the levels we distinguish. Several issues concerning variances at all levels are discussed in this chapter. Partitioning the variance between levels is straight forward in two-level linear models, but more complicated when we consider more than two levels or when our outcome is dichotomous. We discuss ways of clarifying and interpreting the importance of the higher level variance in logistic multilevel regression analysis. This can be done by transforming the difference between the 2.5 and 97.5 centile into an odds ratio or by using the median odds ratio, both of which can be interpreted in the same way as the odds ratio of a specific fixed effect. The higher level variance estimated from multilevel logistic regression models tends to be low leading to the question as to whether this small variance is still important. The clustering of observations within higher level units also informs power calculations. More variance at a higher level means that we need more observations to achieve the same power as when there is little variation at the higher level. The specification of levels is important, both from a theoretical and a statistical point of view. Omitting a relevant level has consequences for the estimation of the amount of variation associated with the remaining levels.

Keywords Multilevel analysis · Variance partitioning · Multilevel logistic regression · Median odds ratio · Power calculation · Design effect · Omitted level bias

One feature of multilevel models that is absent in single-level models is the ability to partition any unexplained variance between levels and hence quantify the importance of different levels. As we explained in Chap. 3, we can develop hypotheses solely concerned with variation in the phenomenon we are studying. In this chapter we give further consideration to the important topic of variance, and we consider interpretation of the variance and expound upon the implications of the variance both for model interpretation and for study design.

Variance Partitioning for Continuous Responses

In Chap. 5 we saw that the intraclass correlation coefficient ρ_{I} was a simple summary of the proportion of the total variance in a two-level random intercept model that was attributable to the higher level.

$$\rho_{\mathrm{I}} = \frac{\sigma_{u0}^2}{\sigma_{u0}^2 + \sigma_{e0}^2} \tag{6.1}$$

There are many situations in which the proportion of variance at a higher level cannot be summarised in such a simple fashion. These include circumstances when we have more than two levels (meaning that σ_{e0}^2 and σ_{u0}^2 are not the only variances), in the presence of heteroscedasticity (non-constant level 1 errors, in which case σ_{e0}^2 is not the only variance at level 1), and when we are fitting a model with random slopes (σ_{u0}^2 is not the only variance at level 2).

In general the proportion of the total variance that is attributable to a particular level in the model, for a given set of compositional and contextual characteristics, is called the variance partition coefficient (VPC; Goldstein et al. 2002). In many cases the VPC must be calculated for specific values of the covariates included in a multilevel regression model. For example, in the case of a two-level random slope model with a continuous outcome written as

$$y_{ij} = \beta_0 + \beta_1 x_{1ij} + u_{0j} + u_{1j}x_{1ij} + e_{0ij} \tag{6.2}$$

where the random part is given by $u_{0j} + u_{1j}x_{1ij} + e_{0ij}$ which depends on x_{1ij}. This means that the total variance, and therefore also the proportion of the variance that is at level 2, varies according to the value of the level 1 characteristic x_{1ij}.

Variance Partitioning for Multilevel Logistic Regression

In a multilevel logistic regression model, the VPC cannot be defined as in Eq. (6.1) even in the simplest variance component model. As detailed in Chap. 12, the observed outcome y_{ij}, a dichotomous response taking the value 1 if true and 0 otherwise, is modelled as a binomial process with denominator 1 and probability π_{ij} such that

$$y_{ij} \sim \text{Binomial}(1, \pi_{ij}) \tag{6.3}$$

In a random intercept model with a series of predictors x_{pij}, the transformed probability π_{ij} is modelled such that

$$\text{logit}(\pi_{ij}) = \log\left(\frac{\pi_{ij}}{1-\pi_{ij}}\right) = \beta_0 + \beta_1 x_{1ij} + \cdots + u_{0j} \tag{6.4}$$

Now because of the assumption of a binomial distribution, the variance of the y_{ij} is given by $\pi_{ij}(1 - \pi_{ij})$. This is dependent on the predicted values π_{ij} and so, in turn, is dependent on all of the covariates x_{pij}. Moreover, the random effects u_{0j}, again assumed to be normally distributed with variance σ^2_{u0}, are on the logit scale, and so it is not possible to make a direct comparison between the level 2 variance σ^2_{u0} and the total variance $\pi_{ij}(1 - \pi_{ij})$.

Goldstein et al. (2002) discuss four approaches to the estimation of the VPC. The first approach, and the most commonly used, is the latent variable method used by Snijders and Bosker (2012, Chap. 17). This entails substituting the constant quantity $\pi^2/3 \approx 3.29$ for the lowest level variance, meaning that for a two-level multilevel logistic regression model with a random intercept,

$$\rho_{\text{I}} = \frac{\sigma^2_{u0}}{\sigma^2_{u0} + \pi^2/3} \tag{6.5}$$

The second is a simulation method that is generalisable and has the advantage of not depending upon approximations. The third uses a Taylor series expansion (a power series approximation of a mathematical function) to provide an algebraic approximation for the VPC. The last method uses a binary linear model; this is a very approximate approach that involves treating the dichotomous responses y_{ij} as though they are normally distributed and fitting a model accordingly and, as such, tends to work better when the probability of the outcome is close to 0.5 rather than close to 0 or 1.

Variance Partitioning for Models with Three or More Levels

In the presence of more than two levels, the VPC details the proportion of unexplained variance that is attributable to the different levels in the model. Merlo et al. (2012) modelled the probability of death using a multilevel logistic regression model with four levels; individuals were nested within households, which were in turn clustered within census tracts and municipalities. The authors estimated variances associated with the three highest levels, denoted by σ^2_{H}, σ^2_{C} and σ^2_{M}, respectively, and used these to calculate the VPCs under the latent variable method (Snijders and Bosker 2012) as

$$\begin{aligned}
\text{VPC}_{\text{M}} &= \sigma^2_{\text{M}} / \left(\sigma^2_{\text{M}} + \sigma^2_{\text{C}} + \sigma^2_{\text{H}} + \pi^2/3\right) \\
\text{VPC}_{\text{C}} &= \left(\sigma^2_{\text{M}} + \sigma^2_{\text{C}}\right) / \left(\sigma^2_{\text{M}} + \sigma^2_{\text{C}} + \sigma^2_{\text{H}} + \pi^2/3\right) \\
\text{VPC}_{\text{H}} &= \left(\sigma^2_{\text{M}} + \sigma^2_{\text{C}} + \sigma^2_{\text{H}}\right) / \left(\sigma^2_{\text{M}} + \sigma^2_{\text{C}} + \sigma^2_{\text{H}} + \pi^2/3\right)
\end{aligned} \tag{6.6}$$

Note that these variance partition coefficients are cumulative, indicating the proportion of unexplained variance at the level in question and at higher levels. This means that they can also be interpreted as the correlation between individuals from the same higher level unit; individuals living in the same household must live in the same census tract and people from the same census tract must live in the same municipality since these are strictly clustered. It is straight forward to calculate the proportion of the total variance associated with a particular level by subtraction. For example, in the null model, estimates of VPC_H and VPC_C were 0.186 and 0.023, respectively, indicating a correlation in mortality between individuals within the same household of 0.186 and suggesting that 16.3% of the total variance in mortality was attributable to differences between households within census tracts.

Interpretation of Variances

In a multilevel model with a random intercept, the interpretation of the variance in terms of the VPC—however estimated—is fairly straightforward. For example, Gonzalez et al. (2012) investigated the clustering of young adults' body mass index (BMI) within families; for a two-level null model, they reported a variance between families (σ_{u0}^2) of 8.92 and a variance between young adults within families (σ_{e0}^2) of 13.92. The variance partition coefficient (which in this simple case is the same as an intraclass correlation coefficient) is therefore

$$\mathrm{VPC} = \sigma_{u0}^2 / \left(\sigma_{u0}^2 + \sigma_{e0}^2\right) = 8.92/(8.92 + 13.92) = 0.391$$

This means that they found 39.1% of the variation in BMI in young adulthood to be attributable to the family level, with the remaining 60.9% being due to differences between young adults within families. The total variance in the sample is 22.84 and so the standard deviation σ is 4.779; with a reported mean BMI of 25.38, we would expect 95% of the young adults to have a BMI of between $(\mu - 1.96\sigma, \mu + 1.96\sigma) = (16.01, 34.75)$. We can also say something about the variation between families; we would expect 95% of families to have a mean young adult BMI of between $\left(\mu - 1.96\sqrt{\sigma_{u0}^2}, \mu + 1.96\sqrt{\sigma_{u0}^2}\right)$ or (16.99, 28.69).

In multilevel logistic regression models, we have less information available—just the higher level variance σ_{u0}^2 in a two-level random intercept model—and our interpretation of the variance is different. We are, however, still able to interpret the random part of a multilevel logistic regression model, and given that it is slightly more complex, this is arguably more important than for the multilevel linear regression model. For example, Esser et al. (2014) examined in-hospital mortality among very low birthweight neonates in Bavaria. Following adjustment for individual casemix (including gestational age, sex and the clinical risk index for babies

[CRIB] score), the authors found a variance between hospitals (σ^2_{u0}) of 0.324. Assuming the latent variable method discussed above, the variance partition coefficient calculated according to Eq. (6.5) is given by

$$\text{VPC} = 0.324/(0.324 + 3.29) = 0.090$$

In other words, 9.0% of the total variation in mortality is attributable to differences between hospitals after adjustment for casemix (with the remaining 91.0% relating to differences between patients within hospitals that have not been accounted for by variables included in the model). The high-level variance σ^2_{u0} is again informative, but this time it is on a log odds scale. We would expect 95% of hospitals to have a log odds ratio of mortality—relative to the typical hospital—of $\left(-1.96\sqrt{\sigma^2_{u0}},\ +1.96\sqrt{\sigma^2_{u0}}\right)$. Converting this to an odds ratio scale (by exponentiating), we would expect 95% of hospitals to have an odds ratio (OR) of mortality associated with being in that hospital, compared to the typical hospital, to be in the interval $\left(\exp\left\{-1.96\sqrt{\sigma^2_{u0}}\right\},\ \exp\left\{1.96\sqrt{\sigma^2_{u0}}\right\}\right)$ or (0.33, 3.05).

Rather than considering the 95% coverage intervals, we can make comparisons between the upper and lower limits of the distribution. Returning to the example of Gonzalez et al. (2012), we would expect the mean BMI of a family at the 97.5 centile to exceed that of a family at the 2.5 centile by $2 \times 1.96\sqrt{\sigma^2_{u0}} = 11.71$ —the difference, save for rounding error, between the upper and lower 95% limits of 28.69 and 16.99 calculated above. So 95% of families should be covered by 11.71 points on the BMI scale. It is possible to do something similar for a logistic regression model; we would expect the odds of mortality for a hospital at the 97.5 centile to be $\exp\left\{2 \times 1.96\sqrt{\sigma^2_{u0}}\right\}$ or 9.31 times the odds of mortality associated with a hospital at the 2.5 centile. Again, apart from rounding error, this is approximately the ratio of the two limits of the coverage interval, 3.05 and 0.33.

The variance estimate from a multilevel logistic regression model can therefore be used as a means of informing us about the variation between higher level units in the dataset. The comparison of the 97.5 and 2.5 centiles is arbitrary; a commonly used alternative that is not dependent on such an arbitrary range and which was introduced by Larsen and Merlo (2005) is the median odds ratio (MOR). The MOR is the median of odds ratios comparing two people with identical covariates chosen randomly from different higher level units (ordered so that the odds ratio is always at least one). It is calculated as

$$\text{MOR} = \exp\left\{\sqrt{2 \times \sigma^2_{u0}}\Phi^{-1}(0.75)\right\} \tag{6.7}$$

$\Phi^{-1}(0.75)$ is the 75th centile of the standard normal density or 0.6745 giving

$$\text{MOR} = \exp\left\{0.954 \times \sqrt{\sigma_{u0}^2}\right\} \tag{6.8}$$

In the example of in-hospital mortality among very low birthweight neonates given by Esser et al. (2014), the variance of 0.342 gives an MOR of 1.72. This calculation has converted the variance to a measure of dispersion on the odds ratio scale, telling us something about the average difference between two random hospitals. Since it is now on the odds ratio scale, this can be compared to any other odds ratio, for example, for any of the fixed effects such as sex.

The MOR is used as a means of transforming the variance onto a meaningful and interpretable scale in multilevel logistic regression; there are equivalent measures for other forms of multilevel analysis. Chan et al. (2011) found a median rate ratio (MRR) of 1.31 between practices for treatment using warfarin among patients with nonvalvular atrial fibrillation using a multilevel modified Poisson regression model. Chaix et al. (2007) reported a median hazard ratio (MHR) of 1.25 between small areas in Sweden when analysing ischaemic heart disease mortality. The calculation of the MRR and the MHR follows the same principles as for the MOR. More details about the MRR can be found in Austin et al. (2018) and details of the MHR in Austin et al. (2017).

The MOR and related measures make use of the distributions of the residuals and are easy to calculate since they depend only on the higher level variance σ_{u0}^2. An alternative measure, the absolute relative deviation (ARD), quantifies the average difference between the effect of each high-level unit and the effect of an average high-level unit (see Martikainen et al. 2003; Tarkiainen et al. 2010). The ARD uses the model residuals u_{0j} and so is more complicated to calculate but may be particularly useful when there are fewer higher level units (and the distribution of these higher level units may not strictly follow a standard statistical distribution).

Zero Variance

Unexplained variance between high-level units may constitute a small proportion of the total variance in the outcome. Unfortunately there is no consensus as to exactly what constitutes a 'small' proportion. Usually the higher level variance is small compared to the lower level variance. The common exception is for repeated measures in which there will typically be less variability between measurement occasions than between the higher level units. For example, in a study of health functioning in a cohort of British civil servants, Stafford et al. (2008) found 57% of the variation in physical functioning and 49% of the variation in mental functioning at baseline to be associated with the level of the individual. Chapter 11 describes the modelling of repeated measures on areas rather than individuals; in that example 82% of the variation in mortality rates is seen to be at the district level.

In some situations, a higher level variance will be estimated to be zero. The suggestion that all of the unexplained variation is at the individual (lowest) level does not mean that the mean outcome is identical for all contexts; rather, this means that there is no more variation between higher level units than we would have expected by chance. But that does not mean that there is no variation, and, at first sight, the differences between high-level units may appear substantial.

To illustrate this concept, we simulate a random assignment of individuals to 25 hospitals, with each hospital comprising between 90 and 120 patients. Each patient has a 'vitality score'; these scores are generated as random draws from a normal distribution with mean 1.64 and variance 1. Figure 6.1a shows the mean scores for the 25 hospitals under one such simulation. There is little variation between the hospital means—the minimum and maximum are 1.45 and 1.77 with the variance of the hospital mean scores (0.007) being very small compared to the individual variance of 1 that was used to generate these data.

If the vitality score is such that a patient with a score of 0 or more denotes life and a score below 0 denotes death, then we can use the individual scores to categorise

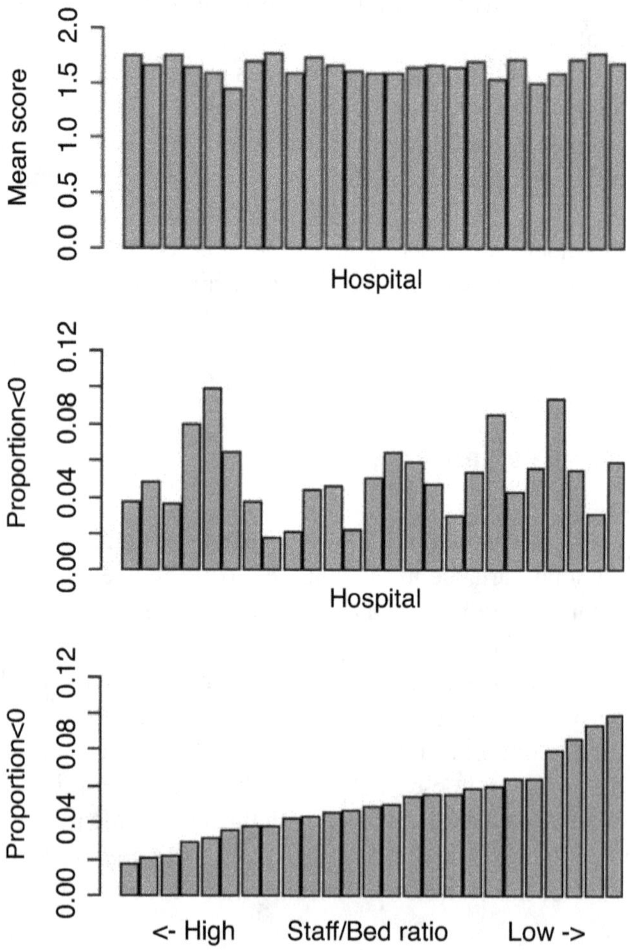

Fig. 6.1 Simulated data of individuals aggregated to hospitals showing (**a**) the variation between hospitals in the mean vitality score; (**b**) the variation between hospitals in the mortality rate (for whom the vitality score <0) and (**c**) the association between the hospital mortality rate and a contextual variable

patients. A score of 0 corresponds to −1.64 standard deviations so about 5% of all patients will be classified as dead. Figure 6.1b shows the results of aggregating the individual patient deaths to the hospital level and expressing these as a proportion. The proportion of deaths in each hospital now ranges between 0.018 and 0.099, but this fivefold difference in mortality rates between hospitals has occurred by chance. We would quite reasonably estimate the variance between hospitals to be zero since there is no more than we would expect by chance.

When there is no variance between higher level units in a two-level model, the intraclass correlation coefficient is 0 and the model effectively collapses to a single-level model. However, in such circumstances Merlo et al. (2009) point out that this should not exclude the possibility of investigating (and indeed discovering) contextual effects. Figure 6.1c shows how the ranking of hospitals in terms of their mortality rates may be correlated with key staffing indicators such as the staff/bed ratio. Despite there being no unexplained variance being associated with the hospitals, we can find a significant relationship with a contextual variable.

Merlo et al. (2012) argue that the general contextual effects (the overall extent to which context influences individual health outcomes, assessed using the variance and VPC) should have greater prominence in research and that such measures are more informative than tests of the significance of small area variation common in spatial epidemiological analysis. The authors further suggested that the small variances typically found at the area level should lead to less importance being placed on administrative areas as a determinant of individual health than is currently the case (see also our discussion of the relevance of contexts in Chap. 2).

Multilevel Power Calculations

Power calculations are an important aspect of study designs involving primary data collection and are often regarded as essential by funders even for the analysis of existing data. When a study includes different levels, it is necessary to take these into account when conducting the power calculation; failure to do so will lead to an overestimation of the power available for the analysis since the lack of independence between observations nested within the same higher level unit reduces the effective sample size.

The focus of the power calculation depends on its purpose. Common uses are to indicate the power that is available to detect a specified effect with a given sample size, the sample size needed to detect a specified effect at a given level of power or an estimate of the effect size that could be detected with a given sample size at a specified level of power. The three quantities power, sample size and effect size are related, and so the unknown quantity can be changed by simple algebraic manipulation. (We have assumed that the significance level used is the common $\alpha = 0.05$.) As is the case for single-level power calculations, two of the three quantities are assumed to be known in order to estimate the third. However, specifying the sample size in a multilevel design is more complicated; in addition to the number of individuals (level 1 units), we need to know the number of level 2 units and the extent of the clustering of the outcome within the level 2 units as expressed by the intraclass correlation coefficient ρ_I.

The calculation of the required sample size n for a single-level problem with power β to detect an effect size of magnitude x/σ at a significance level α is as follows:

$$n = \left[\frac{Z_{1-\alpha/2} + Z_{1-\beta}}{x/\sigma}\right]^2 \tag{6.9}$$

Z_r is the value from the standard normal distribution with the proportion r below it, and so $\alpha = 0.05$, $Z_{1-\alpha/2} = 1.96$. The effect size here is standardised and expressed in terms of the number of standard deviations and assumes that the outcome is normally distributed; equivalent formulae are available when the dependent variable is dichotomous.

The multilevel data structure is taken into account by inflating the variance in Eq. (6.9) by a design effect D

$$D = 1 + (\bar{n}_j - 1)\rho_I \tag{6.10}$$

$\bar{n}_j$ is the average number of individuals (level 1 units) in a cluster. The design effect therefore depends on both the magnitude of the intraclass correlation coefficient and the average cluster size. If $\rho_I = 0$, there is no correlation between individuals within the same high-level unit, $D = 1$, and the power is the same as for a simple random sample. If $\rho_I = 1$ there is no variation within high-level units, $D = \bar{n}_j$, and there is no gain through sampling more than one individual per cluster. Power can only be increased in this instance by sampling more level 2 units. If $\bar{n}_j = 1$, then only one individual is being sampled per cluster, $D = 1$, and the power is the same as for a simple random sample. In general, D will be greater than 1 and the clustering of outcomes within contexts reduces the power of a multilevel model relative to a simple random sample.

The dependence of the power calculation on the design effect means that we need to have an idea of the likely magnitude of the design effect. Design effects can often be calculated based on the reporting of intraclass correlation coefficients in the literature. For example, if we were interested in compliance with a colorectal cancer screening programme, we might base our power calculation on the study by Pornet et al. (2011). They found a variance between geographical areas in France (Ilôts Regroupés pour l'Information Statistique, IRIS) of 0.040 in an empty model. Given that this estimate was derived from a multilevel logistic regression model, the estimated intraclass correlation coefficient calculated using Eq. (6.5) is 0.012. This means that an estimated 1.2% of the variation in uptake of screening is associated with the area. This study was based on the analysis of 8691 individuals in 829 IRISs; if we were to take a similar sample, then the average cluster size would be $\bar{n}_j = 10.48$. Based on Eq. (6.10), the design effect is given by

$$D = 1 + (10.48 - 1) \times 0.012 = 1.11$$

Even with a trivial intraclass correlation coefficient, and a modest average cluster size, the clustering of individuals within areas means that we would need to increase our sample size by 11% to get the same power as a simple random sample of uncorrelated individuals. Note that this increase in sample size needs to be reflected in an increase in the number of areas, since an increase in the number of individuals per area would in turn increase the magnitude of the design effect.

It is possible that a literature search will turn up a relevant research article from which the intraclass correlation coefficient can be found for a multilevel power calculation. There are also resources reporting intraclass correlation coefficients for different study types, such as those for various health outcomes in UK settings (Ukoumunne et al. 1999), cardiovascular disease in primary care practices in Canada (Singh et al. 2015) and BMI, physical activity and diet across countries (Masood and Reidpath 2016). The need for information to perform power calculations is a further argument for the need to report the intraclass correlation or variances in research articles (see Chap. 10 for further discussion of this).

From the above, it would appear that a large intraclass correlation coefficient is the enemy of efficient and economical study design, with even small intraclass correlation coefficients leading to substantial increases in the sample size required (and hence in many cases, the cost involved) to replicate the power of a simple random sample. However, this is design dependent since a repeated measure design—with a large associated intraclass correlation coefficient—can increase the power of an analysis. We can illustrate this by considering two simulated study designs for the evaluation of an area intervention. Figure 6.2a shows how the power available to detect a specific effect size increases with the effect size in a *repeated*

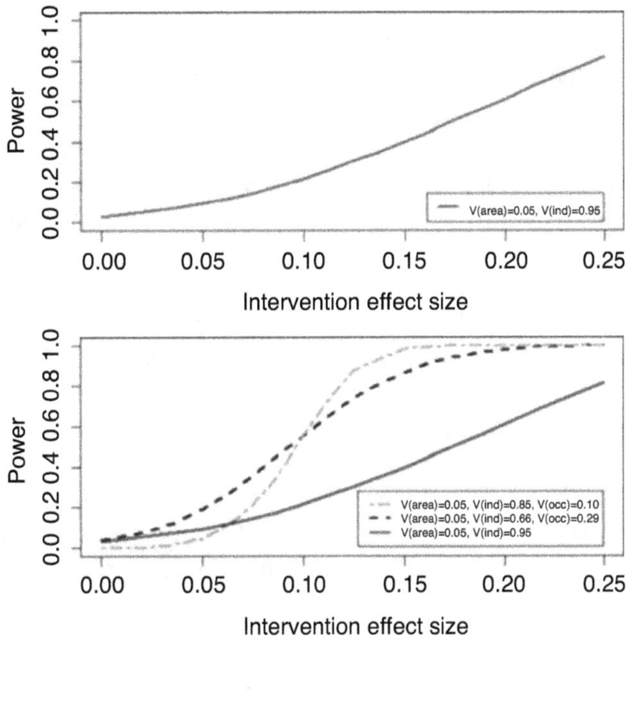

Fig. 6.2 Simulation showing the power to detect an effect of given size for an area-based intervention based on (**a**) a repeated cross-sectional design (40 individuals in 50 areas) and (**b**) a repeated measures design (two observations on 20 individuals in 50 areas)

cross-sectional design. This simulated study has 20 individuals measured before the intervention and 20 after the intervention in each of 50 areas, assuming an intraclass correlation coefficient of 0.05. With this design, the effect size has to be close to 0.25 before the power reaches 0.8. In Fig. 6.2b, the study design is changed to a *repeated measures* design, such that each of 20 individuals is measured before and after the intervention (two measurements per person). This design retains the same total number of measurements as in the repeated cross-sectional design (2000), and the total variance is unchanged, but there is now some variation within as well as between individuals. This study is now more highly powered to detect effects of modest sizes, with power of 0.8 to detect an effect size of 0.11–0.13 based on the same proportion of the variance at the area level as in Fig. 6.1a but with 69–89% of the remaining variance being attributable to differences between individuals. With this study design, the fact that a relatively small proportion of the total variance (10–29%) is associated with the measurement occasion means that any change between the pre- and post-intervention measures is more likely to denote an effect of the intervention.

Power calculations are commonly used to determine whether it will be possible to detect an effect of a certain size; as such they involve the comparison of the magnitude of a parameter estimate to its precision (as measured by its standard error). But the accuracy of different parameter estimates, and their standard errors, may also be dependent on the sample size. Maas and Hox (2005) showed that in general estimates were unbiased in two-level linear multilevel models if there were sufficient (at least 50) level 2 units. With fewer level 2 units, the only estimate that was affected was the standard error of the high-level variance.

Software for Multilevel Power Calculations

In the simplest designs, it may be possible to inflate the sample size required over that needed for a simple random sample using the design effect, as we did for the example on compliance with colorectal cancer screening above. However, this may not be straightforward for more complicated designs such as when there is considerable lack of balance between cluster sizes or when the effect size to be estimated is not at the lowest level (such as the simulated area-based intervention above). For such circumstances, specialist software is available, for example, MLPowSim (Browne et al. 2009), Optimal Design (Spybrook et al. 2011) and PINT (Snijders and Bosker 1993). The topic along with the software has also been covered in some detail by Moerbeek and Teerenstra (2015).

There may be other constraints on the sample size calculation such as cost. In particular, cost may be an important consideration when there is a cost associated with each higher level unit that is sampled over and above the costs of the individuals sampled. This is the case if, for example, we had to organise data collection in more hospitals, needing permissions, time of hospital personnel, field workers, etc. Snijders (2001) gives an example of incorporating cost considerations into a multilevel study design.

Population Average and Cluster-Specific Estimates

The parameter estimates obtained from a multilevel model are sometimes called *cluster-specific* (or *random effect*) estimates. These estimates are conditional on the random part of the model and therefore indicate the effect of the variable in question on two individuals from the same higher level unit. In contrast, *population average* (also called *marginal*) estimates indicate the effect of a covariate on the average person (Diez-Roux 2002). The two estimates are identical for normally distributed responses but will tend to differ for non-linear responses, such as for a logistic regression model, with the differences becoming larger as the variance increases. Population average estimates are usually given as the output from generalised estimating equations (GEEs; see Zeger et al. 1988) whilst cluster-specific estimates are the default output from most multilevel modelling packages. The population average estimate β^* is approximately related to the cluster-specific estimate β as follows (Larsen and Merlo 2005):

$$\beta^* \approx \beta / \sqrt{1 + 0.346\sigma^2_{u0}} \tag{6.11}$$

Note that β and β^* here are parameter estimates on their original scale, i.e. log odds ratios for a logistic regression model. As can be seen from Eq. (6.11), the smaller the variance σ^2_{u0} the smaller the difference between the two estimates. For example, with an estimate of $\beta = 1.40$ (giving an odds ratio OR $= 1.49$), a variance of $\sigma^2_{u0} = 0.05$ leads to a population average estimate of $\beta^* = 0.397$ (OR $= 1.49$) whilst a variance of $\sigma^2_{u0} = 0.50$ gives $\beta^* = 0.369$ (OR $= 1.45$). So if required (e.g. if requested by a journal), population average effects can be obtained from the cluster-specific effects. The distinction between the multilevel and GEE approaches is explored in more detail elsewhere (Burton et al. 1998; Hu et al. 1998; Hubbard et al. 2010).

Omitting a Level

Suppose we have a study which has data on two levels. A theoretical analysis of our research problem might lead us to hypothesise the importance of other levels too. What is the consequence of omitting a theoretically important level for the interpretation of the portioning of variance? A statistical and empirical analysis (using UK Census data) was made by Tranmer and Steel (2001). We distinguish between three situations shown in Fig. 6.3.

To make it more concrete, think of an example in which we are studying episodes of care of patients admitted to hospital departments. The data we have in Fig. 6.3a refer to patients within hospital departments. It may also be important to have information on the hospitals. In Fig. 6.3b, we have data on patients and hospitals, but not on the hospital department. Finally, in Fig. 6.3c, we lack any information at the level of the patient.

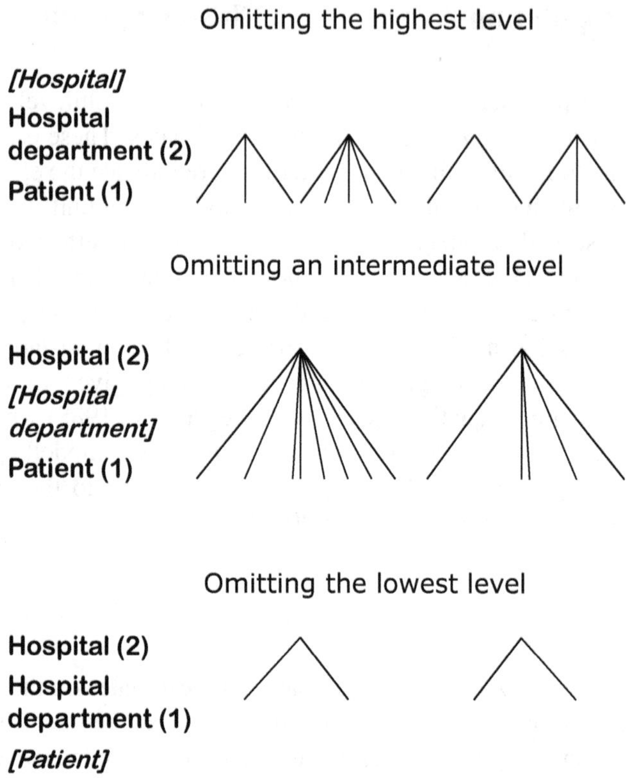

Fig. 6.3 Illustration of omitting different theoretically important levels

What happens to the variance in these situations? The first situation is quite straightforward (although not satisfactory); the variation at the highest level in Fig. 6.3a is combined with the variation at the next level down and is indistinguishable from it. In the example of hospitals, the variance estimated at the level of the department includes variance between hospitals as well as variance between departments within hospitals, but we do not know the proportion of the variance that is associated with each of these two levels. The patient-level variance will, however, be estimated accurately. In Fig. 6.3b, the department level is omitted, and the associated variance is distributed between the patient and hospital levels. Sacker et al. (2006) give an example of such a situation. They studied self-rated health of individuals taken from the British Household Survey at different times. They compared a model with two levels, individuals nested within areas (electoral wards) and a model with three levels where the level of the household is included between individuals and areas. As Fig. 6.4 shows, part of the individual-level variance estimated from the two-level model is actually related to the households people live in and (a smaller) part of the area-level variance estimated from the two-level model turns out to be associated with variation between households within the areas.

Tranmer and Steel (2001) show that for a linear model the proportion of the intermediate-level variance that will be distributed to the highest level is approximately $\overline{n}_{jk}/\overline{n}_k$, where $\overline{n}_{jk}$ and $\overline{n}_k$ are the average cluster size (in terms of level 1 units, e.g. individuals) at the intermediate and highest levels, respectively, with the remainder being distributed to the lowest level. However, if the magnitude of the

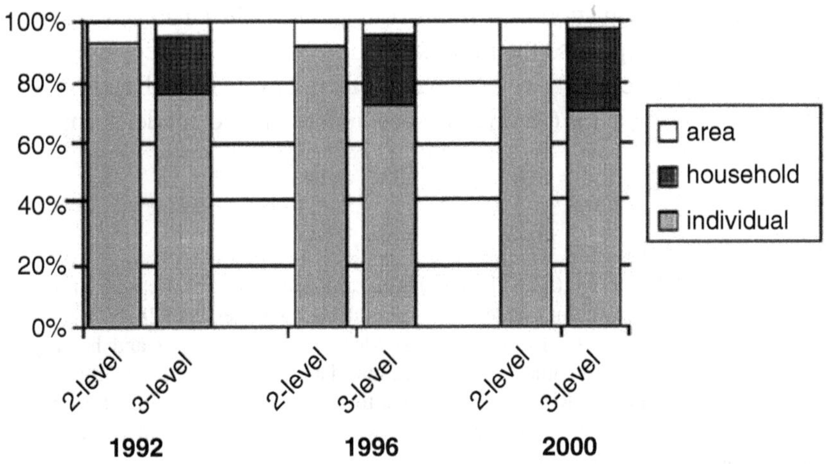

Fig. 6.4 Proportion of variance at each level of a two-level (individuals within areas) and three-level (individuals within households within areas) baseline model of poor general health in the British Household Panel Study. (Reproduced with permission from Elsevier, Health & Place)

variance at the omitted level is unknown, it is impossible to assess the impact of its omission.

When the lowest level is omitted as in Fig. 6.3c, the model is rather different since the analysis is aggregated to the intermediate level (such as hospital department). The variance at the highest level (hospital) is estimated correctly, but the estimated variance at the intermediate level (department) includes a component from the lowest (individual) level. Although the proportion of the lowest level variance that is incorrectly attributed to the intermediate level is likely to be small—Tranmer and Steel (2001) estimate this proportion to be just $1/\overline{n}_{jk}$—this will commonly be a small proportion of a large variance since σ_{u0}^2 is commonly much smaller than σ_{e0}^2. For example, let us assume that in the correctly specified three-level model, 5% of the variance is at the level of the hospital, 5% at the level of the hospital department and the remaining 90% of the variance refers to differences between patients within hospital departments. The fact that σ_{e0}^2 is 18 times σ_{u0}^2 means that, even if there are as many as 100 patients in each hospital department ($\overline{n}_{jk} = 100$), omitting the patient level would result in an 18% inflation of the estimated variance between hospital departments.

Conclusion

The variances at different levels form an important and informative part of the multilevel model and even small variances at higher levels can have a substantial impact on the required sample sizes. Despite their importance for model interpretation, assessment of the importance of contexts and for the conduct of future power calculations, Riva et al. (2007) found in a review that many studies did not report variance components. This is clearly an oversight by authors and journals, and we would hope that this situation will improve over time. In Chap. 10 (Reading and writing), we further emphasise the importance of reporting variances from multilevel studies. We have also seen that when a level is omitted from an analysis, the impact on the variances estimated in the (incorrectly specified) multilevel model is unpredictable.

References

Austin PC, Wagner P, Merlo J (2017) The median hazard ratio: a useful measure of variance and general contextual effects in multilevel survival analysis. Stat Med 36:928–938

Austin PC, Stryhn H, Leckie G, Merlo J (2018) Measures of clustering and heterogeneity in multilevel Poisson regression analysis of rates/count data. Stat Med 37:572–589

Browne WJ, Lahi MG, Parker RMA (2009) A guide to sample size calculations for random effect models via simulation and the MLPowSim Software Package. School of Clinical Veterinary Sciences, University of Bristol, Bristol

Burton P, Gurrin L, Sly P (1998) Extending the simple linear regression model to account for correlated responses: an introduction to generalized estimating equations and multi-level mixed modelling. Stat Med 17:1261–1291

Chaix B, Rosvall M, Merlo J (2007) Assessment of the magnitude of geographical variations and socioeconomic contextual effects on ischaemic heart disease mortality: a multilevel survival analysis of a large Swedish cohort. J Epidemiol Community Health 61:349–355

Chan PS, Maddox TM, Tang F, Spinler S, Spertus JA (2011) Practice-level variation in warfarin use among outpatients with atrial fibrillation (from the NCDR PINNACLE program). Am J Cardiol 108:1136–1140

Diez-Roux AV (2002) A glossary for multilevel analysis. J Epidemiol Community Health 56:588–594

Esser M, Lack N, Riedel C, Mansmann U, von Kries R (2014) Relevance of hospital characteristics as performance indicators for treatment of very-low-birth-weight neonates. Eur J Public Health 24:739–744

Goldstein H, Browne W, Rasbash J (2002) Partitioning variation in multilevel models. Understanding Stat 1:223–231

Gonzalez A, Boyle MH, Georgiades K, Duncan L, Atkinson LR, MacMillan HL (2012) Childhood and family influences on body mass index in early adulthood: findings from the Ontario Child Health Study. BMC Public Health 12:755

Hu FB, Goldberg J, Hedeker D, Flay BR, Pentz MA (1998) Comparison of population-averaged and subject-specific approaches for analyzing repeated binary outcomes. Am J Epidemiol 147:694–703

Hubbard AE, Ahern J, Fleischer NL, Van der Laan M, Lippman SA, Jewell N, Bruckner T, Satariano WA (2010) To GEE or not to GEE: comparing population average and mixed models for estimating the associations between neighborhood risk factors and health. Epidemiology 21:467–474

Larsen K, Merlo J (2005) Appropriate assessment of neighborhood effects on individual health: integrating random and fixed effects in multilevel logistic regression. Am J Epidemiol 161:81–88

Maas CJM, Hox JJ (2005) Sufficient sample sizes for multilevel modeling. Methodology 1:86–92

Martikainen P, Kauppinen TM, Valkonen T (2003) Effects of the characteristics of neighbourhoods and the characteristics of people on cause specific mortality: a register based follow up study of 252 000 men. J Epidemiol Community Health 57:210–217

Masood M, Reidpath DD (2016) Intraclass correlation and design effect in BMI, physical activity and diet: a cross-sectional study of 56 countries. BMJ Open 6:e008173

Merlo J, Ohlsson H, Lynch KF, Chaix B, Subramanian SV (2009) Individual and collective bodies: using measures of variance and association in contextual epidemiology. J Epidemiol Community Health 63:1043–1048

Merlo J, Viciana-Fernández FJ, Ramiro-Fariñas D, the Research Group of the Longitudinal Database of the Andalusian Population (LDAP) (2012) Bringing the individual back to small-area variation studies: a multilevel analysis of all-cause mortality in Andalusia, Spain. Soc Sci Med 75:1477–1487

Moerbeek M, Teerenstra S (2015) Power analysis of trials with multilevel data. Chapman & Hall, Boca Raton

Pornet C, Dejardin O, Morlais F, Bouvier V, Launoy G (2011) Socioeconomic determinants for compliance to colorectal cancer screening: a multilevel analysis. J Epidemiol Community Health 64:318–324

Riva M, Gauvin L, Barnett TA (2007) Towards the next generation of research into small area effects on health: a synthesis of multilevel investigations published since July 1988. J Epidemiol Community Health 61:853–861

Sacker A, Wiggins RD, Bartley M (2006) Time and place: putting individual health into context. A multilevel analysis of the British household panel survey, 1991-2001. Health Place 12:279–290

Singh J, Liddy C, Hogg W, Taljaard M (2015) Intracluster correlation coefficients for sample size calculations related to cardiovascular disease prevention and management in primary care practices. BMC Res Notes 8:89

Snijders TAB (2001) Sampling. In: Leyland AH, Goldstein H (eds) Multilevel modelling of health statistics. Wiley, Chichester

Snijders TAB, Bosker RJ (1993) Standard errors and sample sizes in two-level research. J Educ Stat 18:237–260

Snijders TAB, Bosker RJ (2012) Multilevel analysis: an introduction to basic and advanced multilevel modeling. Sage, Los Angeles

Spybrook J, Bloom H, Congdon R, Hill C, Martinez A, Raudenbush S (2011) Optimal design plus empirical evidence: documentation for the "Optimal Design" software version 3.0. Available from http://www.wtgrantfoundation.org/resources/optimal-design

Stafford M, Gimeno D, Marmot MG (2008) Neighbourhood characteristics and trajectories of health functioning: a multilevel prospective analysis. Eur J Public Health 18:604–610

Tarkiainen L, Martikainen P, Laaksonen M, Leyland AH (2010) Comparing the effects of neighbourhood characteristics on all-cause mortality using two hierarchical areal units in the capital region of Helsinki. Health Place 16:409–412

Tranmer M, Steel DG (2001) Ignoring a level in a multilevel model: evidence from UK census data. Environ Plan A 33:941–948

Ukoumunne OC, Gulliford MC, Chinn S, Sterne JAC, Burney PGJ (1999) Methods for evaluating area-wide and organisation-based interventions in health and health care: a systematic review. Health Technol Assess 3(5):iii-92

Zeger S, Liang K-Y, Albert P (1988) Models for longitudinal data: a generalized estimating equation approach. Biometrics 44:1049–1060

Part 3
Research Presentation and the Process of Modeling

7

Disentangling the Context and Composition

Abstract Individual-level outcomes are influenced by people's individual characteristics and by characteristics of the higher level units or contexts. In the previous chapter, we discussed the apportioning of variation between lower and higher levels. Here we move to explaining this variation. Higher level variation might be explained by variables at that level, known as contextual effects. However, they may also be the effect of the concentration of people with particular characteristics in higher level units. So the variation at higher level might be reduced just by adding individual-level variables. We illustrate how to disentangle the context and composition with an example of the influence of individual social capital and neighbourhood social capital on people's self-rated health.

The chapter ends with a general discussion of issues to take into account when estimating the contextual effects.

Keywords Multilevel analysis · Compositional effects · Contextual effects · Model specification · Model interpretation · Social capital

It is recognised that people's health is patterned by individual characteristics and also by area characteristics. There remains, however, debate as to whether people's health behaviours and health outcomes are influenced by the social and physical environments of the place in which they live (Macintyre et al. 1993) or whether the different health outcomes and health behaviours observed across areas merely reflect the concentration of people living within those areas (Sloggett and Joshi 1994). The first of these—the influence of the characteristics of the environment—are usually termed contextual effects; the second—the characteristics of people within areas and consequent concentration of these characteristics—are called compositional effects. Multilevel modelling presents a natural way of determining the relative importance of compositional and contextual effects and thereby of disentangling their importance. This is easily generalised to other example, such as hospitals, where, for example, we could think of a contextual effect as the influence of a hospital quality system on patient outcomes, and compositional effects might include the concentration of people with a particular stage of the disease. This chapter considers how multilevel modelling can be used to disentangle individual and contextual influences on individual health.

Context or Composition?

To be clear as to the definitions of context and compositional effects, we can refer to their definitions provided in Diez-Roux's (2002) glossary for multilevel analysis:

> *COMPOSITIONAL EFFECTS*
>
> *When inter-group (or inter-context) differences in an outcome (for example, disease rates) are attributable to differences in group composition (that is, in the characteristics of the individuals of which the groups are comprised) they are said to result from compositional effects.*
>
> *CONTEXTUAL EFFECTS*
>
> *Term generally used to refer to the effects of variables defined at a higher level (usually at the group level) on outcomes defined at a lower level (usually at the individual level) after controlling for relevant individual level (lower level) confounders.*

It is important that we should consider the meaning of any contextual variables in an analysis. Once an individual variable is aggregated to a context (e.g. by taking the mean), then its interpretation may change. For example,

> *mean neighborhood income may provide information that is not captured by individual-level income. The mean income of a neighborhood may be a marker for neighborhood-level factors potentially related to health (such as recreational facilities, school quality, road conditions, environmental conditions, and the types of foods that are available), and these factors may affect everyone in the community regardless of individual-level income. Similarly, community unemployment levels may affect all individuals living within a community, regardless of whether or not they are unemployed. (Diez-Roux* 1998*)*

However, the distinction between compositional and contextual characteristics may not be straightforward since individuals may be constrained by their environment. Macintyre and Ellaway explain this idea:

> *Occupation may be determined by the local labor market; housing tenure by the local housing market; education by the available educational system and local provision; income by the prevailing labor market conditions; and car ownership by the density of population, distance to facilities, and local transport networks. Hence, rather than seeing [these] as properties of individuals, we could ... see them as features of the local environment. (Macintyre and Ellaway* 2003*)*

The fact that people with certain characteristics are concentrated in the same neighbourhoods is related to neighbourhood processes, such as selective migration and retention. These neighbourhood processes may be related to the outcome of interest, for example self-rated health, in a direct (less healthy people staying in the area) and indirect way (people with higher education or income moving out, but income and education in part determining individual health). Such neighbourhood processes are important for the interpretation of results of our analyses and pose interesting research questions in themselves (see Sampson 2012).

Using Multilevel Modelling to Investigate Compositional and Contextual Effects

We can illustrate the ways in which MLA makes it possible to investigate compositional and contextual impacts on health using an example based on an investigation of the influences of individual and neighbourhood social capital on self-rated health. This study used data from the Dutch Housing and Living Survey (Mohnen 2012; Mohnen et al. 2015). For this example, we concentrate on one measure of individual social capital that was used: whether or not the respondents had contact (including by telephone) at least weekly with friends, people whom they knew very well or family members (who did not live in the same household). The authors also created a neighbourhood social capital score using ecometric techniques (see Chap. 8) based on respondent views as to whether people in the neighbourhood knew each other, whether neighbours were nice to each other and whether there was a friendly and sociable atmosphere in the neighbourhood. (In this study, the neighbourhoods comprised on average 2500–3000 addresses and about 4000 residents. The total analytic sample of 53,260 lived in 3273 neighbourhoods giving an average of 16.3 respondents per area.) Individual social capital is therefore a dichotomous variable (72.7% reported at least weekly contact with friends and family, subsequently referred to as high individual social capital) whilst neighbourhood social capital is a score ranging from −0.78 to 0.46 (mean = −0.10, standard deviation = 0.20). Positive scores indicate greater social capital. Self-perceived health is dichotomised with 79.0% rating their health as good or better; as such, multilevel logistic modelling is appropriate for these data.

We can investigate the importance of the compositional (individual) and contextual (area) social capital on good or better self-rated health by comparing the following series of random intercept models:

Model	Description
M0	Null model
M1	Individual social capital
M2	Neighbourhood social capital
M3	Individual and neighbourhood social capital
M4	Individual and neighbourhood social capital and their interaction

All models adjust for a range of individual socio-demographic confounders: sex, age, ethnic background, education, employment, income, home ownership and length of residence. Furthermore, all models include three neighbourhood variables: the proportion of respondents with income in the lowest twenty percent, an average measure of perceived home maintenance and urban density. So the null model M0 above is not empty; it consists of the eight individual and three neighbourhood variables listed above (as do all of the other models), but coefficients of these are not relevant to our interest in the relative importance of individual and area social capital. For each model, we will examine the interpretation of the effects of interest

Table 7.1 Coefficients (log odds ratios) exploring associations between social capital and good or better self-rated health for models M0 (null), M1 (individual), M2 (area), M3 (individual and area) and M4 (individual, area and interaction) (Mohnen 2012)

Model	Individual social capital	Area social capital	Interaction: individual*area
M0			
M1	0.081		
M2		0.230	
M3	0.076	0.203	
M4	0.065	0.257	−0.135

by plotting the predicted log odds. This series of models is a good way of disentangling context and composition (more on developing a modelling strategy can be found in Chap. 9).

Table 7.1 presents the estimated coefficients for the social capital variables for each of the models. The following sections interpret these coefficients and detail the implications of the specified model for the association of individual and area social capital with self-rated health.

Model M0: Null Model

Since we are not interested in other covariates, we omit them and describe this model algebraically as

$$\begin{aligned} y_{ij} &\sim \text{Binomial}(1, \pi_{ij}) \\ \text{logit}(\pi_{ij}) &= \log\left(\frac{\pi_{ij}}{1-\pi_{ij}}\right) = \beta_0 + u_{0j} \end{aligned} \tag{7.1}$$

The logit of the probability of reporting good or better self-rated health for individual i in neighbourhood j is modelled using a mean or intercept and a random effect for each area. The estimate of β_0 is the estimated log odds of good health for an individual living in the average area, conditional on having certain baseline characteristics of both individual and area. (The exact characteristics depend on the precise coding of variables and how age is centred, etc., but these are not of interest to our substantive research question regarding the relationship between social capital and health.) The estimates from this model are plotted in Fig. 7.1. Figure 7.1a plots the predicted log odds of good or better health separately for those with high (solid grey line) and low (solid black line) individual social capital across the observed range of values of area social capital on the horizontal axis. In this instance, the lines coincide since we have not included a term differentiating between high and low individual social capital in model M0, and the lines are flat since there is no effect of neighbourhood social capital (again this is not included in M0). Figure 7.1b plots the predicted log odds of good or better health separately for areas with high (solid

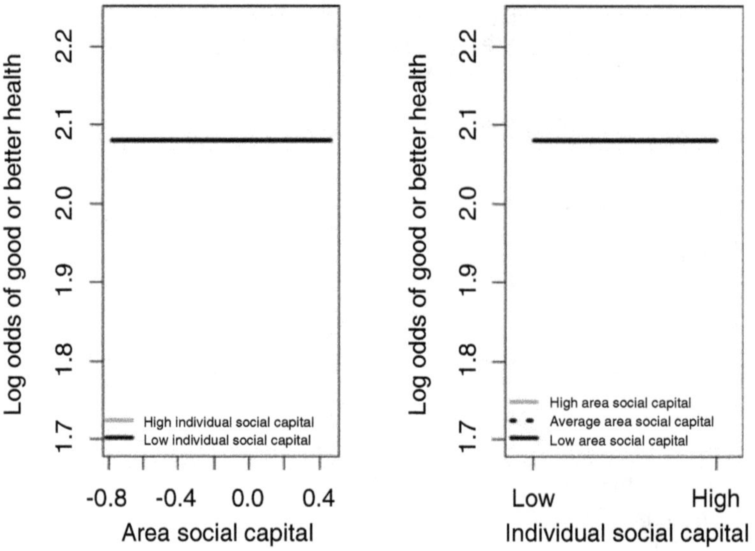

Fig. 7.1 Predicted log odds of good or better health obtained under model M0 (null model) across (**a**) area and (**b**) individual social capital

grey line), average (dotted black line) and low (solid black line) social capital across individual social capital on the horizontal axis. (We have used areas with a social capital score of 0.23, −0.10 and −0.43 to indicate high, average and low social capital, respectively.) Again all three lines overlap because there is no term in M0 denoting area social capital, and the lines are flat because there is no difference in the estimated log odds of good or better health between those with high or low individual social capital.

Model M1: Individual Social Capital

This time our model includes individual social capital, x_{1ij}, and its associated parameter estimate β_1:

$$\text{logit}(\pi_{ij}) = \beta_0 + \beta_1 x_{1ij} + u_{0j} \tag{7.2}$$

Parameter estimates from this model are used to create Fig. 7.2. From Fig. 7.2a we can see that those with high individual social capital are now more likely to report being in good health (or better) than those with low individual social capital. Since neighbourhood social capital is not included in M1, the predicted log odds of good health are constant regardless of the extent of neighbourhood social capital. Figure 7.2b illustrates this another way; we are unable to distinguish between areas with high, average or low neighbourhood social capital (the lines lie on top

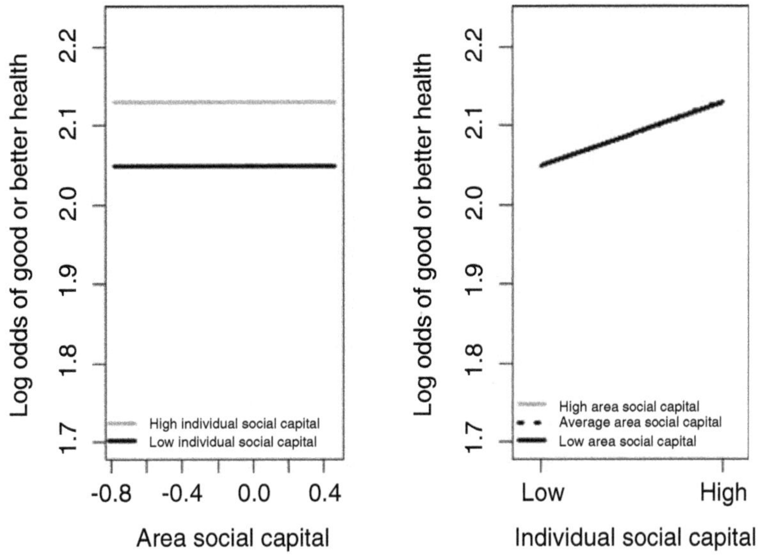

Fig. 7.2 Predicted log odds of good or better health obtained under model M1 (containing individual social capital only) across (**a**) area and (**b**) individual social capital

of each other) but, regardless of the extent of neighbourhood social capital, respondents with high individual social capital are more likely to report good health than those with low individual social capital.

Model M2: Neighbourhood Social Capital

Our model this time includes neighbourhood social capital, x_{2j}, and its associated parameter estimate β_2:

$$\text{logit}(\pi_{ij}) = \beta_0 + \beta_2 x_{2j} + u_{0j} \tag{7.3}$$

Parameter estimates this time have been used to create Fig. 7.3. Figure 7.3a shows that there are no differences between those with high or low individual social capital since individual social capital is not included in Eq. (7.3). What we do see, regardless of individual social capital, is a gradient corresponding to area social capital; respondents living in areas with high social capital are more likely to report being in good health than those living in areas with average social capital who are, in turn, more likely to report being in good health than those living in areas with low social capital. Figure 7.3b shows again no difference between individuals with high or low individual social capital; there is a distinction in the likelihood of reporting being in good health that is dependent on the social capital of the area of residence but which is not affected by individual social capital as this is not included in Eq. (7.3).

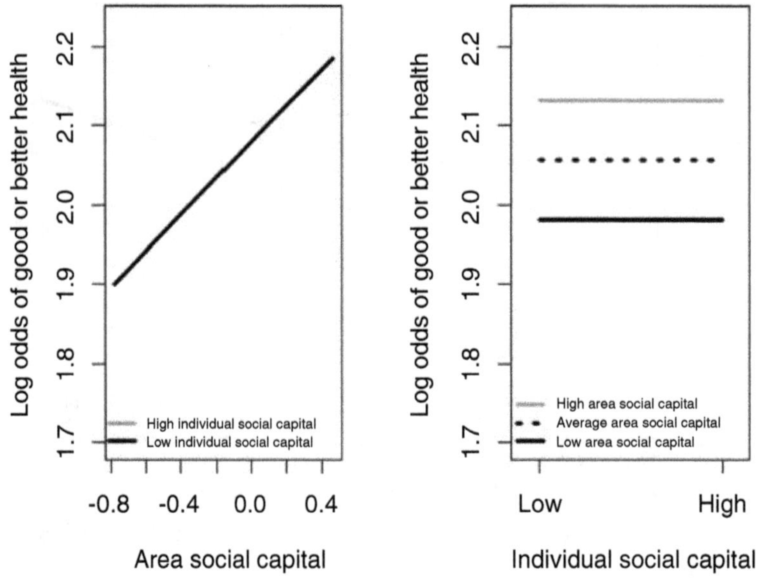

Fig. 7.3 Predicted log odds of good or better health obtained under model M2 (containing area social capital only) across (**a**) area and (**b**) individual social capital

It is worth noting at this stage that in terms of Diez-Roux's definition we could argue that in this case area social capital (x_{2j}) is not strictly a contextual variable (Diez-Roux 2002) since there is an important individual-level confounder missing from Eq. (7.3), namely individual social capital. It is possible that the relationships discovered in model M2 and described in Fig. 7.3 reflect a relationship between individual social capital and health combined with a tendency for those with high (low) individual social capital to cluster in neighbourhoods which therefore have high (low) area social capital. We can explore this in models M3 and M4 when both individual and area social capital are included in the same model. In general, it is important to ensure that the lowest level in a model is as complete as possible when we are interested in contextual effects to ensure that we are interpreting these appropriately and not incorrectly assigning individual characteristics, for which we have not fully controlled, to the area level.

Model M3: Individual and Neighbourhood Social Capital

This time the model is expanded to include both individual and neighbourhood social capital:

$$\text{logit}(\pi_{ij}) = \beta_0 + \beta_1 x_{1ij} + \beta_2 x_{2j} + u_{0j} \tag{7.4}$$

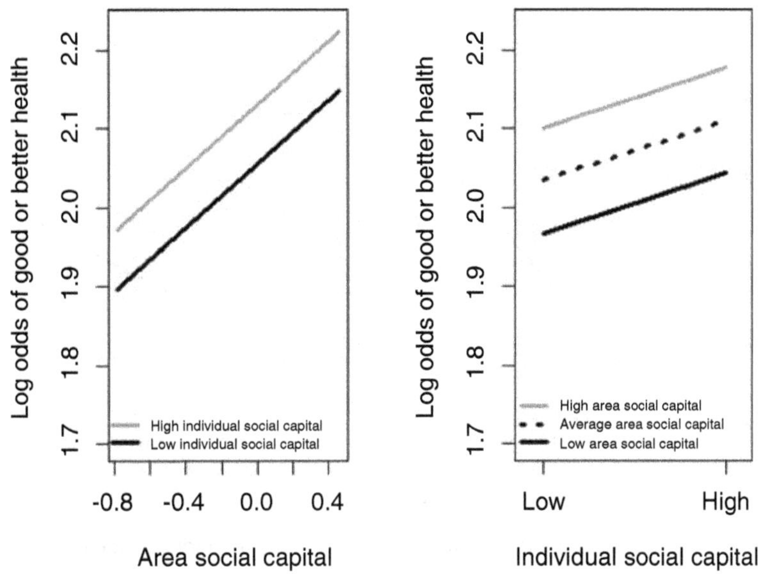

Fig. 7.4 Predicted log odds of good or better health obtained under model M3 (containing individual and area social capital) across (**a**) area and (**b**) individual social capital

The parameter estimates from this model are used to plot the predicted log odds of good or better health in Fig. 7.4. It is clear that the likelihood of reporting good health increases as area social capital increases, but individuals with weekly contact with friends and family were also more likely to report good health. The two effects are independent (there is no interaction included in M3); the predicted difference between people with high and low individual social capital is the same (on the log odds scale) regardless of the area social capital. This is reflected in the lines in Fig. 7.4a being parallel. Similarly, the fact that the lines in Fig. 7.4b are parallel indicates that the impact of area social capital is the same regardless of whether an individual is classified as having high or low individual social capital.

Model M4: Individual and Neighbourhood Social Capital and Their Interaction

Model M4 develops M3 by including the interaction between individual and neighbourhood social capital:

$$\text{logit}(\pi_{ij}) = \beta_0 + \beta_1 x_{1ij} + \beta_2 x_{2j} + \beta_3 x_{1ij} x_{2j} + u_{0j} \tag{7.5}$$

The inclusion of the interaction term between individual and area social capital—$x_{1ij}x_{2j}$ in Eq. (7.5)—and its associated parameter estimate β_3 means that the assumption of independence of the compositional and contextual effects has been dropped.

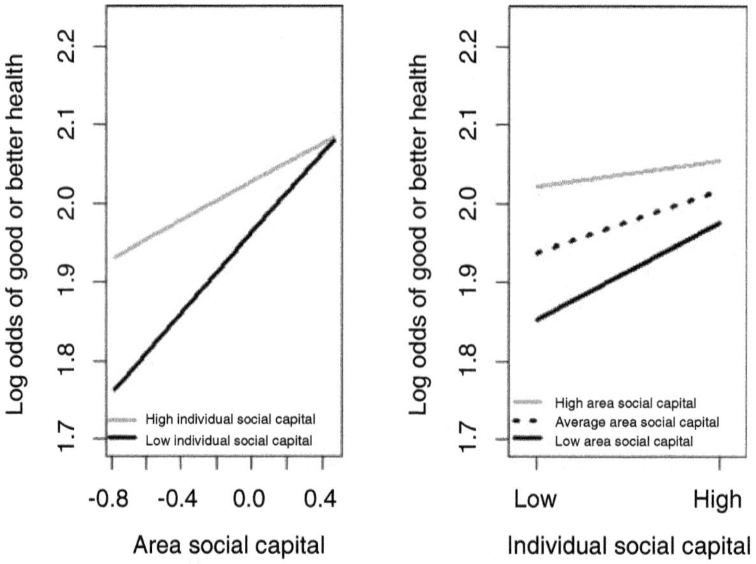

Fig. 7.5 Predicted log odds of good or better health obtained under model M4 (containing individual and area social capital and their interaction) across (**a**) area and (**b**) individual social capital

Figure 7.5 illustrates the impact of this on the predicted log odds of good health or better. Whilst it is still clear that there is a gradient across area social capital, with an increase in the probability of reporting being in good health increasing with increasing area social capital, from Fig. 7.5a we can see that the gradient is stronger (i.e. the impact of area social capital is more pronounced) for those with low individual social capital than with high individual social capital. Figure 7.5b suggests that individual social capital has a greater impact on self-reported health in low social capital areas than in average social capital areas, and more in average social capital areas than in high social capital areas. Despite this, people in high social capital areas tend to report better health than those in average or low social capital areas irrespective of their individual social capital. Note that the presence of the interaction means that the lines in Fig. 7.5 are no longer parallel; the magnitude of the individual effect (the distance between the lines) depends on the context, and the magnitude of the contextual effect depends on individual circumstances.

Random Slopes and Cross-Level Interactions

A quick comparison of the illustrations in Fig. 7.4 (parallel lines) and Fig. 7.5 (in which the lines are no longer parallel) brings to mind the comparison between the models for random intercepts and random slopes in Fig. 5.5. The same principle applies: if the lines are not parallel, then this indicates that the relationship between an individual variable and the outcome varies between contexts. In a random slopes model, we do not know the reason for the relationship varying between contexts, just the fact that this variation exists. In the example used in the previous section relating to individual and area social capital, the authors could have tested for the existence of a random slope by expanding model M3 to enable the coefficient of individual social capital x_{1ij} to vary between neighbourhoods (let us call this model M3A).

$$\text{logit}(\pi_{ij}) = \beta_0 + \beta_1 x_{1ij} + \beta_2 x_{2j} + u_{0j} + u_{1j} x_{1ij} \qquad (7.6)$$

The coefficient of individual social capital is now given by (β_1 + u_{1j}). This varies between contexts but not in a way that is determined by known area characteristics. For each neighbourhood j, we would estimate a slope residual u_{1j} which would determine the nature of the relationship between individual social capital and health in that neighbourhood. With a cross-level interaction, we are able to describe the contextual circumstances associated with this relationship. From Eq. (7.5) we can see that the coefficient of x_{1ij} is given by (β_1 + $\beta_3 x_{2j}$); this again varies between contexts but this time in a predictable way. (We saw from Fig. 7.5 that the impact of individual social capital was more pronounced in areas with low social capital.) In this way, it is possible to use random slope models as a means of hypothesis generation in exploratory analyses. Inspection of the values of the slope residuals u_{1j} may reveal an apparent association with a known contextual factor. A cross-level interaction is generally to be preferred to a random slope since the former provides a means to describe how relationships differ between contexts (thus providing the potential for an explanation of the mechanism) rather than simply noting that such variation exists.

Impact of Compositional and Contextual Variables on the Variances

We have emphasised the important information that can be conveyed by the variances at different levels in a multilevel model. It is also worth reflecting on changes to the variances that occur during the modelling process.

When any variable is added to a multilevel model, as with an ordinary least squares (single level) regression model, we would expect to see a reduction in the total variance—the additional term is explaining some of the variability in outcomes. When compositional characteristics are added, we may see a reduction in the variance at any level of the model; patient characteristics, for example, may explain some of the differences between hospitals in patient outcomes. A hospital serving an elderly community, for example, may achieve worse patient outcomes than average solely due to the difference in the ages of the patients they see compared to other hospitals. And of course we would expect individual characteristics to explain some of the differences in outcomes between individuals.

The situation is slightly different when we consider contextual variables. Whilst this will still produce a reduction in the total unexplained variance (or no change in the total variance if the variable is not related to the outcome), a variable describing contexts cannot explain variation *within* those contexts. If we consider the impact of individual and neighbourhood income on self-reported health, then individual income could account for some of the variations between individuals within neighbourhoods as well as between the neighbourhoods themselves, whilst mean neighbourhood income could only explain some of the variation between neighbourhoods. Mean neighbourhood income does not differ between individuals in the same neighbourhood and therefore cannot explain differences in individual outcomes within neighbourhoods.

We should note here that a cross-level interaction between a level 1 and a level 2 variable will behave like a level 1 variable. In the above example, the interaction between individual and area income will vary between individuals living in the same neighbourhood and so may explain part of the variation within neighbourhoods.

Although the addition of a variable defined at a certain level should reduce the total variance, and the variance in the outcome attributed to that level, there may be circumstances under which the addition of a variable may increase the variance at higher levels. For example, the addition of a compositional variable (such as the patient's age) may increase the variance between hospitals whilst decreasing the total (hospital plus patient) variance. There are three possible reasons for this phenomenon which we outline below.

Firstly, we should note that we are dealing with estimates, and there is uncertainty around these estimates. This is particularly true in the random part of the model and particularly at higher levels where there are fewer observations. So when noting a small increase in a high-level variance following the addition of a compositional characteristic, it is worth considering whether such an increase is important or whether this may reflect a lack of precision in the estimated variances. Certainly if the total variance appears to increase following the addition of a variable, this can only be due imprecision in the estimates.

Secondly, there may be a genuine increase in the variance between contexts following the addition of a compositional characteristic. In these circumstances, the omission of a compositional variable in effect masks existing variation between contexts. An unadjusted analysis of patient outcomes may show little variability between hospitals when the patient's age is ignored. However, if outcomes deteriorate with increasing age, then the inclusion of individual age within a multilevel model may increase the variance between hospitals as those hospitals with a greater proportion of elderly patients are in fact performing better than average, given the age of their patients, and those with a smaller proportion of elderly patients are actually performing worse than would be expected. An example of this is given by Aakvik et al. (2010) who consider the contributions of patient, GP and municipality to certified sickness absence. They find that upon the addition of patient-level covariates to a null model, the total variance in the number of days of sick leave for females decreases from 5828 to 5650. However, they indicate an increase in the variance attributable to the GPs from 46.7 to 47.4.

Finally, multilevel logistic regression is a special case in which the reported variance at the higher level may appear to increase following the addition of a variable measured at a lower level. An explanation as to why this may happen is provided by Snijders and Bosker (2012), but briefly this reflects the link between the variance and the probability of an outcome described in Chap. 6, with the variance of the y_{ij} being given by $\pi_{ij}(1 - \pi_{ij})$ when the outcome follows a binomial distribution. As we saw from Eq. (6.5), the variance partition coefficient in a multilevel logistic regression model can be approximated by

$$\rho_{\mathrm{I}} = \frac{\sigma_{u0}^2}{\sigma_{u0}^2 + \pi^2/3} \tag{7.7}$$

If we add a compositional variable to a two-level multilevel logistic regression, then we might reasonably expect to see this explain a greater proportion of the variance within contexts (level 1) than between contexts (level 2), in which case the variance partition coefficient (the proportion of unexplained variance attributable to differences between contexts) should increase. Since $\pi^2/3 \approx 3.29$ is fixed, the only way to increase the variance partition coefficient is to increase the level 2 variance σ_{u0}^2. This means that, in a multilevel logistic regression model, σ_{u0}^2 can increase even though the variance between level 2 units decreases. Jat et al. (2011) provide such an example in their analysis of maternal health service use in India. They show that the district-level variance associated with the receipt of postnatal care increases from 0.389 in the empty model to 0.480 when a variety of individual, community and district variables are included. As a consequence, the proportion of the unexplained variance associated with the districts increases from 8.5 to 11.1%.

Model Specification and Model Interpretation

The exact specification of the model that is fitted can impact on the estimates that are obtained and hence on the interpretation of the model. It is not surprising to find that regression coefficients can differ depending on whether certain terms are included in a regression model or not, but in a multilevel model regression coefficients can also differ depending on the terms that are included in the random part of the model. We will illustrate this with an example.

A reanalysis of 1930 US Census data considered levels of illiteracy by race/nativity (with the population classified into 'native whites', 'foreign-born whites' and 'blacks') and, importantly, whether the relationship between illiteracy and race varied between states (Subramanian et al. 2009). The two models of interest shown in Table 7.2, derived from Table 2 of the original paper, compare a two-level variance components model with a model in which the coefficients for the three racial groups are allowed to vary.

Table 7.2 Odds ratios (OR) and 95% credible intervals (CI) for illiteracy by race/nativity under different models

	M3		M4	
	OR	(95% CI)	OR	(95% CI)
Native white (ref)	1.00		1.00	
Foreign-born white	13.63	(13.58–13.67)	5.71	(5.18–6.29)
Black	5.86	(5.84–5.88)	5.95	(5.42–6.53)

For full table see Subramanian et al. (2009)

$$\text{M3}: \text{logit}(\pi_{ij}) = \beta_0 + \beta_2 x_{2ij} + \beta_3 x_{3ij} + u_{0j} \tag{7.7}$$

$$\text{M4}: \text{logit}(\pi_{ij}) = \beta_0 + \beta_2 x_{2ij} + \beta_3 x_{3ij} + u_{1j}x_{1ij} + u_{2j}x_{2ij} + u_{3j}x_{3ij} \tag{7.8}$$

The probability of illiteracy π_{ij} for racial group i in state j is modelled in terms of three dummy variables indicating race/nativity, x_{1ij}, x_{2ij} and x_{3ij}, denoting 'native whites', 'foreign-born whites' and 'blacks', respectively.

The odds ratio indicating average illiteracy among the 'foreign-born white' group compared to the 'native white' group decreased from 13.63 (95% CI 13.58–13.67) to 5.71 (95% CI 5.18–6.29) when this coefficient is allowed to vary between states. These are derived from the coefficients β_2 in Eqs. (7.7) and (7.8), respectively, and the substantial difference between these odds ratios indicates the dependence of the fixed parameters on the specification of the random part of the model. The substantial reduction in the deviance information criterion (DIC)—an indicator of the fit of a model (Spiegelhalter et al. 2002)—shown in Table 7.2 suggests that model 4 provides a better fit to the data. In this case inappropriate specification of the random part of the model has a sizable impact on the estimate of illiteracy among the 'foreign-born white' group. The reasons for this difference relate to the relationship between the fixed part coefficients and the higher level variance detailed in the section 'Population Average and Cluster-Specific Estimates' in Chap. 6.

Sources of Error Affecting the Estimation of Contextual Effects

Blakely and Woodward (2000) identified six limitations in study design and sources of error that affected the estimation of contextual effects. This paper remains relevant, and these limitations should be borne in mind when fitting or interpreting a multilevel model that includes one or more variables at the macro level.

Lack of Variation in the Contextual Variable

The variation present in an individual-level variable will be reduced when aggregated to a contextual level. For example, there will be more variation in individual income than in mean neighbourhood income. Such a reduction in variability between contexts, combined with there often being few contexts (there will certainly be fewer contexts than individuals in a multilevel model), means that there will be less power to detect a contextual effect than there is to detect the effect of an individual-level variable. Given the reduction in the range of values that a contextual variable can have (because of the reduced variability), it is worth bearing in mind that fairly modest contextual effects may be important.

Precision of Estimates and Study Design

Since there will always be fewer contexts than lower level units (individuals), contextual effects will be estimated with less precision. If the estimation of contextual effects is an essential part of your research, then this should be taken into account through the research design; an increase in the precision of the contextual effects will generally be achieved by increasing the number of higher level units (possibly at the expense of the number of lower level units included, as discussed in Chap. 3).

Selection Bias

If the individuals sampled for or otherwise included in a study are not representative of the population (such as would be achieved through a random sample), then the study is said to suffer from selection bias. The concern is that the association between a variable of interest and the outcome in the analytical sample differs from that seen in the eligible population (Hernán et al. 2004). In a multilevel study, particularly when we are interested in estimating contextual effects, the potential for selection bias exists at all levels of the model. We therefore have to consider representativeness at all levels (not just at the individual level) and should report response levels and any consideration of bias at all levels.

Confounding

Confounding occurs when one variable is associated with a key variable (such as the exposure of interest) and also influences the outcome. Contextual factors may suffer from both within-level confounding (confounding by other contextual factors) and cross-level confounding (confounding by individual characteristics). It is also possible that a contextual variable will confound the relationship between an individual-level variable and the outcome. The solution to the presence of such confounding variables is generally to adjust adequately for such variables in the analysis (Royston et al. 2006).

Information Bias

The estimation of contextual effects may be affected both by misclassification or mismeasurement of the contextual variable and by the incorrect assignment of individuals to the contexts. If either occurs in a systematic way, then there is a potential for biased results. Whilst misclassification and mismeasurement issues are also present for individual-level variables, the incorrect assignment of individuals to contexts introduces further potential for bias, particularly in the case when contextual variables are subsequently created by aggregating individual variables to their (incorrectly assigned) contexts.

Model Specification

The exact specification of the multilevel model may influence the estimation of contextual effects for several reasons. The contexts used may impact on the magnitude of the effect detected (with smaller areas more closely approximating individual circumstances) but may also be important in terms of the mechanism through which the contextual variable operates (e.g. with areas defined by political or other administrative boundaries). Cross-level effect modification and indirect cross-level effects are often overlooked; the presence of a cross-level interaction, for example, may mean that the interpretation of a contextual effect depends on the circumstances of the individual. The nature of a contextual effect may be complex and may not be linear. It is therefore important to consider different functional forms or multiple categories for the contextual effects although the lack of variation in the contextual variable noted above, and in some cases a restricted number of contexts, may make this difficult. Finally, multicollinearity is likely to be more problematic for contextual variables than for individual variables which may in turn make it impossible to estimate independent effects for several contextual variables.

Conclusions

Both the characteristics of the individuals themselves (compositional factors) and those of the relevant contexts in which individuals operate (contextual factors) may influence individual outcomes. In order to be able to judge the importance of contextual variables, it is important that full and appropriate adjustment has been made for potential differences in composition between the higher level units. Multilevel analysis provides a useful tool to explore the impact of compositional and contextual factors, and the interpretation of potentially complex models can be aided by relatively simple figures. The analysis of contextual effects can introduce a further dimension of complexity into regression modelling.

References

Aakvik A, Holmås TH, Islam MK (2010) Does variation in general practitioner (GP) practice matter for the length of sick leave? A multilevel analysis based on Norwegian GP-patient data. Soc Sci Med 70:1590–1598

Blakely TA, Woodward AJ (2000) Ecological effects in multi-level studies. J Epidemiol Community Health 54:367–374

Diez-Roux AV (1998) Bringing context back into epidemiology: variables and fallacies in multilevel analysis. Am J Public Health 88:216–222

Diez-Roux AV (2002) A glossary for multilevel analysis. J Epidemiol Community Health 56:588–594

Hernán MA, Hernández-Díaz S, Robins J (2004) A structural approach to selection bias. Epidemiology 15:615–625

Jat TR, Ng N, San Sebastian M (2011) Factors affecting the use of maternal health services in Madhya Pradesh state of India: a multilevel analysis. Int J Equity Health 10:59

Macintyre S, Ellaway A (2003) Neighborhoods and health: an overview. In: Kawachi I, Berkman LF (eds) Neighborhoods and health. Oxford University Press, Oxford

Macintyre S, MacIver S, Sooman A (1993) Area, class and health: should we be focusing on places or people? J Soc Policy 22:213–234

Mohnen SM (2012) Neighborhood context and health: how neighborhood social capital affects individual health. Utrecht University, Utrecht

Mohnen SM, Völker B, Flap H, Subramanian SV, Groenewegen PP (2015) The influence of social capital on individual health: is it the neighbourhood or the network? Soc Indic Res 121:195–214

Royston P, Altman DG, Sauerbrei W (2006) Dichotomizing continuous predictors in multiple regression: a bad idea. Stat Med 25:127–141

Sampson RJ (2012) Great American city: Chicago and the enduring neighborhood effect. Chicago University Press, Chicago

Sloggett A, Joshi H (1994) Higher mortality in deprived areas: community or personal disadvantage? Br Med J 309:1470–1474

Snijders TAB, Bosker RJ (2012) Multilevel analysis: an introduction to basic and advanced multilevel modeling. Sage, Los Angeles

Spiegelhalter DJ, Best NG, Carlin BP, van der Linde A (2002) Bayesian measures of model complexity and fit (with discussion). J R Stat Soc Ser B 64:583–639

Subramanian SV, Jones K, Kaddour A, Krieger N (2009) Revisiting Robinson: the perils of individualistic and ecologic fallacy. Int J Epidemiol 38:342–360

8

Latent Variable Analysis in MLA

Abstract Multilevel analysis can be used to construct characteristics of higher level units. This is done on the basis of systematic observations by several observers or of perceptions of respondents who describe, for example, their neighbourhood. By using MLA, we solve a number of problems associated with simple aggregation of data from the individual level to the higher level. The chapter starts by identifying these problems and then works step by step towards more elaborate models to measure latent characteristics of higher level units. Latent variable analysis in MLA is also called 'ecometrics', a new term for methods to measure characteristics of ecological units on the basis of multiple observations or responses.

Keywords Multilevel analysis · Ecometric analysis · Aggregation · Contextual variables · Latent variable analysis · Reliability · Patient safety

In Chap. 3, in the section on hypotheses, we mentioned different types of variables that can characterise higher level units. They could be either directly measured at the higher level or aggregated from characteristics of lower level units (such as individuals). Examples of variables that are measured at the higher level are the specialty of a hospital ward, or the total surface of green areas in a neighbourhood. Other characteristics can be measured by aggregation from individual-level characteristics, such as the average age or income of the inhabitants of a neighbourhood. Sometimes we are not dealing with separate variables but with composite scores, based on several variables or responses. Examples are questionnaires that ask people about neighbourhood contacts and that could be combined into a social capital measure or questionnaires to doctors and nurses in hospitals that ask about dealing with issues of safety which could be combined into a measure of patient safety culture.

We could just aggregate the individual variables or responses to items in questionnaires to the appropriate higher level. However, there are problems associated with doing this, and we can overcome these problems by applying MLA to construct our higher level variables. We then use MLA to estimate the higher level effect—e.g. a neighbourhood effect or a hospital effect—net of the individual variation at other levels. When applied to composite scores, this approach is now known as ecometrics or latent variable analysis in MLA (Raudenbush 2003; Raudenbush and Sampson 1999).

The use of ecometrics in public health and health services research is becoming more frequent. It is therefore important to pay attention to this application of multilevel research. Following its name—ecometrics as the measurement of ecological characteristics—it is currently mainly used to construct variables to characterise neighbourhoods, such as social capital (Mohnen et al. 2011; Nyqvist et al. 2014; Prins et al. 2012). It is much less frequently used for other ecologies of humans, such as work places (Oksanen et al. 2013), schools (Gilreath et al. 2012) or healthcare institutions (van Schoten et al. 2014).

This chapter is based around an example of patient safety culture in hospital departments. We will discuss the multilevel model and its interpretation in ecometric analysis, and we will compare ecometrics with traditional methods. We end the chapter with a discussion of ecometric properties (comparable to psychometric properties), such as reliability.

Problems with Simple Aggregation

Simple aggregation of individual variables to a higher level unit is not wrong, but there can be a couple of problems with doing this. First, our individual-level variables are often derived from a sample of individuals. When we group these individuals into higher level units, the sample sizes may vary. Some higher level units might have many more individual observations than others, and this is especially likely to be the case when the study was not originally designed as a multilevel study. If we simply aggregate an individual-level variable using such data, our aggregated variable is then based on different numbers of observations. However, if we aggregate the data and use this aggregated variable in our model, all aggregated observations are treated in the same manner, irrespective of whether they were based on say 100 individual observations or just ten. The solution to this has already been presented in Chap. 3; the multilevel approach to estimating higher level effects or residuals takes into account whether the number of observations differs between higher level units. The estimated values for units with few observations are shrunk towards the overall mean.

The second problem is particularly important when the individual variables contain a subjective element. Examples are people's responses to questions about their neighbourhood ('how safe is your neighbourhood?') or the hospital in which they were treated ('were you treated with respect during your visit to this hospital?'). The responses to such questions supposedly indicate a characteristic of the higher level unit—the neighbourhood or the hospital—but part of the response is determined by individual differences in how people perceive their neighbourhood or hospital. The response may also be determined in part by incidental circumstances, such as what they read in the newspaper that morning. What we are really interested in is the common component in all responses about the same unit, net of the individual component. We can obtain this by partitioning the variance in individual responses into that attributable to higher level units and that attributable to individuals. We do this using MLA as detailed in Chap. 6. Related to this is the argument that using ecometrics the effect of same source bias is reduced (as noted by de Jong et al. 2011). Same source bias originates from the fact that in survey research often both the independent variables and the dependent variables are asked from the same respondent in the same questionnaire.

A third problem is that the sample of individuals in higher level units may differ between these units as a result of selective non-response. Selective non-response might lead to there being more elderly respondents or more highly educated respondents in some hospitals or neighbourhoods. If these characteristics are related to the variables that we want to aggregate, simple aggregation would lead to the creation of a biased contextual variable. This might be the case if elderly people have a higher level of response in some neighbourhoods in a survey looking at neighbourhood safety, since we know that elderly people perceive their neighbourhood as less safe than younger people. Again the solution is to use MLA to control for the effects of differential neighbourhood composition. The idea that the estimation of contextual effects should take into account relevant compositional factors was discussed in Chap. 7.

Finally, there is a specific problem when the responses at the individual level form a scale where several questions or items together are supposed to measure a characteristic of the higher level unit. For example, rather than simply asking people who were treated in a hospital whether they were treated with respect, we could design some questions that when combined measure the unobserved variable ‘respectful treatment’. We could construct the scale at the individual level in a single-level model. However, if we did this we would lose information about the fact that the items are not only nested within the individuals that complete the questionnaire but also within the higher level units that we want to characterise. The solution here is to analyse the data using a multiple response model with items at the lowest level, nested within individuals and higher level units (latent variable analysis). We have described such data structures in Chap. 4.

This means that we can use MLA to construct a contextual variable, because we want to say something about higher level units, based on individual-level observations. We can use either a single variable (using a two-level model) or a number of variables collected at the individual level (using a three-level model) and combine these into a higher level variable. The first step is to construct a multilevel model including the variable(s) that we want to use to describe our higher level units as dependent variable(s). In the second step we then take the higher level residual (the higher level effect) and use this as an independent variable in a subsequent multilevel analysis, relating this to a dependent variable (such as self-rated health).

Single Variables

We can use MLA both when we want to construct a characteristic of a higher level unit based on a single individual variable and when we wish to combine information from several related individual variables. We begin by considering the single-variable case. From the problems that we discussed in the previous section, we can see that it is possible to make another distinction. Some individual variables indicate objective information, such as household income, whilst others indicate perceptions or evaluations of characteristics of the higher level units, such as perceived safety or the extent to which treatment was respectful.

When using objective information, such as household income per neighbourhood, we may have access to population data from municipalities or national statistical sources. However, this information is not always available, especially not when we have good reasons to deviate from a standard administrative definition of neighbourhoods (as discussed in Chap. 2). In such a case, we may have to use sample data. As discussed above, the sample size might differ between neighbourhoods, and we would have more confidence in an aggregated variable which is based on more information than one based on fewer observations. The estimated neighbourhood-level income from a multilevel analysis will be closer to the overall mean when the sample size (and thus the number of observations) in that neighbourhood is smaller.

When analysing individual perceptions or evaluations, multiple questions are often used. However, for research into patient experiences with healthcare providers, single questions are also often used. These could be used to compare healthcare providers, or they could be used as independent variables at the provider level in the analysis of an individual-level dependent variable. Research with the so-called consumer quality index on GP care showed very strong clustering of the single item from the questionnaire about privacy at the reception desk ('Can people in the waiting room hear what is being discussed at the reception desk?'; Meuwissen and De Bakker 2008). They found the intra-class correlation to be 0.29; nearly a third of the variation in responses was associated with the level of the GP practice. Although there is still a lot of variation between the individual patients in how they answered this question, the answers clearly say something about the contexts. The GP practice residuals could subsequently be used in a separate analysis to predict individual satisfaction with GP care.

Composite Variables: The Traditional Method

As we said, usually perceptions will be based on composite variables. We will discuss both the 'traditional approach' and the ecometric approach. The example we will use is based on data from a study on patient safety culture in hospital wards (Smits 2009). Patient safety culture could be seen as an independent variable at the level of the hospital ward to predict adverse events among patients. Patient safety culture is measured by several items in a questionnaire for hospital personnel.

Other examples for comparable data structures and approaches in analysing data could be a questionnaire about social capital for inhabitants of neighbourhoods (Mohnen et al. 2011) or observations that are made concerning the disorderliness of streets within neighbourhoods, including items such as people drinking outside, graffiti and broken windows (Raudenbush and Sampson 1999).

The items from the patient safety questionnaire that we will be using relate to 'feedback and learning from error'. The items are:

- We are informed about errors that happen in this unit.
- We are given feedback about changes put into place based on event reports.
- In this unit, we discuss ways to prevent errors from happening again.
- Mistakes have led to positive changes here.
- After we make changes to improve patient safety, we evaluate their effectiveness.
- We are actively doing things to improve patient safety.

The traditional approach would be to perform a psychometric analysis and combine the items into a scale, all within a single-level model. This would involve undertaking an analysis of the characteristics of the items, their inter-correlations, item total correlation and so on. We would calculate Cronbach's alpha as a measure of the reliability of the scale. Finally we would actually calculate the scale and aggregate the individual scale values to ward level. This would be our independent variable for subsequent multilevel analysis of individual-level outcomes such as the occurrence of adverse events.

We will not go deeply into the psychometric properties of this scale (for more details, see Smits et al. 2008). The scale average in an analysis of 583 employees in four hospitals was 3.34; Cronbach's alpha was 0.78; and the correlation of the scale with a grading of patient safety from excellent to failing was 0.40.

After aggregating the individual scale values to the level of hospital wards, we can rank the wards in terms of their patient safety culture. Some hospitals can be seen to have a more favourable patient safety culture than others.

Composite Variables: A Simple Multilevel Model

In this section we will take the analysis one step further but do not stray too far from the traditional approach: we will analyse the individual scale values in a multilevel model. In the following section, we will introduce the ecometric approach in which we treat the separate items that form the scale as the lowest level, with these responses nested within the individual.

In our example, we are not interested in individual variation in perceived safety culture, but only in the common variance at the ward (or hospital) level. When we theorise about patient safety culture, our hypothesis about variation would be that if something approximating patient safety culture exists, we should find significant clustering at the level of hospitals or wards since this is almost certain to vary between units. Culture as a concept implies a shared definition of the situation. And if we want to characterise the wards or hospitals, then we need to remove the individual variation.

In this example, the sample size varies between wards. The average sample was 22, but there was a minimum of only seven questionnaires and a maximum of 53. In this case we estimate a three-level model with the data structure shown in Fig. 8.1.

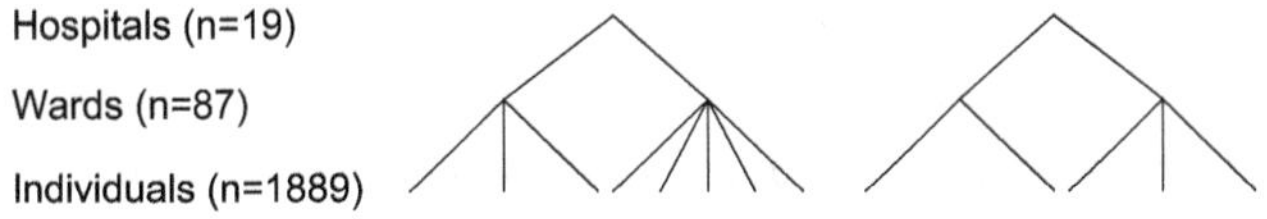

Fig. 8.1 Data structure illustrating the example of a simple composite variable model

Table 8.1 Estimates from a multilevel analysis of the individual scale values for the scale 'feedback and learning from error'; empty model (simple multilevel model)

Parameter		Coefficient	(SD)
	Fixed part		
Constant		3.372	(0.045)
	Random part		
Hospital-level variance		0.021	(0.013)
Ward-level variance		0.052	(0.012)
Individual-level variance		0.293	(0.010)

We use a three-level model because the hospital wards are themselves nested within hospitals, and the hospital itself may affect the safety culture within its wards. When analysing social capital in neighbourhoods, we could work with a two-level model involving neighbourhoods at the highest level and scale values for a social capital scale as the dependent variable at the level of the individual. The social capital scale would have been constructed from individuals who answered questions about their neighbourhood. In our example of patient safety culture, the minimum number of observations on a ward is relatively small (only seven observations in one ward). The question then is: how confident would we be about an estimate of the population parameter 'patient safety culture' derived from the ward that had this small sample size? How confident can we be of any difference from the population mean given the small sample size? This is the rationale for using an estimator that shrinks the estimate for this ward a bit closer to the overall mean.

The multilevel model we estimate is described in Eq. (8.1).

$$\begin{aligned} y_{ijk} &= \beta_0 + v_{0k} + u_{0jk} + e_{0ijk} \\ v_{0k} &\sim N\left(0, \sigma_{v0}^2\right) \\ u_{0jk} &\sim N\left(0, \sigma_{u0}^2\right) \\ e_{0ijk} &\sim N\left(0, \sigma_{e0}^2\right) \end{aligned} \tag{8.1}$$

Here y_{ijk} is the response 'feedback and learning from error' for respondent (nurse or doctor) i in ward j and hospital k, measured on a scale from 0 to 5 (the answers to the six items forming the scale were given values 0 through 5, then added and divided by the number of items). The random intercept model described partitions the variance between the individual, ward and hospital levels. The resulting estimates from this model are shown in Table 8.1.

The constant gives the scale average. In addition we have estimated three variance components: at hospital, ward and individual level. It is important to note that there is a significant variation at ward level, which is what we would expect given that the item in question is measuring an aspect of patient safety culture.

An advantage of the multilevel analysis over and above the traditional approach of simply aggregating the individual scale values is that we can adjust for compositional effects by including individual independent variables that may have an impact on individual responses but not necessarily hospital culture. The adjusted model is described in Eq. (8.2).

$$\begin{aligned} y_{ijk} &= \beta_0 + \beta_1 x_{1ijk} + \beta_2 x_{2ijk} + \beta_3 x_{3ijk} + v_{0k} + u_{0jk} + e_{0ijk} \\ v_{0k} &\sim N(0, \sigma^2_{v0}) \\ u_{0jk} &\sim N(0, \sigma^2_{u0}) \\ e_{0ijk} &\sim N(0, \sigma^2_{e0}) \end{aligned} \tag{8.2}$$

In addition to the constant, this model includes three variables enabling adjustment for the number of years an individual has worked in the ward, the number of hours he or she work per week and whether the respondent is a physician or a nurse. The estimates from this model are detailed in Table 8.2.

Although the adjusted model fits the data better than the empty model, in this dataset the variance components of the adjusted model are nearly the same as for the null model. This is of course not necessarily the case. Apparently employee characteristics, in this case the composition of our samples according to length of employment on this ward, the number of hours they work and whether they are nurses do not vary much enough between wards or hospitals to influence the results. In other datasets, there might be bigger effects of composition; it is not possible to know whether these will exist before undertaking the analysis.

As we have two higher levels, wards and hospitals, we can also calculate two variance partition coefficients for each model (see Table 8.3).

Table 8.2 Estimates from a multilevel analysis of the individual scale values for the scale 'feedback and learning from error'; empty model and adjusted model (simple multilevel model)

		Empty model		Adjusted model	
Parameter		Coefficient	(SD)	Coefficient	(SD)
	Fixed part				
Constant		3.372	(0.045)	3.373	(0.046)
Years in this ward				0.028	(0.010)
Hours per week				−0.050	(0.025)
Nurse (reference: physician)				0.011	(0.004)
	Random part				
Hospital-level variance		0.021	(0.013)	0.023	(0.013)
Ward-level variance		0.052	(0.012)	0.051	(0.011)
Individual-level variance		0.293	(0.010)	0.290	(0.010)
−2*log likelihood		3080.7		3059.5	

Table 8.3 Variance partition coefficients at hospital and ward level (simple multilevel model)

Level	Empty model	Adjusted model
Hospital	0.058	0.063
Ward	0.142	0.140

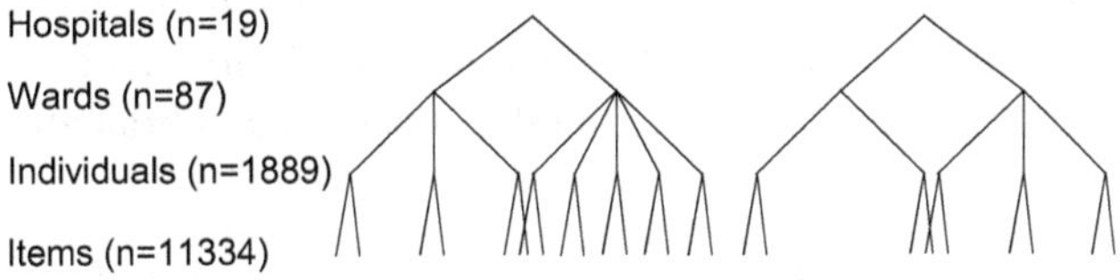

Fig. 8.2 Data structure illustrating the example of an ecometric model

Twenty per cent of the total variation in this scale is above the level of the individual; this is a relatively strong clustering effect. The scale apparently measures something at the level of the contexts, as should be the case given that we intended to measure culture.

This all looks fine, but as we mentioned in the introduction to this chapter, there is still a problem with this approach. The items are nested within individuals, wards and hospitals. We should take ward-level correlations between items into account and because we want the scale to say something about wards, we would also like to know how reliable a measure it is of 'feedback and learning from error' at the ward level. For this reason, in the next section we move beyond the traditional approach or the simple multilevel model based on the individual scale values to a full ecometric approach.

Ecometric Approach

In the ecometric approach, we will estimate a more complicated model: a multiple response model with items at the lowest level, nested in individuals and higher level units. The data structure then looks as in Fig. 8.2.

The term 'ecometrics' was coined by Raudenbush. He describes ecometrics as a statistical method to evaluate the validity and reliability of imperfect measures of contextual properties (Raudenbush 2003). The term is analogous to psychometrics, the difference being that it does not aim to measure latent psychological characteristics of individuals but latent characteristics of ecological units. The data used in ecometrics are multiple observations on an ecological unit, made by trained observers or individuals (e.g. respondents in a survey) who are able to give information about characteristics of these units. As in psychometrics, the aim is to combine these multiple observations into a single scale or latent variable and to analyse the characteristics of the scale such as its reliability and validity. Mujahid et al. (2007) have illustrated the ecometric approach by using survey data to construct a number of scales that are relevant for health and health behaviour.

They include respondents' perceptions of the walking environment, the availability of healthy food and social cohesion. An example based on observers' evaluations of neighbourhood environment is given by Gauvin et al. (2005).

The basis of an ecometric analysis is a three-level model: the items or observations are the lowest level, nested within observers or individual respondents, and these nested again in higher level units. (In our example, the higher level units of interest are the hospital wards, but these are in turn nested within the hospitals to take the particular data structure and the possibility that hospitals influence the culture on wards into account.) The model is shown algebraically in Eq. (8.3).

$$y_{ijkl} = \beta_0 + \beta_2\left(x_{2ijkl} - \frac{1}{6}\right) + \beta_3\left(x_{3ijkl} - \frac{1}{6}\right) + \beta_4\left(x_{4ijkl} - \frac{1}{6}\right) + \beta_5\left(x_{5ijkl} - \frac{1}{6}\right)$$

$$+\beta_6\left(x_{6ijkl} - \frac{1}{6}\right) \quad +f_{0l} + v_{0kl} + u_{0jkl} + e_{1ijkl}x_{1ijkl} + e_{2ijkl}x_{2ijkl} + e_{3ijkl}x_{3ijkl}$$

$$+e_{4ijkl}x_{4ijkl} + e_{5ijkl}x_{5ijkl} + e_{6ijkl}x_{6ijkl}$$

$$f_{0l} \sim N\left(0, \sigma^2_{f0}\right)$$

$$v_{0kl} \sim N\left(0, \sigma^2_{v0}\right)$$

$$u_{0jkl} \sim N\left(0, \sigma^2_{u0}\right)$$

$$e_{mijkl} \sim N\left(0, \sigma^2_{\text{em}}\right), \quad m = 1\ldots6 \tag{8.3}$$

In this formulation, β_0 is the scale average and $\beta_2 \cdots \beta_6$ are the deviance scores for items 2–6, respectively. With six items, and therefore six responses per individual, we include only five dummy variables $x_{2ijkl}\ldots x_{6ijkl}$ coded 1 if the response relates to that item and 0 otherwise. We subtract the reciprocal of the number of items—in this case $\frac{1}{6}$—from each of the dummy variables to ensure that we obtain the deviance scores. This amounts to scoring each variable equal to $\frac{5}{6}$ if the response relates to that item and $-\frac{1}{6}$ otherwise, meaning that each of these variables has a mean of 0. By doing so, the value obtained for β_0 is comparable to the scale value of the original single-level model (between 0 and 5). Otherwise the scale value would be the average of the item that was left out. The response y_{ijkl} refers to item i for respondent j in ward k and hospital l. There are variances associated with the hospital, ward and individual levels, whilst each of the six items is assumed to be independently normally distributed with its own variance $\sigma^2_{e1} \ldots \sigma^2_{e6}$.

Application of the Ecometric Approach

Applying this model to our data gives the results presented in Table 8.4.

We can start by pointing out the differences between the simple multilevel model shown in Table 8.1 and the model shown in Table 8.4. Apart from the constant, which is the scale average, we now have fixed effects for the different items. We did not have that for the simple model because the scale was first constructed at the individual level, and the scale value for each individual was taken as the dependent variable. There is also a difference in the random part. In addition to the individual-, ward- and hospital-level variances, we now also estimate a variance for each item.

When it comes to interpreting the model shown in Table 8.4, we first note that the average scale value obtained is almost identical whether we use the ecometric or the simple approach. This is because we use the item weights for the fixed effects as explained above. This is only necessary when we want an easily interpretable and comparable scale average.

The other fixed effects give the weights of the scale items. The average score of item 2, for example, is 3.375 + (0.394∗5/6) = 3.703. The fixed effects indicate how frequently individuals tend to agree with a statement, something called item difficulty in psychometric analysis. Item 3 was the item for which agreement was most common: 'In this unit, we discuss ways to prevent errors from happening again'. Agreement was least common for item 6: 'We are actively doing things to improve patient safety'. It appears to be easier to agree with item 3 than with item 6.

Then we move on to the variance components or the random part of the model. Each item has its own variance, indicating the measurement error. Item 1 has the biggest variance: 'We are informed about errors that happen in this unit'. The ecometric analysis has separated the individual variance in the traditional approach

Table 8.4 Estimates from a multilevel analysis of the scale 'feedback and learning from error'; empty model (ecometric approach)

Parameter		Coefficient	(SD)
	Fixed part		
Constant		3.375	(0.044)
Item 1 (reference)			
Item 2		0.394	(0.026)
Item 3		0.643	(0.024)
Item 4		0.328	(0.025)
Item 5		0.265	(0.024)
Item 6		−0.020	(0.026)
	Random part		
Hospital-level variance		0.019	(0.012)
Ward-level variance		0.049	(0.011)
Individual-level variance		0.201	(0.009)
Item 1 variance		0.716	(0.026)
Item 2 variance		0.536	(0.020)
Item 3 variance		0.354	(0.014)
Item 4 variance		0.450	(0.017)
Item 5 variance		0.354	(0.014)
Item 6 variance		0.516	(0.019)

into item-specific measurement error and variance associated with the individual. The item variance is used to calculate the reliability of the scale (see next section). The other variances can be used to calculate variance partition coefficients.

As with the simple model, we can estimate an ecometric model (Fig. 8.2) in which we adjust for individual characteristics. However, once again the empty and adjusted models do not differ much and so we have not shown these results.

Table 8.5 shows the variance components for the model presented in Table 8.4 and for a model adjusted by the number of years spent working on that ward, the number of hours worked per week and the type of employee (nurse or physician). As a consequence of removing the measurement error (item variance) from the individual variance, the intra-class correlations are higher compared to those obtained under the simple approach and shown in Table 8.3. The percentage of the variance at ward and hospital levels combined has increased from 20 to 25%.

So far we have analysed the scale 'feedback and learning from error', and we have estimated the variances at the ward and hospital levels. The final step is to calculate and save the ward residuals or effects. Whilst the hospital level is still in the analysis, the ward residuals show the departure from the hospital mean. The ward residuals can be used as an independent variable at ward level in a new analysis. Figure 8.3 shows the ranking of the hospital wards according to how they score on the scale 'feedback and learning from error'.

Table 8.5 Variance partition coefficients at hospital and ward level (ecometric approach)

Level	Empty model	Adjusted model
Hospital	0.072	0.078
Ward	0.183	0.180

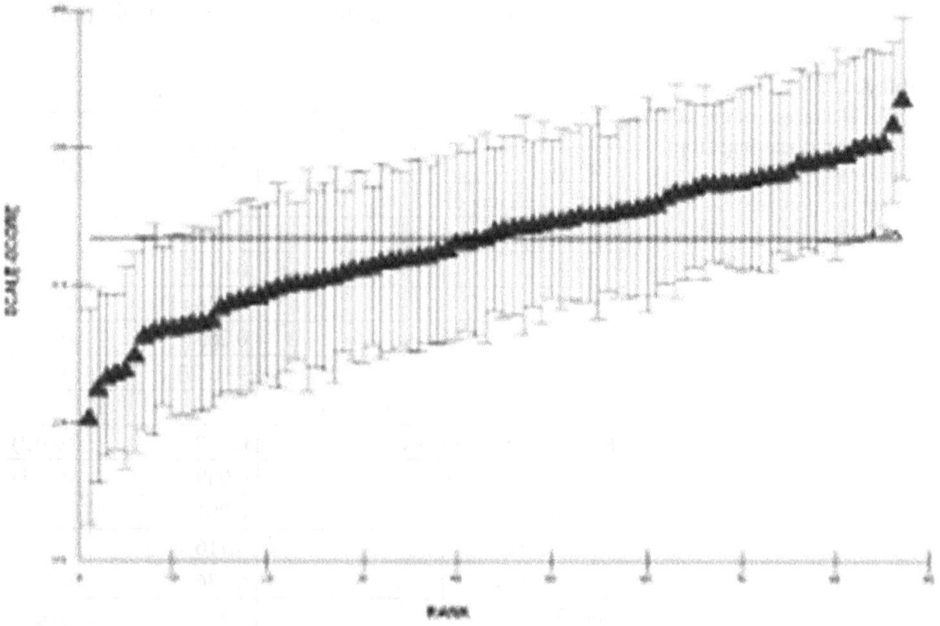

Fig. 8.3 Ranking of hospital wards on the scale 'feedback and learning from error'. Ward residuals from the empty model (including the hospital level + mean scale value)

The point estimates of the ward residuals can be used as an independent variable in a new analysis. We then have the ward effect, net of the individual variation in the perceptions of employees about patient safety culture. Some wards score significantly lower on patient safety culture, and some score significantly higher within their hospital. If we want an overall ward effect, we can omit the hospital level from the analysis meaning that the hospital-level variance would all go to the ward level (as described in Chap. 6: Apportioning variation in multilevel models).

Comparison of the Traditional and Ecometric Approach

In an analysis of neighbourhood disorder, Steenbeek (2011) compared simple aggregation of the individual-level scale values and ecometric analysis. In his analysis of 71 Dutch neighbourhoods, only 6% had exactly the same rank. Nearly 30% of neighbourhoods moved ranks between the two analyses by more than five positions. With some exceptions, agreement between the two methods was greatest at the extremes, and there were notable differences in 'average' neighbourhoods. In a similar manner, we can compare two sets of rankings of the wards in our example, one based on the simple aggregation of scale values and the other based on the ecometric analysis. Figure 8.4 compares the ranks obtained under the two methods.

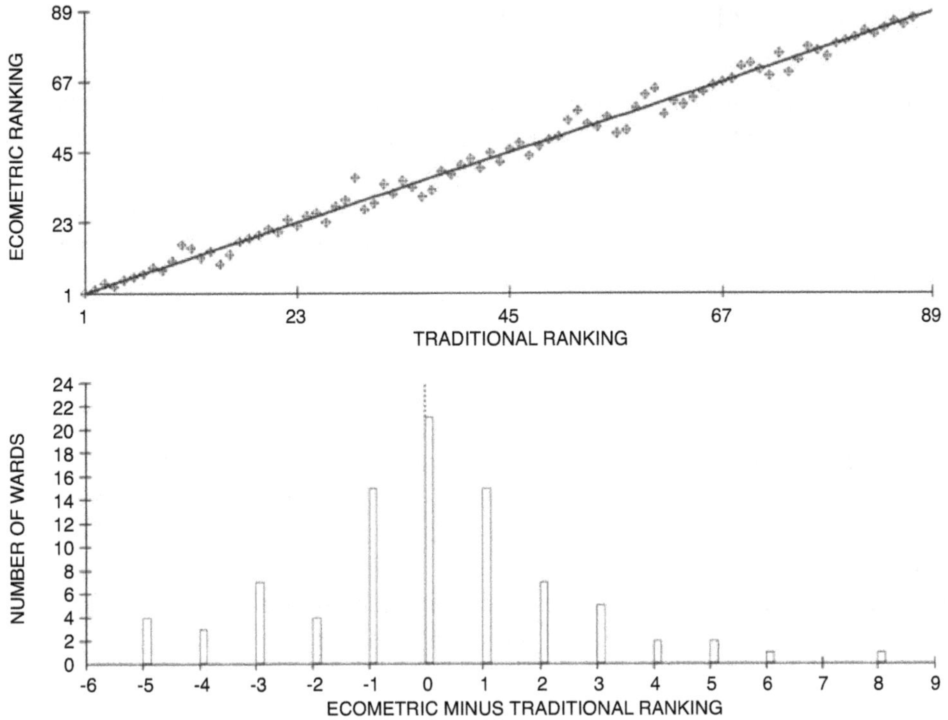

Fig. 8.4 Comparison of ranking of hospital wards based on ecometric analysis and the traditional method (aggregated scale values)

The top panel of Fig. 8.4 shows on the horizontal axis the ranking of the wards based on the aggregated scale values, or the 'traditional method', and on the vertical axis the ranking based on the ecometric analysis. We note from the top panel that in this particular example the two rankings are fairly consistent. Most of the hospital wards are very close to the diagonal, and this is true at the extremes more than in the middle. Secondly, the lower panel shows the distribution of the differences of the rankings, with the number of wards on the vertical axis and the difference between the ecometric and the traditional ranking on the horizontal axis. In approximately a quarter of the wards, the ranking is the same. In 40% of the wards the difference is two or more ranks out of the 87 wards. The correlation between the scores produced by the traditional method and the ecometric approach is consequently very high. As yet little has been published that cites the correlation between the two approaches. Steenbeek et al. (2012) also found high correlations between the two methods (over 0.90), and Mohnen et al. (2011), in an analysis of neighbourhood social capital, found a correlation of $r = 0.80$. These differences are not very big, but if these were to be used for information relating to public performance, especially when the results are presented by grouping constituents into three or five categories, then even a difference of one or two ranks could move a unit from an 'average' category to one described as performing 'below average'.

Further Ecometric Properties of the Scale

In psychometric analysis, reliability is usually expressed by means of Cronbach's alpha. There is an equivalent to Cronbach's alpha in ecometric analysis which takes into account how much agreement there is between observers or respondents evaluating the same ecological unit (the extent of inter-subject agreement), the number of informants or respondents sampled, and the number of items. This is shown in Eq. (8.4).

$$\text{Reliability} = \frac{\sigma_{v0}^2}{\sigma_{v0}^2 + \sigma_{u0}^2/\overline{n}_J + \sum_{m=1}^{n_I}\sigma_{\text{em}}^2/n_I\overline{n}_J} \tag{8.4}$$

In our example σ_{v0}^2 is the ward-level variance, σ_{u0}^2 the individual-level variance, $\sum_{m=1}^{n_I}\sigma_{\text{em}}^2$ is the item consistency (the sum of the error variances at item level, also known as the measurement error), $\overline{n}_J$ is the average number of individual respondents in a ward, and n_I is the number of items. As the model still includes the hospital level, the ward-level variance relates to the departure from the hospital means.

Using Eq. (8.4), the reliability of the scale 'feedback and learning from error' at the ward level can be calculated as follows.

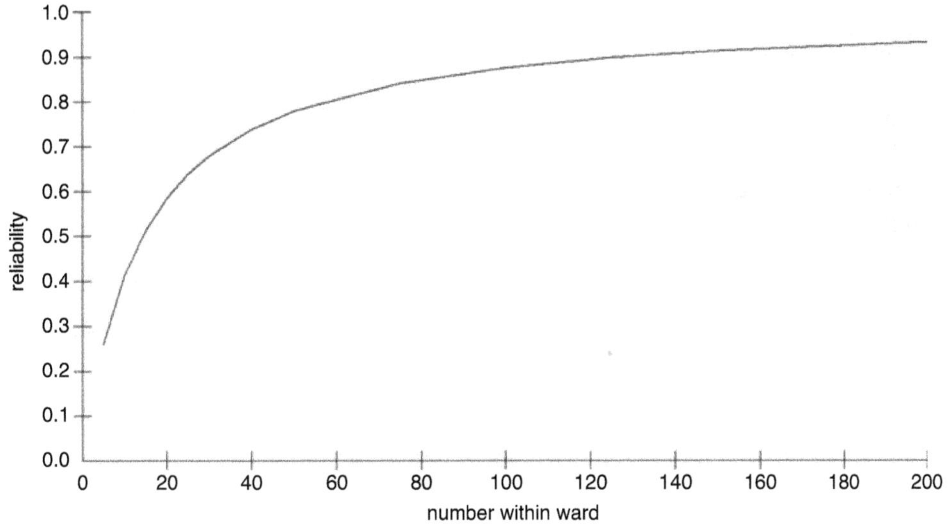

Fig. 8.5 The relationship between reliability and average sample size per higher level unit

$$\text{Reliability} = \frac{0.049}{0.049 + 0.201/22 + 2.926/(6 \times 22)} = 0.61$$

This reliability is adequate but not very high. It is a lower reliability than Cronbach's alpha at the level of the employees which would be calculated using a traditional approach (which was 0.78). It is also much lower than the ward-level reliability, which we would calculate by first aggregating the individual items to ward level and then performing a reliability analysis, giving a value of Cronbach's alpha of 0.90. This means that a failure to take into account the structure of the data would result in an overestimation of reliability at the ward level.

From Eq. (8.4) it is clear that the average number of observers or respondents per higher level unit is an important determinant. We can see this relationship in Fig. 8.5; reliability increases sharply with the number of observers or respondents per ecological unit. Raudenbush and Sampson (1999), Steenbeek (2011) and, in the field of public health research, Corsi et al. (2012) give graphs like this based on their own data. The form of the relationship is the same. Such graphs can inform us as to the appropriate number of observers or respondents per ecological unit when we want to apply an ecometric analysis. At about 30–40 respondents per ecological unit, the reliability is usually above 0.70. An important cause of low reliability is a small sample size; see, for example, Riva et al. (2011).

The item inter-correlations inform us about whether some of the items might be redundant; very high item inter-correlations suggest that we could have done with fewer items since they appear to measure the same thing. If the item inter-correlations are very low, then the items do not appear to relate to the same latent variable meaning that we could increase reliability by omitting uncorrelated items when constructing the scale. In an ecometric analysis, we can compare the item inter-correlations at the individual level and at the ward level. In our example, these range between 0.61 and 0.94 at ward level and between 0.26 and 0.49 at the level of the individual employees within the wards. Judging from the ward-level item inter-correlations, we could probably have used fewer items. However, we could not have known this in advance. If we were to develop a measurement instrument for use at an ecological level, the development of this instrument would include an analysis of the item inter-correlations. Based on the results of this analysis, we would be in a position to reconsider the items measured.

We can assess the construct validity of the scale at ward level by examining associations with other contextual measures. As an example, we calculated the correlation of the scale with self-reported frequency of event reporting at ward level. This correlation is 0.63, a moderately high correlation. In wards that have higher scores on the scale 'feedback and learning from error', more people tend to say that they frequently report events. However, these are not necessarily the same people who (at individual level) say that they receive feedback about errors. The correlation at the individual level between the scores on the scale 'feedback and learning from error' and the self-reported frequency of event reporting is only 0.36.

Conclusions

Ecometrics is a statistical method used to combine multiple data items collected from individuals, be these respondents in a survey or trained observers, about higher level units. This combination of individual responses is used to ascertain properties of the higher level units. We can take into account varying sample sizes associated with the higher level units and consequent reliability, shrinking the estimates for units with few observations towards the overall mean. We can also take into account the composition of the sample and adjust for compositional differences. Ecometrics also allows us to analyse interesting properties of the data, such as the extent of clustering at different levels, and the reliability and difficulty of items.

References

Corsi DJ, Subramanian SV, McKee M, Li W, Swaminathan S, Lopez-Jaramillo P, Avezum A, Lear SA, Dagenais G, Rangarajan S, Teo K, Yusuf S, Chow CK (2012) Environmental Profile of a Community's Health (EPOCH): an ecometric assessment of measures of the community environment based on individual perception. PLoS One 7:e44410

Gauvin L, Richard L, Craig CL, Spivock M, Riva M, Forster M, Laforest S, Laberge S, Fournel MC, Gagnon H, Gagné S, Potvin L (2005) From walkability to active living potential: an "ecometric" validation study. Am J Prev Med 28(suppl 2):126–133

Gilreath TD, Chaix B, King G, Matthews S, Flisher AJ (2012) Multi-level influence of school norms on tobacco use in South Africa: an ecometric consideration of group differences. Cancer Causes Control 23(suppl 1):27–36 de Jong K, Albin M, Skärbäck E, Grahn P, Wadbro J, Merlo J, Björk J (2011) Area-aggregated assessments of perceived environmental attributes may overcome single-source bias in studies of green environments and health: results from a cross-sectional survey in southern Sweden. Environ Health 10:4

Meuwissen LE, De Bakker DH (2008) [CQ-index GP care: development of the measurement instrument]. NIVEL, Utrecht

Mohnen SM, Groenewegen PP, Völker B, Flap HD (2011) Neighborhood social capital and individual health. Soc Sci Med 72:660–667

Mujahid MS, Diez-Roux AV, Morenoff JD, Raghunathan T (2007) Assessing the measurement properties of neighborhood scales: from psychometrics to ecometrics. Am J Epidemiol 165:858–867

Nyqvist F, Nygård M, Steenbeek W (2014) Social capital and self-rated health amongst older people in Western Finland and Northern Sweden: a multi-level analysis. Int J Behav Med 21:337–347

Oksanen T, Kawachi I, Kouvonen A, Takao S, Suzuki E, Virtanen M, Pentti J, Kivimäki M, Vahtera J (2013) Workplace determinants of social capital: cross-sectional and longitudinal evidence from a Finnish cohort study. PLoS One 8:e65846

Prins RG, Mohnen SM, van Lenthe FJ, Brug J, Oenema A (2012) Are neighbourhood social capital and availability of sports facilities related to sports participation among Dutch adolescents? Int J Behav Nutr Phys Act 9:90

Raudenbush SW (2003) The quantitative assessment of neighborhood social environments. In: Kawachi I, Berkman LF (eds) Neighborhoods and health. Oxford University Press, Oxford

Raudenbush SW, Sampson RJ (1999) Ecometrics: toward a science of assessing ecological settings, with application to the systematic social observation of neighborhoods. Sociol Methodol 29:1–41

Riva M, Bambra C, Curtis S, Gauvin L (2011) Collective resources or local social inequalities? Examining the social determinants of mental health in rural areas. Eur J Public Health 21:197–203

van Schoten SM, Baines RJ, Spreeuwenberg P, de Bruijne MC, Groenewegen PP, Groeneweg J, Wagner C (2014) The ecometric properties of a measurement instrument for prospective risk analysis in hospital departments. BMC Health Serv Res 14:103

Smits M (2009) Unintended events in hospitals: causes and the role of patient safety culture. PhD thesis (Free University, Amsterdam). NIVEL, Utrecht

Smits M, Christiaans-Dingelhoff I, Wagner C, van der Wal G, Groenewegen PP (2008) The psychometric properties of the 'Hospital Survey on Patient Safety Culture' in Dutch hospitals. BMC Health Serv Res 8:230

Steenbeek W (2011) Social and physical disorder: how community, business presence and entrepreneurs influence disorder in Dutch neighbourhoods. PhD thesis, ICS, Utrecht

Steenbeek W, Völker B, Flap H, van Oort F (2012) Local businesses as attractors or preventers of neighborhood disorder. J Res Crime Delinq 49:213–248

9

Modeling Strategies for Multilevel Analysis

Abstract When devising a modelling strategy, researchers determine the steps they will take to answer their research question or test their hypothesis. Two general principles are important. Firstly, most of the steps that you would take in a single-level regression analysis are also relevant for MLA. Secondly, start with simpler models, for example in terms of the number of levels, and add further complexity as required. The statistical model used depends on the measurement level of the dependent variable. In a baseline model, the variances are estimated at each level. After that we can start to analyse the fixed effects in a more exploratory manner or a specific hypothesis can be tested. Disentangling context and composition and providing an indication of their relative importance are often the aims of the modelling strategy. As the number of higher level units is often small, it may not be possible simultaneously to analyse several contextual variables. We end this chapter by discussing the interpretation of results in the light of a number of common assumptions.

Keywords Multilevel analysis · Modelling strategy · Measurement level · Exploratory research · Hypothesis testing · Sample size · Assumptions

Before you actually start analysing your data, it is important to define a strategy for your analysis or modelling strategy. The modelling strategy describes what you intend to do when analysing the data and takes the form of a sequence of steps that lead to an answer to your research question. The modelling strategy naturally comes somewhere in the middle of the research cycle (Fig. 9.1). It is determined by the research questions of your study, the hypotheses (where these exist) and the nature of the data; as such, it reflects the logic of your research. After you have determined your modelling strategy, you will undertake the analysis and write up the results in tables and figures as necessary and in the main body of your report. The way that you write up your research should follow the steps of your modelling strategy (see also Chap. 10).

Many of the decisions you make when defining your modelling strategy are not specific to multilevel analysis but are appropriate for data analysis in general.

Fig. 9.1 The place of the modelling strategy in the research cycle

- research question
- hypotheses
- description of research design
- available data
- *modelling strategy*
- *selection of models to be reported*
- tables and interpretation
- conclusions

Everything that you have learned about single-level regression analysis is likely to be important when you undertake a multilevel regression analysis.

Some important general advices are to start simple and only make your analysis more complicated when you are happy that you have a clear understanding of the results of your simpler analysis. This is not to say that we would argue in favour of using inadequate statistical models purely on the grounds of simplicity. But, as an approach to improve your understanding of the data and the research problem, it is a useful step. How can you expect to understand and explain a complex model if you do not have an understanding of a simpler underlying model?

Define the Data Structure

We discussed multilevel data structures in Chap. 4. The simplest multilevel data structures are strict hierarchies with only two levels. Often our data structures in the real world are more complicated, but again it is useful to start simple.

Simplification could be based on the frequencies of the occurrence of certain combinations in the data. For example, although in reality your data might contain a level below individual patients, such as that of the separate contacts patients make with the health service, it may be that in your data 99% of patients only had one contact. Or, if we were analysing pregnancy outcomes in different hospitals, we would want to take into account that pregnancies are nested in women, with one woman possibly having more than one pregnancy. However, if we have hospital data from only 2 years, it could be that there is a very small number of women with more than one pregnancy in the data set. A way of keeping things simple would be to select initially only the first pregnancy that occurred of any women with two pregnancies in the data set or to select one at random. That would result in a two-level analysis instead of a three-level analysis with limited power to differentiate between the levels of women and pregnancies. After conducting the analysis for a two-level model, and once you are satisfied that the conclusions for this model are clear, you can run a three-level model to check whether that alters the results. Given that there would be little additional data—just the additional pregnancies of the few women who had more than one pregnancy during the 2-year study period—we would not expect substantial differences between the models. The most important additional information is likely to be the ability to partition the variation between that attributable to unexplained differences between women and that due to differences between pregnancies within women. This means that it would probably make more sense to report the results of the three-level analysis rather than the two-level analysis. However, the sparsity of the data structure (the vast majority of women only having one pregnancy during the study period and virtually no women with more than two) may cause computational problems and a need to resort to reporting the results from a two-level model.

The decision to simplify might also be based on a preliminary analysis of variation, if this were to show that the variation at one of the levels in your dataset was trivial. With simple hierarchical data, the inclusion of additional levels is not a big problem, but with the more complicated data structures (such as cross-classified and multiple membership models), it might be a wise first step at least to consider leaving out levels that do not really contribute to the variation in the outcomes.

Often there are also deviations from strict hierarchies. A multiple membership model could be simplified if only a few cases belong to more than one higher level unit. If most patients usually see their own GP and only occasionally another GP, you could assign them to their usual GP. (If there is a list system, then this would be the GP to whose list that patient belongs.) Doing this simplifies the data structure to a strict hierarchy and keeps the analysis simple.

The first steps in the analysis of a cross classified data structure could be to analyse the two hierarchies separately first, as was done for example by Chum and O'Campo (2013). They studied the determinants of cardiovascular disease in residential neighbourhoods and the neighbourhoods where people worked. This gave a first impression of the variation at different levels. The prevalence of CVD clustered more strongly in residential than in work neighbourhoods. Their strategy was to estimate the variance attributable to each level in three models (individuals nested in residential neighbourhoods, work neighbourhoods and the cross classification of the two). Their next step was then to analyse the fixed effects associated with the characteristics of the two contexts in this cross-classified structure.

The information that can be gained through the use of a cross-classified data structure depends to some extent on the degree of overlap between the two hierarchies. If there is considerable overlap, then the results from the two-level models are unlikely to differ since there would be little difference between the hierarchical data structures used in each. However, when there is less overlap, the results may differ if one context is more important than the other. In either case, using a cross-classified model will help to gain an understanding of the relative importance of the contexts, which may in itself relate to one of your research questions.

Measurement Level and Distribution of the Dependent Variable

The measurement level and the distribution define the statistical model that should be used. If the dependent variable is continuous and approximately normally distributed, then linear regression is appropriate. It may be that a transformation is necessary to make the outcome follow an approximate normal distribution; you should remember that such transformations make your job of explaining the model and the parameter estimates more difficult. With a dichotomous variable, you will normally choose logistic regression. Often an ordinal dependent variable, such as self-rated health, can be dichotomised to make the analysis simpler. It should be noted, however, that this results in a loss of information. It is up to you as the researcher to decide whether this loss of information is acceptable; this will in part depend on the field of research and what is currently seen as 'good practice'. Often we only find out whether this loss of information is important after comparing the analysis of a dichotomised dependent variable with, for example, an ordered logit analysis. Such analyses are often best undertaken as a form of sensitivity analysis (in this case it is the sensitivity to the choice of analytical model that you are testing). When the results of two competing analyses are not materially different, it can be enough to say so in a sentence or two. The choice of which set of results to present as your main results then amounts to a trade-off between the need to explain a more complex model and the added information that such a model may bring.

The results of a linear regression model are often not seriously affected by violations of the distributional assumptions. As a consequence, a first step in your analysis could again be to use a simpler model, such as linear regression, and only when you have a fuller understanding of your data and the relationships between variables progress to more complicated models, such as ordered logits in the case of ordinal variables or Poisson models in the case of count variables.

The Baseline Model

Defining the baseline model comes early in your modelling strategy. It is often called the null model or empty model. This suggests that the baseline, against which we will evaluate further models, is always a model that contains no individual variables. This is, however, not necessarily the case. For example, if the main focus of your analysis is the relationship between income and access to specialised care, and if you know that access to specialised care is also dependent on age, you might decide to use a model including only age as the baseline.

In a study of body mass index (BMI) among women in nearly 33,000 communities in 57 countries, Corsi et al. (2012) adjusted their baseline model for the age of the women. Given that BMI is known to be related to age, and the countries studied have a range of rather different demographic profiles (and there are probably even greater differences between the communities within those countries), it is only possible to interpret the variation in BMI at the levels of communities and countries after accounting for differences in the age structure.

It often makes sense to adjust the baseline model for age and sex when studying health outcomes. For example, Voigtländer et al. (2010) made such an adjustment to their baseline model when analysing the influence of regional and neighbourhood deprivation on self-rated health. Another example is provided by Deraas et al. (2014) who fitted a baseline model including age and sex in their study of the influence of primary care on unplanned hospital admissions.

Cole et al. (2009) studied mental health outcomes and musculoskeletal disorders in a cohort of healthcare workers. They had five measurements per worker. They adjusted their baseline model for year of observation to take changes in the prevalence of health problems over time into account when estimating the variance at hospital and regional level.

The baseline model consists of limited information such as the overall average of the dependent variable (and relationships with key variables of interest such as age and sex) and the variances at the different levels. In previous chapters, we have discussed how to interpret the variation at the different levels in the study (see Chap. 6: Apportioning variation in multilevel models).

Exploratory Research and Hypothesis Testing

The modelling strategy differs according to the aims of the research and the research questions. We distinguish here between exploratory research and hypothesis testing research.

In *exploratory research*, the research question is only partly specified. The dependent or outcome variable is specified, but the independent variables are not. An example of an exploratory research question would be: does hospital length of stay vary between hospitals and which characteristics of hospitals explain this variation? The dependent variable is length of stay and the independent variables are not specified. A useful modelling strategy in a case like this would be as follows:

1. Estimate a random intercept model to verify if there is indeed variation between hospitals in length of stay of the patients. This null or baseline model might already include some basic patient characteristics that are known to be related to length of stay and without which any analysis would be deemed to be incomplete: perhaps the patient's age and sex. In an exploratory analysis, it may be more appropriate not to include any covariates in the null model.
2. Then add the individual-level variables, such as diagnosis, comorbidities or treatment. Adding the individual-level variables might reduce the variation between hospitals because of differences in case-mix (differences in the composition of the patient population) between hospitals.

3. The next step is to add hospital characteristics to see which variables at this level relate to length of stay. These could include the size of the hospital or the degree of specialisation.
4. At this stage, it might be interesting to explore random slopes for some of the individual-level variables. For example, the relationship between the age of the patients and length of stay might vary between hospitals. In an exploratory analysis, the slope variation can be a source of new hypotheses about how hospitals influence length of stay.
5. Finally, you could consider introducing selected cross-level interactions. Your choice of the interactions to include might be informed by your findings regarding the random slopes. If, for example, you have seen that the effect of age on length of stay varies between contexts, then you could explore whether this was due to an interaction between the patient's age and a hospital characteristic such as the size of the hospital. Alternatively you may have a particular interest in examining cross-level interactions involving pre-specified individual or contextual variables. If this were the case, then these key variables would usually be mentioned in your research question, and it might be more appropriate to undertake this analysis *before* looking for random slopes in step 4.

Changes in the amount of variation at the different levels should be evaluated at each step. In an exploratory analysis, you might want to use a stepwise procedure, selecting those variables that matter for the outcome of your study, such as forward or backward selection of significant variables. As with any exploratory analysis, you should be aware that performing multiple tests at a given level of significance means that you are likely to encounter statistically 'significant' results by chance.

In *hypothesis testing research*, we specify not only the dependent variable but also one or more independent variables. An example of a research question related to a hypothesis could be: is more social capital in neighbourhoods related to better self-rated health among the people who live there? The first step is the same as in exploratory research: estimate an appropriate baseline model to see how the variation in self-rated health is apportioned between individuals and neighbourhoods. Again, this baseline model might include some variables that are known to be correlated with self-rated health. At this point you can either introduce the contextual variable of interest (social capital in this example) or the individual variables. In the following sequence, we start with the contextual variable(s) of interest.

1. Add the contextual variable to the baseline model and see if there is a significant relationship with the outcome variable. If not the hypothesis is refuted. However, its effect could be masked by differences in the composition of the population of neighbourhoods. Hence, it might be worthwhile checking what happens to the effect if individual-level variables are added.
2. Add the relevant individual-level variables to the previous model and see whether the effect of the contextual variable stays the same or disappears. If there was an effect of the contextual variable and that disappears when individual variables are taken into account, then the apparent contextual effect was the result of differences in the composition of the neighbourhood populations.

3. In hypotheses testing research, you might also have specific ideas about cross-level interactions. Your hypothesis might be that the effect of social capital is stronger for people who have lived in their neighbourhood for a longer time. We would assume that the length of residence (an individual level variable) would already have been included in the model in step 2, in which case the next step would be to include the cross-level interaction between neighbourhood social capital (the contextual variable) and length of residence. It is not necessary first to fit a random slope model to test whether the effect of length of residence varies randomly between contexts.

Context and Composition

In Chap. 7 we discussed a very common modelling strategy, aimed at disentangling contextual effects and compositional effects. As is clear from the previous section, an attempt to make a distinction between contextual and compositional influences is a goal common to many modelling strategies in multilevel research.

Modelling the Effects of Higher Level Characteristics

In Chap. 3 we defined higher level units as units that can be sampled. Sample size is thus an issue not only at the lowest level but also at the higher levels. We have many lower level units nested within fewer higher level units. The number of higher level units is often restricted by the fact that in reality they form an entire population. Think of neighbourhoods within a city; the number of neighbourhoods is restricted by the size of the city and perhaps the administrative definitions with which we are working. The number of EU member states is equally restricted at any one time to the number of countries that are in the EU. Another restriction is more pragmatic; when the higher level units are organisations, such as schools, and you want to study students nested in schools, the effort needed to include more schools in a study is often considerable.

The number of higher level units has consequences if the focus of the research is on the effect of higher level characteristics. This number should then be sufficient to estimate a mean, a variance and the effect of the relevant variables of interest at that level. As a rule of thumb, the number of units that you need is approximately ten times the number of variables you want to include in the analysis. This means that if you want to include ten variables to test your hypothesis about the characteristics of hospitals and how they influence an outcome at patient level, you would need at least a hundred hospitals. Alternatively, if you want to analyse the effect of characteristics of the healthcare systems of EU member states on access to healthcare, the maximum number of higher level units (at the time of writing) is 28. As such, the number of country-level variables that could be included in an analysis is only two or three.

This limitation on the number of contextual variables that can be included in an analysis has consequences for the design of studies and for the modelling strategy. For the design of a study where the effects of higher level characteristics are important, it is more important to increase the number of higher level units (if this is possible) than the number of lower level units (Snijders and Bosker 2012). In terms of a modelling strategy, this means that we have to be careful not to include too many independent higher level characteristics at the same time. In the example of the analysis of 28 EU member states in which we wish to study the effect of healthcare systems on access to healthcare, we would probably want to include one confounder, such as the wealth of a country, along with one characteristic of the healthcare system at a time. We could repeat the analysis several times using each relevant healthcare system characteristic individually and compare the results. We would not be able to analyse the effects of several characteristics at the same time. This also excludes the possibility of adding a contextual variable with several categories since this would be operationalised by introducing a series of dummy variables. We would consequently have to be more careful in formulating our conclusions which would be based more on weighting the results against our hypotheses and background knowledge than on strict statistical criteria.

In Chap. 10 we will give some examples of studies where the authors were not sufficiently aware of this problem and, as a consequence, introduced more contextual variables than the available number of higher level units could support.

Random Effects at Higher Levels

In all of the models considered in this book, we have assumed that the higher level effects are all normally distributed. (This may be after an appropriate transformation; for example, in a multilevel logistic regression, we assume that the log odds ratios associated with membership of the higher level units are normally distributed.) This assumption is convenient but not always appropriate. Austin (2005, 2009) has considered the impact of this assumption and found that an inappropriate assumption of normality at the higher level does not appear to have implications for the estimation of fixed effects, but it may lead to biased or incorrect estimates of the variances. This then has consequences for assessment of the importance of different levels in a model or for studies in which the residuals themselves are of some importance (such as studies of institutional performance).

One way in which the distribution of higher level residuals may appear non-normal is due to the presence of outliers. Multilevel data may contain outliers in the same way that the data for traditional regression models may be outlying; the difference is that in a multilevel model, the outliers may be at any level in the model. Methods have been developed for the detection and treatment of outliers at higher levels (Langford and Lewis 1998; Lewis and Langford 2001). These essentially rely on including a fixed effect for a context regarded as outlying; this removes the impact of this unit on the estimation of the higher level variance whilst including the lower level units (such as individuals) in the analysis.

Interpreting the Results in the Light of Common Assumptions

As we said at the beginning of this chapter, a number of assumptions are the same as in single-level regression analysis. We will briefly illustrate this with an example of a hypothetical intervention study. We have chosen the example of an intervention study to be able to address some assumptions that are typically made in such studies. The example is the evaluation of an intervention to reduce BMI. Individuals have been randomised to the intervention and control groups, and we have pre- and post-intervention measures for everyone in the study. Individuals are nested within communities (e.g. neighbourhoods or schools). A slightly different study design of a community intervention would be possible, in which it would be the communities (and all individuals within them) rather than the individuals that would be randomised to the intervention and control groups. The structure of the data is that of a three-level model with measurement occasions nested in individuals, clustered within areas (a repeated measures design). To make the intervention and control groups comparable, we adjust for age, sex and educational status (basic/higher). Algebraically the model can be written as shown in Eq. (9.1).

$$
\begin{aligned}
y_{ijk} &= \beta_0 + \beta_1 x_{1jk} + \beta_2 x_{2jk} + \beta_3 x_{3jk} + \beta_4 x_{4jk} + \beta_5 x_{5ijk} + \beta_6 x_{4k} x_{5ijk} + v_{0k} + u_{0jk} + e_{0ijk} \\
v_{0k} &\sim N\left(0, \sigma^2_{v0}\right) \\
u_{0jk} &\sim N\left(0, \sigma^2_{u0}\right) \\
e_{0ijk} &\sim N\left(0, \sigma^2_{e0}\right)
\end{aligned}
\tag{9.1}
$$

Here y_{ijk} is the primary outcome, BMI, at measurement occasion (pre- or post-intervention) i for individual j in community k. x_{1jk}, x_{2jk} and x_{3jk} are individual-level covariates relating to the person's baseline age, sex and educational status; these do not change between measurement occasions. x_{4jk} denotes whether the individual is in the intervention (coded 1) or control (coded 0) groups, and x_{5ijk} indicates whether the measurement occasion was pre- (coded 0) or post- (coded 1) intervention. The term $x_{4jk}x_{5ijk}$ is then the cross-level interaction picking out the post-intervention measurement occasion in the intervention group. The coefficient associated with this term, β_6, is the parameter of interest, indicating the success or otherwise of the intervention. In addition to the individual characteristics, the model takes into account that there may have been a baseline difference in BMI between the intervention and control groups and that there may be a population change in BMI between the two

Table 9.1 Parameter estimates for the evaluation of a hypothetical intervention on BMI

Parameter		Coefficient	(SD)
	Fixed part		
Constant		25.155	(0.052)
Age		−0.510	(0.015)
Male		0.315	(0.042)
Higher education		−1.015	(0.042)
Intervention		−0.048	(0.044)
Time = post		0.018	(0.018)
Intervention ∗ (time = post)		−0.195	(0.025)
	Random part		
Community-level variance		0.090	(0.019)
Individual-level variance		1.961	(0.044)
Measurement occasion variance		0.396	(0.008)

measurement occasions; neither of these events should mistakenly be ascribed to an intervention effect. We also model the variances at the three levels.

First of all we will consider some assumptions underlying the fixed part of the model that was used to make the groups comparable. For these assumptions, it is irrelevant whether we are discussing an intervention study or an observational study. The parameter estimates are given in Table 9.1.

One assumption made in the model described in Eq. (9.1) is that the effect of age on BMI is linear for all ages. This is an assumption that can be tested easily by comparing this model with one where we also add age squared or a model where we recode age into a number of categories. Another assumption is that the effect of age on BMI is the same regardless of sex or education level and that the effect of education is the same for men and women. These assumptions can be tested by using interaction terms between these variables. Alternatively, if the study is powered for this, we could consider stratified analyses by key variables such as gender. Often a stratified analysis will give you a better impression of the size and direction of the interaction effect and whether this differs between groups. (This is at the cost of power; there will obviously be fewer observations in each of the strata than in the overall analysis.) However, as the stratified analysis takes more space in the tables, you may decide to report the version with the interaction effect and use the stratified analysis as a valuable step in your own interpretation of the interaction.

Next consider the impact of the intervention itself. An assumption here is that the intervention is equally effective regardless of age, sex or education level. It is conceivable that, and may be worth testing whether, the intervention is differentially effective for older and younger people, men and women or more and less educated people. Knowing not just whether an intervention has worked but for which groups it appears to be more or less successful is important if we subsequently want to improve or tailor the intervention and if we are interested in the impact of the intervention on inequalities. We can examine differential impacts on subgroups by introducing the appropriate interaction terms (between the intervention and the subgroup of interest) into the model.

There are also some assumptions implicit in the way the random part of the model has been formulated. In this model we have assumed that the variance in BMI is the same regardless of age, sex and educational level. This can be tested by estimating the variances separately for age groups, men and women and educational categories. Another assumption is that the variance is unchanged by the intervention. The model that was estimated, shows a decrease in mean BMI in the intervention group, but it is possible that the intervention has changed the variance. An example would be if the intervention had a greater impact on those with higher BMI; this would result not just in the decrease in BMI seen in the intervention group following the intervention but also a reduction in variance in the same group.

All of the above assumptions may be reasonable and may be supported by the data. But if the data does not support these assumptions, then fitting the alternative models may impact on estimates in unpredictable ways. In an example such as this, we have an extremely important single parameter—the intervention effect—and cannot say with certainty that changes to the model would not alter the magnitude or statistical significance of this estimate. In short, it is unlikely that your modelling strategy will test every aspect of your model, but it is important that you are aware of your underlying assumptions.

Conclusions

The modelling strategy for a multilevel analysis begins with the research question and hypothesis that the study is addressing. Simplifications to the model that you are fitting will help you to gain a better understanding of the data and an idea of your answer, with further detail being provided by the complexity that you subsequently add. There will inevitably be assumptions underlying any choices that we make during the construction of a modelling strategy, including which models we consider and which we do not. Whilst it may not be necessary formally to test every assumption, it is important that we are aware of the assumptions that we have made and what their consequences might be—even if the answer is that their consequences may be unpredictable.

References

Austin PC (2005) Bias in penalized quasi-likelihood estimation in random effects logistic regression models when the random effects are not normally distributed. Commun Stat Simul Comput 34:549–565

Austin PC (2009) Are (the log-odds of) hospital mortality rates normally distributed? Implications for studying variations in outcomes of medical care. J Eval Clin Pract 15:514–523

Chum A, O'Campo P (2013) Contextual determinants of cardiovascular diseases: overcoming the residential trap by accounting for non-residential context and duration of exposure. Health Place 24:73–79

Cole DC, Koehoorn M, Ibrahim S, Hertzman C, Ostry A, Xu F, Brown P (2009) Regions, hospitals and health outcomes over time: a multi-level analysis of repeat prevalence among a cohort of health-care workers. Health Place 15:1046–1057
Corsi DJ, Finlay JE, Subramanian SV (2012) Weight of communities: a multilevel analysis of body mass index in 32,814 neighborhoods in 57 low- to middle-income countries (LMICs). Soc Sci Med 75:311–322
Deraas TS, Berntsen GR, Jones AP, Førde OH, Sund ER (2014) Associations between primary healthcare and unplanned medical admissions in Norway: a multilevel analysis of the entire elderly population. BMJ Open 4:e004293
Langford IH, Lewis T (1998) Outliers in multilevel data. J R Stat Soc Ser A 161:121–160
Lewis T, Langford IH (2001) Outliers, robustness and the detection of discrepant data. In: Leyland AH, Goldstein H (eds) Multilevel modelling of health statistics. Wiley, Chichester, pp 75–91
Snijders TAB, Bosker RJ (2012) Multilevel analysis: an introduction to basic and advanced multilevel modeling. Sage, Los Angeles
Voigtländer S, Berger U, Razum O (2010) The impact of regional and neighbourhood deprivation on physical health in Germany: a multilevel study. BMC Public Health 10:403

10

Research Articles and MLA: Reading and Writing

Abstract This chapter focuses on two issues. Firstly, we consider the critical reading of research articles that use MLA, and secondly we explore the standards for writing up research that has used MLA. Critical reading is important both for people who do not regularly use MLA themselves and for those who are regular users. The irregular users need to be able to assess the methodology of studies using MLA, whilst regular users may find inspiration for new ways and strategies of data analysis and for ways to write up and present their own research, particularly the methods and results sections. So the reading and writing parts of this chapter are related. When a method of analysis is used that is relatively new to its field, there are no clear standards as to what should be included in the methods section or how the tables might be laid out.

Keywords Multilevel analysis · Critical reading · Reporting

Communication is an important part of the research process. Research results are important in themselves, but will only be used if they are communicated to the relevant audiences. In public health and health services research, we usually have two types of audiences: the research community and the users of research in policy and practice (Bensing et al. 2003).

The 'end users' of research probably will not read the research papers themselves, but intermediaries certainly will. Such intermediaries might be health scientists and epidemiologists who work in policy development positions within (public) health authorities. It is crucial that we as researchers should write up our research in a way that makes our methodological and statistical approach as clear as possible.

The research community enters the process when we submit a paper for publication. Some reviewers will be selected for their specialised statistical knowledge, whilst others will be selected for their substantive knowledge about the subject of the research. We cannot guarantee that the latter will be completely up-to-date with MLA. We therefore need to write about our approach and to present our results in a way that is understandable to many audiences.

Critical Reading

An increasing number of research articles in the area of public health and health services research are being published that use multilevel analysis. We have simply counted the number of articles that used the term 'multilevel' in a Pubmed search of the journals *Social Science and Medicine*, *Journal Epidemiology and Community Health* and *European Journal of Public Health* (see Fig. 10.1). This simple search may have missed some articles that used slightly different terminology such as 'hierarchical' instead of 'multilevel'. However, the picture is clear and that is one of a huge increase in the use of multilevel analysis in our area of research: from 5 articles in 1998 to 65 articles in 2015 in just these three journals.

In the past the alternatives to multilevel analysis that we described in Chap. 3 were often used. However, it is now rare to see a published paper that analyses clustered data and does not use multilevel analysis. In fact, as early as 1998 we came across an article the authors of which—in a foot note—said that they initially submitted a 'naïve' (as they called it themselves) single-level analysis, but were asked by the reviewers to repeat the analysis using MLA (Matteson et al. 1998).

Given that currently so many research articles use MLA, it is important that researchers, even if they do not apply MLA themselves, are able to understand and critically appraise the work of others. When reading an article, we are inclined to focus more on the substantive results and less on the methodology, to the extent that we sometimes take the methodology for granted and skip the methods section. When relatively new and complicated methods are used, and we can still count MLA as such, the tendency to skip the methods section might be even stronger. However, it is also more dangerous to do so when the methods are new (Bingenheimer 2005). With new methods there will be no clear standards for reporting research results (see later in this chapter), researchers may make mistakes or debatable choices in their methodology, and reviewers are not always able to judge exactly what was done. It is therefore important for researchers and for users of research results to develop a way to read critically research articles that use MLA.

To help new users to read research articles critically and to understand the multilevel design employed, we have formulated a number of questions. You can

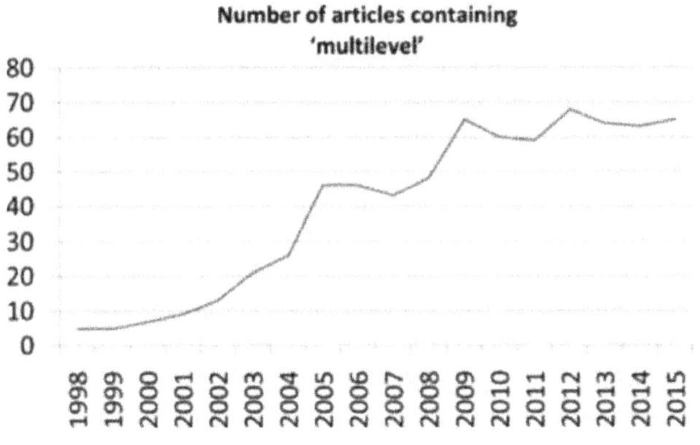

Fig. 10.1 Number of articles containing the term 'multilevel' in a Pubmed search of the journals Social Science and Medicine, Journal Epidemiology and Community Health and European Journal of Public Health

use these questions when reading and abstracting research articles. We will briefly elucidate them.

What Is the Research Question?

It might seem superfluous to draw attention to the research question. It is not, for two reasons. Firstly, we still occasionally stumble across published research articles that have no clear formulation of a research question or hypothesis at all. That means that as a reader you have to reconstruct the question yourself *after* reading the paper. Secondly, the research question determines the choice of method. It is therefore important to have a clear picture of what question the authors want to answer.

Increasingly researchers formulate an objective or aim instead of a research question. Usually an objective or aim will be less specific. Verstappen et al. (2005) formulated their objective in the abstract as *'To describe the variation in the numbers of imaging investigations requested by general practitioners (GPs) and to find likely explanations for this variation'*. In the introduction to the article they are a bit more specific without, however, making clear what the 'likely explanations' might be.

> *The present study measured the variation of imaging investigations among a large group of GPs and investigated the influence of professional and contextual determinants at three levels: the individual GP, local GP groups, and the region.*

Compare this with an example of an explicit research question, as formulated by Turrell et al. (2007):

> *What is the relation between area-level socioeconomic disadvantage and mortality before and after adjusting for within area variation in individual level occupation? Does the relationship between mortality and individual level occupation differ by area level disadvantage? What is the variation in mortality at different geographical levels?*

Research questions also differ regarding how specific they are. Some research questions ask whether there is a relationship between two variables, without specifying the direction. Others ask whether a particular relationship will be found. These are basically hypotheses formulated as research questions. An example of this is a study by Van Stam et al. (2014) on Sexual and Reproductive Health (SRH). They tested the hypothesis that the relationship between educational attainment and SRH differed according to the level of globalisation of the region where the subjects live (effect moderation). Hence, their research question can also be formulated as: Is this hypothesis confirmed or refuted in our data?

The combination of a research objective and a concrete hypothesis is also specific enough to guide the remainder of an article. For example, Agyemang et al. (2009) formulated as their objective '*to assess the effect of neighbourhood income and unemployment/social security benefit (deprivation) on pregnancy outcomes*'. Their hypothesis was '*that low neighbourhood income and deprivation [are] associated with poor pregnancy outcomes after adjustment for individual-level characteristics*'.

In a general analysis of research questions, Mayo et al. (2013) discussed the use of language, suggesting that words such as 'explore' and 'describe' should be avoided when formulating a research question because of the difficulty such words pose in determining whether or not the question has been answered. They stress how the correct formulation of the research question will assist the researcher in the choice of the optimal design for the study.

In many cases the multilevel nature of the problem is already indicated by the research question, such as when the question is about the relationship between variables at different levels. An example is the research question posed by Jat et al. (2011): *what are the effects of individual, community and district level characteristics on the utilisation of maternal health services?*

Which Levels Can Be Distinguished Theoretically?

It is important to be aware of the difference between the levels that one would like to be able to distinguish in an ideal situation and the reality with which one actually has to work. If the research question is to explain differences between hospitals in patients' judgements about quality of care, the most obvious levels are probably patients at the lower level and hospitals at the higher level. However, if we analyse the research problem in terms of the actors involved and the opportunities and constraints they experience (see Chap. 2), we might come to the conclusion that the physician responsible for the treatment and the ward in which the patients are treated are likely to be the drivers of patients' experiences. That might imply a three-level model of patients, physicians and hospitals, or possibly four levels with physicians nested within wards (or a cross-classification of physicians and wards, depending on the hospital structure).

Often the introduction of an article uses a theoretical notion of a relevant higher-level unit, connected to a mechanism that relates this context to individual behaviour or outcomes. The 'data and methods' section then moves to an operational definition of higher-level units, often chosen for practical reasons of data availability. This pragmatically chosen definition of the higher-level units might be different from the units implied by the theoretical reasoning in the introduction of the article. The results are therefore based on units that do not correspond to what was intended and this may lead to less clear effects. Returning to the previous example regarding patients' judgements of quality of care, if the physician is the true driver of the patients' experiences but this level is unobservable, then the extent to which there will be differences between hospitals will depend on the degree to which physicians assessed as providing high or low quality cluster within the same hospitals. Often in the discussion the emphasis moves back from the pragmatic context of the available data that were used in the analysis, to the theoretical notions from the introduction.

We illustrate this with research examples that have studied the effect of neighbourhood characteristics on health or health behaviour. Ball et al. (2007) moved from 'local neighbourhoods' in the abstract to suburbs of between 4000 and 30,000 inhabitants in the methods section, and back to neighbourhoods in the last paragraph of the discussion. In a study on obesity in New York City, Black et al. (2010) used United Hospital Funds areas as neighbourhoods. NYC has 34 of these areal units. Given the population of the city (over eight million people), these must be huge areas and it is doubtful that we could really call them neighbourhoods. The article gives the average sample size per area, but not the number of inhabitants. Sellström et al. (2008) studied environmental influences on smoking during pregnancy. Citing the importance of peer groups in adolescent smoking, they state that social influences are apparently important in explaining why pregnant women keep on smoking. The actual units they use in their analysis to capture these social influences are neighbourhoods with between 4000 and 10,000 inhabitants. This is quite far from the idea of peer group influences that they brought up in their theoretical reasoning.

Another example of the connection between the theoretical reasoning in the introduction of an article and the definition of spatial units in the methods section is provided in a paper by Karvonen et al. (2008) on smoking patterns. They state: '*An ideal spatial context for an exploration of smoking patterns by small area would comprise a reasonably stable and homogeneous population with relatively low variation of disadvantage*'. Subsequently in the methods section, they rationalise their use of 107 neighbourhoods in Helsinki: '*These areas are of the size that most residents could walk across them in 15–20 min and have an average population of 4000*'.

These examples—and there are many more—illustrate the importance of theorising the contexts that are being used as higher-level units and of being aware of the fact that there is often a gap between the theoretically interesting units and what is actually available or used. This gap may be part of the explanation for the finding that the influences of contextual variables on individual outcomes are sometimes weak, and it is important that any such gap should be acknowledged in the paper.

What Is the Structure of the Actual Data Used?

Apart from the issue discussed in the previous section, there are often reasons why there is a discrepancy between the levels that would be relevant on theoretical grounds and those actually used. One reason is that information may be lacking on some relevant levels.

In the example of patients' judgements about quality of hospital care that we gave at the end of Chap. 2, the researchers might for pragmatic reasons have chosen hospitals to be their higher level. For some indicators of quality of care this may be appropriate (such as those that reflect hospital policies) but for others—think of whether the treatment by hospital personnel is polite—the more appropriate level might be wards, teams or even individual nurses and doctors. One reason to use only the hospital level is that there is no information available about the levels in between (Hekkert et al. 2009; Sixma et al. 2009).

Another reason might be that the numbers at a certain level are too small. The extreme case is when there is only one unit at one level within each higher-level unit. The household might be a relevant level from a theoretical point of view, but if only one member of each household has been interviewed then the household and individual levels are indistinguishable. In the example dataset used in the tutorial in Chap. 12, the authors collapsed four levels into two for pragmatic reasons, concentrating on patients and GPs but leaving out the practice level (most GPs were single-handed) and the episode of care level (most patients had only one episode of care during the study period). Researchers might also simplify their data structure by choosing only one observation from a (theoretically larger) dataset. For example, Jat et al. (2011), in their study of environmental influences on pregnancy outcomes, only chose the last pregnancy of each woman in their sample. In so doing the level of the women who gave birth and the level of the newborn infants collapsed into one level. Another example is Van Berkestijn et al. (1999) who only used the first consultation in each episode of care. This meant that they could restrict their model to just two levels: the GPs in their study and the episode of care which coincides with the consultation.

A good reason to opt for fewer levels than are actually available is that this may make the analysis less complicated. It is, however, important to be aware that leaving out a higher level is less problematic than leaving out an intermediate level. In the former case, the variation at the omitted level is simply added to that at the new highest level. When an intermediate level is omitted, the variation will in general be split between the higher and lower levels (see Chap. 6 and also the section on variation at different levels later in this chapter).

Whatever the reason for omitting levels, it is important to be aware of the difference between the levels that were theoretically postulated and the levels that were actually used. It is elucidative to draw a simple diagram of the levels and the numbers used at all levels. Chapter 4 on multilevel data structures gives examples of such diagrams.

It is also important to consider the numbers at the different levels and the average number of lower-level units per higher-level unit. The number of higher-level units is sometimes quite small. As we pointed out in Chap. 3, the higher-level units are treated as a sample and there should be sufficient numbers of units at this level for it to make sense to estimate an average and variance. The number of units is also important if authors want to include characteristics of these units in their analysis. If so, the numbers should be sufficient to estimate the coefficients associated with these characteristics in addition to the mean and variance. We have come across several examples where the authors (and reviewers) were apparently not aware of this. Some of these studies are international comparisons with the countries as higher-level units and a characterisation of welfare state regimes in the form of a set of dummy variables as independent variables. Even though the welfare state regime might be seen as a single concept, it is usually operationalised as a series of dummy variables. Eikemo et al. (2008) included 23 countries, their higher-level units, but added

4 dummy variables at this level. Witvliet et al. (2012) had 46 countries and 6 dummy variables for welfare state regimes. And Rathmann et al. (2015) analysed data for 27 countries and included 4 dummy variables indicating welfare state typology.

The problem of trying to include more contextual variables than the data can support is, however, not restricted to the analysis of welfare states. Friele et al. (2006) had one analysis with 80 hospitals and another with 40 hospitals which included 7 independent variables at the hospital level. With a simple rule of thumb of 10 cases for each independent variable, the first analysis was reasonable but not the second. For the estimation of contextual effects, the number of lower-level units becomes irrelevant; the authors were attempting to estimate 9 quantities (a mean, 7 regression coefficients and a variance) from 40 contextual observations. Further examples include Huizing et al. (2007) who had 15 wards in nursing homes and included 6 independent variables at this level, and Nicholson et al. (2009) who included four independent contextual variables with just 22 higher-level units.

What Statistical Model Was Used?

Most statistical models that can be run as single-level analysis can also be used in MLA (see Chap. 4). Questioning what statistical model was used and whether this was appropriate is therefore as relevant when reading a multilevel article as when reading about a single-level analysis. If the authors specify the algebraic form of their model in the article or in a technical appendix, a useful check is to see whether the subscripts correspond to the levels that have been included.

To as great an extent as possible (within the space constraints imposed by journals), the methods section of a paper should provide sufficient information to enable other researchers to reproduce the analysis reported in an article. This includes the type of model (linear, logistic, Poisson, etc.), details of the levels used (including the specification of any which are cross-classified or multiple membership), the variables included in each model in the fixed and random parts (including interactions), and details of the software and estimation procedures used. Published descriptions of the model used and estimation techniques are sometimes so brief that these cannot even be deduced from the software that was used.

Some authors have compared their results of MLA with a single-level model. As we argued in Chap. 3, in cases where the units for whom the outcomes are measured are nested within higher-level units, MLA is the preferred approach. The examples provided here illustrate again that using a single-level model in circumstances that indicate that a multilevel model is appropriate may lead to false conclusions about the effect of higher-level variables. In Chap. 3, we discussed the example of an intervention study in GP practices (Renders et al. 2001) where the intervention effect was significant in a single-level (patients) model, but not in a multilevel model. We also referred to Mauny et al. (2004) who analysed the occurrence of the malaria parasite in blood samples taken from people living in villages in Madagascar. In the single-level model, they found a significant coefficient for the size of villages which they did not find in a MLA. This was due to the misestimated precision when the village size was assigned to all individuals and treated as a series of independent individual-level observations. A similar example that we have previously mentioned in this chapter is the article by Matteson et al. (1998). In a footnote they state that, in the single-level analysis which they initially submitted, more county variables were significant.

What Was the Modelling Strategy?

This relates to the steps that the authors say they are going to take when analysing their data in order to answer their research question and/or to test their hypotheses. Ideally the modelling strategy should follow on from the research question and hypotheses. One typical sequence might be to start by examining the variation at different levels in a null model and reporting the intraclass correlation. The next step would be to introduce individual-level variables, evaluating the changes in variation at all levels. A reduction in the higher-level variation at this stage indicates compositional effects. The next step may then be to introduce higher-level variables and evaluate the decrease in variation at that level. Of course, the modelling strategy should reflect the hypotheses that one wants to test.

It is important that the modelling strategy is a systematic and logical sequence of steps and that the modelling strategy as described in the methods section is indeed executed and reported in the results section. Many research papers do not include a modelling strategy at all or else report their results in a different order to that suggested by the strategy. Tables should reflect the modelling strategy as far as possible; however, it is often not necessary to document every step in the tables. This might easily lead to large and unclear tables (for example, see the four page landscape table in Béland et al. 2002).

Examples of clear modelling strategies accompanied by results sections that follow the steps outlined in the methods section include those presented by Van Yperen and Snijders (2000), Ball et al. (2007) and Merlo et al. (2005).

Van Yperen and Snijders studied Karasek's job demand-control model. The main hypothesis of this model is that the job stress that workers experience depends on the interaction between the demands that are made of them and the amount of control they experience over their own job. Strong demands lead to particularly high levels of job stress when workers have less control over their work. They test this hypothesis and look at demand and control both at the individual level and the group level. Removing the group effects (by including them) means that individual-level demands and control are then relative to those experienced by co-workers. Their modelling strategy neatly follows the hypotheses.

Ball et al. studied educational variation in walking for women and whether this can be explained by intrapersonal and social characteristics and by perceived and objectively assessed facets of the physical environment. Their modelling strategy consisted of four steps. In the first step, only education was included in the model. In subsequent steps, environmental variables, social variables and finally personal variables were added.

Merlo and colleagues studied differences between hospitals in neonatal mortality for low risk and high risk pregnancies against the background of regionalisation and concentration of services. They used four steps, starting with an empty model; they then added characteristics of the hospitals where the deliveries took place. In step 3, maternal and delivery characteristics were added. In the final model, these characteristics were replaced by a propensity score to take confounding by indication into account.

A more specific issue when evaluating the modelling strategy is the completeness of the individual-level model. This is particularly important in studies of composition and context and when forming league tables. In studies of context and composition, the researcher may wish to explore whether variation at the higher or contextual level remains when relevant individual characteristics have been taken into account. The range of individual variables available is often quite small, especially when using routinely collected or register data. In a study on the use of tranquillizers by Groenewegen et al. (1999), only the age and sex of the users were known. In a study of the socio-economic determinants of compliance to colorectal cancer screening (Pornet et al. 2011), the individual model consisted of only age, sex and insurance type. The risk is then that the clustering of people with, for example, a low socio-economic status in certain neighbourhoods leads to apparent neighbourhood-level variation that would have disappeared if socio-economic status had been measured at the individual level.

The completeness of the individual-level model is especially important when creating 'league tables' as a measure of institutional performance. The individual characteristics then act as a means of correcting for differences in case-mix. With good case-mix correction, the higher-level residuals reflect, to as great an extent as possible, the 'true' differences between higher-level units such as nursing homes. Patients or their representatives can use that information to inform their choice of care site (Arling et al. 2007).

Does the Paper Report the Intercept Variation at Different Levels?

Sometimes researchers only report fixed effects. In this case, they are apparently only using MLA in order to have appropriate estimates of the confidence intervals or other measures of uncertainty around the regression coefficients. This may for example be the case when the data are collected using a two-stage sample and the authors want to adjust for that. Nevertheless, it would be interesting to see the extent to which the dependent variable clusters within higher-level units. As we discussed in Chap. 6, an estimate of the higher-level variance is necessary for power calculations. We usually obtain these estimates from published research about similar problems or data sets. However, some of the estimation procedures used (such as generalised estimating equations—GEE) will only correct the standard errors of the estimates without explicitly estimating the variance at the different levels.

Sometimes the variation is of central importance to the research question at hand; even if this is not the case, the reporting of variation can be seen as a service to the academic community because of its potential interest to readers of the article. As such, the intercept variance should be reported as well as the individual variance, enabling the reader to calculate the intraclass correlation coefficient if this was not reported in the article. In some cases the intercept variance is reported for the empty model, whilst in other cases it is more relevant to report the intercept variation only after taking into account some individual-level variables. If treatment outcomes in different hospitals are analysed, and the hospitals differ in composition according to the age, sex and severity of illness of the patients treated, it might be more relevant to report the between-hospital variation after these case-mix variables have been taken into account.

If slope variance is also important, this should be reported alongside the covariance between the intercept and the slope. Remember that the variance of the intercept and the covariance are dependent upon where the slope variable has been centred, so any non-standard centring (that is if the location has been changed so that a value of 0 on the transformed slope variable does not correspond to a value of 0 on the original variable) should also be reported as an aid to interpretation. We provided an introduction to random slopes in Chap. 5 along with a guide to the interpretation of different patterns of covariance.

Cross-Level Interactions

If there is an explicit hypothesis about the interaction between variables at different levels, this can be tested by introducing a cross-level interaction. In a more exploratory analysis or when the hypothesis is about variation in the slopes, one would estimate the slope variance and the covariance between the slope and the intercept. You will, however, have more power to test for a specific cross-level interaction than for a random slope.

In general, interaction terms are not always easy to interpret. It may be helpful to illustrate them using a figure. Several nice examples can be found in the published literature; for example, see any of Turrell et al. (2007), Joshu et al. (2008), Stafford et al. (2008) and Mohnen et al. (2012). From this last publication, we show the interaction between neighbourhood social capital (higher level) and household composition (individual level) on self-rated health (Fig. 10.2).

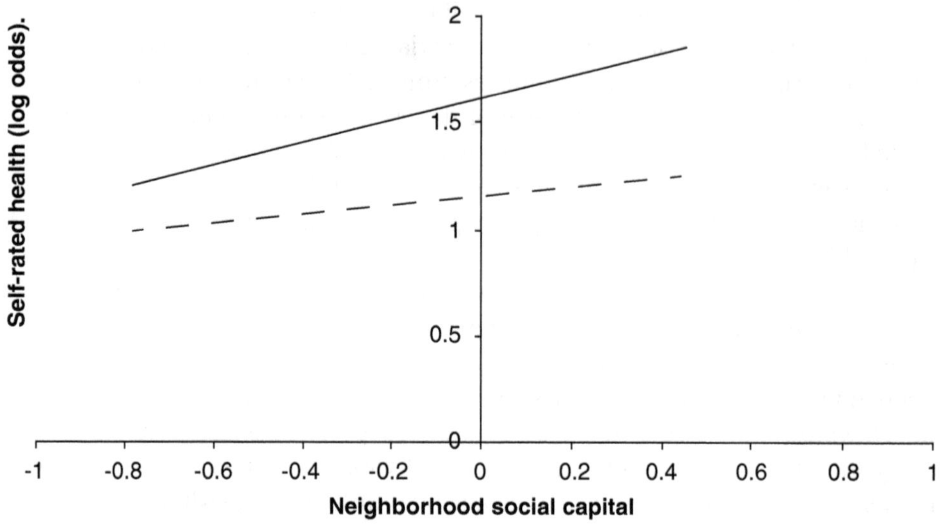

Fig. 10.2 Interaction of neighbourhood social capital and whether (black line) or not (dashed line) there are young children in the household on self-rated health (reproduced with permission from Oxford University Press, the European Journal of Public Health)

What Are the Shortcomings and Strong Points of the Article?

Try to summarise the points of criticism and try to weigh their consequences for the value of the results of the analysis that was presented. Try also to identify a number of positive points from the article you have been reading. The shortcomings are important in critical reading and they are very important in forming your overall judgement as to how confident you can be that the results of the study are indeed a valuable addition to our knowledge. However, the strong points of an article may help you in improving the formulation of your own research.

Writing Up Your Own Research

It is impossible to come up with a single form of presentation that will suit all types of analysis. The information that you need to show depends on your research question (and this is another reason for considering study design carefully before starting). Moreover, all general advice about how to write a research paper applies to papers that report on MLA and this will not be repeated here.

The Introduction or Background Section

The introduction or background section of your research paper should contain a clearly formulated research question—a grammatically well-formed sentence that ends with a question mark. In the 'reading' part of this chapter, we noted the tendency of some research papers only to state an objective, which is often less clearly specified than a research question or a hypothesis.

Previous literature, where available, should be used to develop your research question and the hypotheses you intend to test. As an aid to focusing your arguments when writing the introduction, it is advisable to consider using 'what is known about this subject?' bullet points as required by some journals. It is important to identify the gaps in current knowledge and not just to tread a well-worn path.

Specifically when writing an article using multilevel analysis, the introduction should contain a theoretical argument as to why different levels or contexts are relevant to the particular research question. We started Chap. 1 by stressing the importance of context as an influence on people's health, well-being, health behaviour and healthcare utilisation. This should be reflected in the attention that is given to discussing the relevant aspects of the context. In some cases the context might seem self-evident, such as in a study of health outcomes among hospitalised patients. The relevant context would then be the hospital. Even so, health outcomes are probably more strongly influenced by the particular department in which a patient was treated than the hospital as a whole. In the case when the context is a geographical unit, the link between geographical scale and area type on the one hand and the mechanism that is supposed to cause the outcome at the individual level is particularly important. If, for example, we want to analyse the relationship between social capital and health, the way in which we conceptualise social capital and the type of mechanism that we assume will influence the areal unit that we would want to use. When we conceptualise social capital as the social networks of people living in the same area, supplying each other with emotional and instrumental support, we would require smaller areal units than for a conceptualisation of social capital in terms of community resources, norms and trust (Moore et al. 2005). When the discrepancy between the size of the units used and the supposed mechanism that links the units to the outcomes is too large, it becomes increasingly difficult to draw conclusions based on your analysis of the data.

The Methods Section

The methods section firstly makes the step from the theoretical and conceptual discussion of context as it appears in the introduction or background to the concrete levels actually to be used in the data analysis. Especially when you use existing data at any of the levels, it is likely that there will be discrepancies between the theoretical context and the levels that you use in practice. It is important to describe this discrepancy and to discuss the consequences in the final section of the paper.

In the methods section, you should detail the units or levels used and the data structure. These provide the rationale for the use of MLA. The relevant numbers (for example, the population of the areas and sample drawn from these) should be detailed.

The nature of the statistical model that you use will largely be determined by the dependent variable that you are analysing. As in any other empirical research paper, it should be clear at what scale the dependent variable has been measured and consequently what the statistical model will be. Software packages that handle MLA differ and you should identify which package you have used.

In the days when MLA was relatively new to public health and health services research, authors used to give a general algebraic formulation of their multilevel model. Although by now more researchers are familiar with these models, it may still be useful to detail the actual model used. Particularly if the model that you are using is more complicated or in some way non-standard, providing the full formulation of the model used either in the methods section or in an appendix will aid other researchers understanding of your work and enhance its reproducibility.

The interpretation of the average outcome, variances and regression coefficients sometimes depends on the point of reference taken. Meaningful interpretation can be facilitated by centring independent variables around the mean or another relevant value. Studies do not always state whether or not they centred the data, but this should of course be mentioned.

An important element of the methods section is the description of the modelling strategy. The modelling strategy gives the steps that you are going to take in order to answer your research question or test your hypotheses. A sensible null model should be defined, and you should detail which variables are included in subsequent models and how these variables were selected.

The modelling strategy is not just a summary of the steps taken; it should contain a logical line of reasoning. Chapters 7 and 9 have discussed modelling strategies and working through the example datasets you can see modelling strategy in practice. Snijders and Bosker (2012) give helpful guidance in developing the modelling strategy.

The first step is the definition of your reference model. This might be either an empty model that only estimates the variances or a model including a few basic variables that are deemed necessary to give a fair picture of higher-level variance. The following steps introduce individual-level and/or higher-level variables. These steps are typically evaluated with reference to the first modelling step.

The methods section should enable the reader to replicate the study (at least in principle if not in reality).

The Results Section

The results section reports the findings from your study. You should give the necessary interpretation of your results, but you should also facilitate the reader's own interpretations. Consider, for example, that if variables are on different scales then the interpretation may be difficult. Some variables may be dummies, for example urbanicity may be coded as 0 (non-urban) and 1 (urban), and in the same regression analysis the proportion of the population over 65 may be included, ranging perhaps from 0.12 to 0.25. The coefficients for the two variables are then not comparable; whilst one provides an estimate of the difference between outcomes in urban and non-urban areas, the other gives an estimate of the difference between two non-existent contexts containing no people over the age of 65 and one containing only people over 65.

In quantitative studies, tables play an important part. There are many very different ways of putting the results of an analysis into a table, without a gold standard for reporting multilevel analysis. A table (in general) should be self-contained and give an easy overview. If you want to show several consecutive models in the table, you might wish to avoid an empty column for the reference model by including the variance components in a separate table or as a footnote. If the emphasis is mainly on the higher level and you have a large number of individual-level variables, it might not be necessary to repeat this long list for each modelling step that only involves new higher-level independent variables. The coefficients of the individual-level variables may be largely invariant and could be included in a separate table or in an appendix.

The layout of any table should mirror the modelling strategy. However, it is not always necessary to present each and every step of your modelling strategy in the table. This is particularly the case if steps in the modelling process turn out not to add much information; it may be better to mention that you conducted the steps as intended but, for example, that the results or their interpretation do not differ from other reported models. This is particularly likely to be the case for sensitivity analyses. Again, full results may be reported in appendices or reported as being available from the author.

You should report the variance at the different levels. Even if variation is not at the heart of your study's research questions, it is important for other studies' power calculations. It may also be helpful for readers if you report the intraclass correlation. If your modelling strategy describes a number of subsequent models, you should probably detail changes in variance between models. If you are using logistic regression, you could consider converting variances to a meaningful scale (such as the median odds ratio or MOR; see Chap. 6).

If you report cross-level interactions, it is usually very helpful to your readers if you are able to present these graphically. An example was given earlier in this chapter in Fig. 10.2.

As the presentation of the results in tables is such an important element in terms of enabling your readers to follow and understand your results, we will give a few examples of how your results could be presented in tables. The best advice we can give is to take note when you find articles with a particularly nice presentation.

The first example is the presentation of a table for a two-level linear regression with (for example) an index of health as the dependent variable and independent variables at the individual level (such as age and gender) and at the context level (perhaps neighbourhood social capital). The table columns show the coefficients of the series of models that have been tested, starting from an empty model. The following models are one including only the individual-level variables (model 1), a model with only the contextual variables (model 2) and finally a model with both individual and contextual variables (model 3). Whether or not you need this particular sequence of models depends on your research question and hypotheses and the modelling strategy developed from your research question.

Table 10.1 Example of table layout for a two-level linear regression model

	Model 0 (empty model)	Model 1 (individual-level variables)	Model 2 (context variables)	Model 3 (individual + context variables)
Fixed part				
Intercept	x	x	x	x
Individual variables				
(e.g.) age		x		x
(e.g.) gender		x		x
Context variables				
(e.g.) social capital			x	x
Random part				
Individual-level variance	x	x	x	x
Higher-level variance	x	x	x	x

The table rows show first of all the fixed effects, starting with the overall intercept, followed by the regression coefficients for the variables at individual level and the regression coefficients at higher level. The lower part of the table shows the random part of each model. In the empty model, only the overall intercept and the two variances are estimated. The variances are the unexplained variance in our dependent variable. You could consider adding another row that shows the (change in) model fit. For a linear regression model, this could be the percentage of variance explained in subsequent (nested) models (Table 10.1).

In some cases, it might be convenient to display the random effects in a separate table. This might be the case when your model includes random slopes. The random part will then contain the variance of the slope and the covariance between the slope and the intercept in addition to the variance of the intercept. In the event of a random slope being estimated for a categorical independent variable (such as gender), a useful option is to show the higher-level variance separately for the different categories. Table 10.2 provides an illustration of models showing different formulations of the random part. Note that if variances are shown for the different categories, in this example for men and women, the higher-level intercept variance is not estimated.

The Conclusion and Discussion Section

The conclusion and discussion section should start with a concise description of your main results and, if the study tests a hypothesis, whether or not the hypothesis was refuted. It is important to relate your results to the relevant literature, particularly

Table 10.2 Example of table layout for the random part in different models

Random part	Model 0 (empty model)	Model 3 (individual + context variables) + age random	Model 3 (individual + context variables) + gender random
Individual-level variance	x		
Higher-level intercept variance	x	x	
Slope variance for age		x	
Covariance between age and intercept		x	
Higher-level variance for males			x
Higher-level variance for females			x
Covariance between males and females			x

focusing on differences in results between your study and previous studies and the likely causes of such differences. Some journals ask for a few bullet points on 'what this paper adds'. Even if the journal does not ask for these, it is often helpful to come up with these bullet points for yourself to help to focus the discussion.

This is normally followed by the strengths and weaknesses of the study; you may want to pay particular attention to your data, study design and analytical strategy. Of course, these should be seen against the background of the strengths and weaknesses of other studies in the fields. The strengths and weaknesses should be balanced; there is no reason why this should be an exercise in masochism. If there is a long list of weaknesses and only a few strong points, the authors should probably have undertaken a different (better) study.

It is important for you to provide an interpretation of the meaning of the study. You may come back to your theoretical framework as set out at the beginning of the article and you can discuss the mechanisms underlying the results that you have found and any implications for policy or practice. Finally, it may be worth pointing out any questions that remain unanswered and make suggestions for future research.

None of the above is specific to writing up a multilevel analysis. It is generic to well written research articles and based on an article in the British Medical Journal on structuring the discussion section of a research paper (Docherty and Smith 1999).

Specifically in relation to the discussion section of a multilevel study, it is important to return to the appropriateness of units (and the question as to whether the units that you have used are indeed relevant contexts) and the levels that you have included and excluded.

Conclusions

In this chapter, we have brought two subjects together: critical reading of papers written by others and writing up your own multilevel research. Even if you are only using the results of other people's research, it is important to understand the basics of the methods used. We have developed a number of questions that can help you to get to grips with the multilevel methods applied in published articles. As is true for our advice about writing up your research, our advice on reading other people's research is only in part specific to multilevel analysis. Whatever the methods used, the research questions should be clear and there should be a logical modelling strategy related to the research questions and hypotheses. However, there are also specific issues such as those related to the different levels that one may hypothesise in theory and those encountered in the actual data. When it comes to writing up your research, we have also given some examples of tables. However, there is also a link between reading and writing: look for the things you like about published research, such as understandable ways of putting complicated results into tables or concise ways of formulating conclusions, and avoid forms of presentation on which you are not so keen, such as a surfeit of regression models that add little to the conclusions.

References

Agyemang C, Vrijkotte TGM, Droomers M, Van der VWal MF, Bonsel GJ (2009) The effect of neighbourhood income and deprivation on pregnancy outcomes in Amsterdam, the Netherlands. J Epidemiol Community Health 63:755–760

Arling G, Lewis T, Kane RL, Mueller C, Flood S (2007) Improving quality assessment through multilevel modelling: the case of nursing home compare. Health Serv Res 42:1177–1199

Ball K, Timperio A, Salmon J, Giles-Corti B, Roberts R, Crawford D (2007) Personal, social and environmental determinants of educational inequalities in walking: a multilevel study. J Epidemiol Community Health 61:108–114

Béland F, Birch S, Stoddart G (2002) Unemployment and health: contextual-level influences on the production of health in populations. Soc Sci Med 55:2033–2052

Bensing JM, Caris-Verhallen WMCM, Dekker J, Delnoij DMJ, Groenewegen PP (2003) Doing the right thing and doing it right: toward a framework for assessing the policy relevance of health services research. Int J Technol Assess Health Care 19:604–612

Bingenheimer JB (2005) Multilevel models and scientific progress in social epidemiology. J Epidemiol Community Health 59:438–439

Black JL, Macinko J, Dixon LB, Fryer GE (2010) Neighborhoods and obesity in New York City. Health Place 16:489–499

Docherty M, Smith R (1999) The case for structuring the discussion of scientific papers. Br Med J 318:1224–1225

Eikemo TA, Bambra C, Joyce K, Dahl E (2008) Welfare state regimes and income-related health inequalities: a comparison of 23 European countries. Eur J Public Health 18:593–599

Friele RD, Coppen R, Marquet RL, Gevers JKM (2006) Explaining differences between hospitals in number of organ donors. Am J Transplant 6:539–543

Groenewegen PP, Leufkens HG, Spreeuwenberg P, Worm W (1999) Neighbourhood characteristics and use of benzodiazepines in The Netherlands. Soc Sci Med 48:1701–1711

Hekkert KD, Cihangir S, Kleefstra SM, Van den Berg B, Kool RB (2009) Patient satisfaction revisited: a multilevel analysis. Soc Sci Med 69:68–75

Huizing AR, Hamers JPH, De Jonge J, Candel M, Berger MPF (2007) Organisational determinants in the use of physical restraints: a multilevel approach. Soc Sci Med 65:924–933

Jat TR, Ng N, San Sebastian M (2011) Factors affecting the use of maternal health services in Madhya Pradesh state of India: a multilevel analysis. Int J Equity Health 10:59

Joshu CE, Boehmer TK, Brownson RC, Ewing R (2008) Personal, neighbourhood and urban factors associated with obesity in the United States. J Epidemiol Community Health 62:202–208

Karvonen S, Sipilä P, Martikainen P, Rahkonen O, Laaksonen M (2008) Smoking in context—a multilevel approach to smoking among females in Helsinki. BMC Public Health 8:134

Matteson DW, Burr JA, Marshall JR (1998) Infant mortality: a multi-level analysis of individual and community risk factors. Soc Sci Med 47:1841–1854

Mauny F, Viel JF, Handschumacher P, Sellin B (2004) Multilevel modelling and malaria: a new method for an old disease. Int J Epidemiol 33:1337–1344

Mayo NE, Asano M, Barbic SP (2013) When is a research question not a research question? J Rehabil Med 45:513–518

Merlo J, Gerdtham U-G, Eckerlund I, Håkansson S, Otterblad Olausson P, Pakkanen M, Lindqvist P (2005) Hospital level of care and neonatal mortality in low and high risk deliveries: reassessing the question in Sweden by multilevel analysis. Med Care 43:1092–1100

Mohnen SM, Völker B, Flap H, Subramanian SV, Groenewegen PP (2012) You have to be there to enjoy it? Neighbourhood social capital and health. Eur J Public Health 23:33–39

Moore S, Shiell A, Hawe P, Haines VA (2005) The privileging of communitarian ideas: citation practices and the translation of social capital into public health research. Am J Public Health 95:1330–1337

Nicholson A, Rose R, Bobak M (2009) Association between attendance at religious services and self-reported health in 22 European countries. Soc Sci Med 69:519–528

Pornet C, Dejardin O, Morlais F, Bouvier V, Launoy G (2011) Socioeconomic determinants for compliance to colorectal cancer screening: a multilevel analysis. J Epidemiol Community Health 64:318–324

Rathmann K, Ottova V, Hurrelmann K, de Looze M, Levin K, Molcho M, Elgar F, Gabhainn SN, van Dijk JP, Richter M (2015) Macro-level determinants of young people's subjective health and health inequalities: a multilevel analysis in 27 welfare states. Maturitas 80:414–420

Renders CM, Valk GD, Franse LV, Schellevis FG, van Eijk JT, Van der Wal G (2001) Long-term effectiveness of a quality improvement program for patients with type 2 diabetes in general practice. Diabetes Care 24:1365–1370

Sellström E, Arnoldsson G, Bremberg S, Hjern A (2008) The neighbourhood they live in—does it matter to women's smoking habits during pregnancy? Health Place 14:155–166

Sixma H, Spreeuwenberg P, Zuidgeest M, Rademakers J (2009) [Consumer Quality Index hospital stay]. NIVEL, Utrecht

Snijders TAB, Bosker RJ (2012) Multilevel analysis: an introduction to basic and advanced multilevel modeling. Sage, Los Angeles

Stafford M, Gimeno D, Marmot MG (2008) Neighbourhood characteristics and trajectories of health functioning: a multilevel prospective analysis. Eur J Public Health 18:604–610

Turrell G, Kavanagh A, Draper G, Subramanian SV (2007) Do places affect the probability of death in Australia? A multilevel study of area-level disadvantage, individual-level socioeconomic position and all-cause mortality, 1998-2000. J Epidemiol Community Health 61:13–19

van Berkestijn LG, Kastein MR, Lodder A, de Melker RA, Bartelink ML (1999) How do we compare with our colleagues? Quality of general practitioner performance in consultations for non-acute abdominal complaints. International Journal for Quality in Healh Care 11:475–486

Van Stam M-A, Michielsen K, Stroeken K, Zijlstra BJH (2014) The impact of education and globalization on sexual and reproductive health: retrospective evidence from eastern and southern Africa. AIDS Care 26:379–386

Van Yperen NW, Snijders TAB (2000) A multilevel analysis of the demands-control model: is stress at work determined by factors at the group level or the individual level? J Occup Health Psychol 5:182–190

Verstappen W, ten Riet G, van der Weijden T, Hermsen J, Grol R (2005) Variation in requests for imaging investigations by general practitioners: a multilevel analysis. J Health Serv Res Policy 10:25–30

Witvliet MI, Kunst AE, Stronks K, Arah OA (2012) Assessing where vulnerable groups fare worst: a global multilevel analysis on the impact of welfare regimes on disability across different socioeconomic groups. J Epidemiol Community Health 66:775–781

Part 4
Multilevel Analysis using MLwiN

11

Multilevel Linear Regression through a Specialist Multilevel Modeling Software

Abstract In this chapter, the reader becomes a user. This chapter contains the first of three tutorials that readers can work through, using the specialist multilevel modelling software MLwiN. We introduce MLwiN as a package; this software will also be used in the other two tutorials. This tutorial introduces practical linear multilevel analysis. It uses data on mortality in England and Wales over time. The dependent or outcome variable is the standard mortality ratio in a given year between 1972 and 1996, for districts which are nested within counties.

Because this is the first tutorial, we go into some detail regarding the use of MLwiN, and how to use it to manipulate and explore the data. The tutorial starts with the estimation of a single-level model, then moves on to a two-level and three-level model. We begin with a random intercept model and progress to a random slope model. Throughout the tutorial graphs are used to enable visualisation of the results of the analyses. At the end of this tutorial, we detail an alternative analysis of the data using a multilevel Poisson model.

Keywords Tutorial · Multilevel analysis · Linear regression · Poisson regression · Mortality

This chapter is based on training materials created by Leyland and McLeod (2000). The training materials in this chapter and the two chapters that follow are designed to be used either constituting part of a formal course or as a self-learning aid. They provide an introduction to the ideas behind multilevel modelling and a guide to analysis using the software package MLwiN. Further details on multilevel modelling and MLwiN are available from the Centre for Multilevel Modelling http://www.bristol.ac.uk/cmm/. The materials have been written for MLwiN v3.01. The teaching version of the software is available from https://www.bristol.ac.uk/cmm/software/mlwin/download/.

When working through the examples in this book, the user should periodically save the worksheet. Throughout these materials the instructions to the user appear in boxes. Selections to be made by the user appear in **bold type**, and variable names are given in CAPITALS. If you have to click on a term in an equation, this is presented in ***bold and italics***.

Introduction to the Dataset

The data are taken from the local mortality datapack and detail deaths from all causes in England and Wales in the period 1979–1992. These data can be found at the UK Data Service. The raw data comprise two files: one containing information on deaths over this time period and the other detailing the populations of the relevant areas (districts in England and Wales) in each year. For further information on this and other available datasets, the user should visit the UK Data Service website https://discover.ukdataservice.ac.uk/.

Research Questions

In this tutorial, we will answer the following research questions:

1. What is happening to mortality rates over time?
2. How much variation in mortality rates is there between districts of England and Wales?
3. Is this variation just between districts, or are there also differences between the mortality rates of counties?
4. Does mortality vary according to the type of area?
5. What is happening to the variation in mortality rates over time?

Introduction to MLwiN

Opening a Worksheet

MLwiN files are known as worksheets and these store all the data and model settings from the last saved version. We will start by opening the file '*lmdp.wsz*'—an MLwiN worksheet that has already been prepared for analysis.

In MLwiN, go to the **File** menu
Select **Open worksheet**
Navigate to the folder containing the data file
Open the worksheet called **lmdp.ws**

The name of the current file appears in the bar at the top of the MLwiN window.

Names Window

We can view a summary of this worksheet using the **Names** window. This will automatically appear when a worksheet is opened in MLwiN; at other times, the **Names** window can be called up as follows:

> Go to the **Data manipulation** menu
> Select **Names**

This shows a list of all the variables stored in the worksheet together with some summary information. The worksheet contains 8 variables; these are at the beginning of the worksheet in columns number 1–8. Each column contains 5639 data points and no missing values. Each data point (observation) corresponds to the annual number of deaths in a given district in England and Wales for 1 year in the period 1979–1992. COUNTY, DISTRICT and REGION are area identifiers; there are 403 county DISTRICTs (coded from 101 to 6820) which are nested within 54 COUNTYs (coded from 1 to 68), and these in turn lie within 1 of 10 REGIONs. The data cover 14 YEARs from 1979 to 1992 inclusive. Note that there are only 5639 data points rather than the 5642 that might be expected (403 DISTRICTs with an observation for each of 14 years); 3 data points have been removed because extreme outlying values made them implausible. The next two columns show the number of DEATHS observed in each district at each time point—ranging from 16 to 12,775—and the number that would be EXPECTED. The EXPECTED number of deaths has been calculated on the basis of the age and sex structure of that area's population in each year by applying the 1992 national age- and sex-specific mortality rates. This worksheet has been constructed using the two raw data files contained in the local mortality datapack—the number of deaths and the populations. The OBSERVED and EXPECTED deaths are combined to form the standardised mortality ratio (SMR) for each year in each district. This is calculated as

$$\text{SMR} = \frac{\text{observed deaths}}{\text{expected deaths}} \times 100$$

and reflects the excess deaths in an area, standardised for age and sex, over the national average mortality rate in 1992 (average = 100). The standardisation means that differences between areas in the age and sex structures of their populations are taken into account. The range from 75 to 179 implies a minimum mortality rate for one area in 1 year 25% below the 1992 average and a maximum 79% above the average. Finally, the variable FAMILY is a classification of districts into six groups devised by the UK's Office for National Statistics: 1—Inner London, 2—Rural areas, 3—Prospering areas, 4—Maturer areas, 5—Urban centres, 6—Mining and industrial areas. All of the remaining columns are empty; the default name for such columns is 'C' followed by the column number.

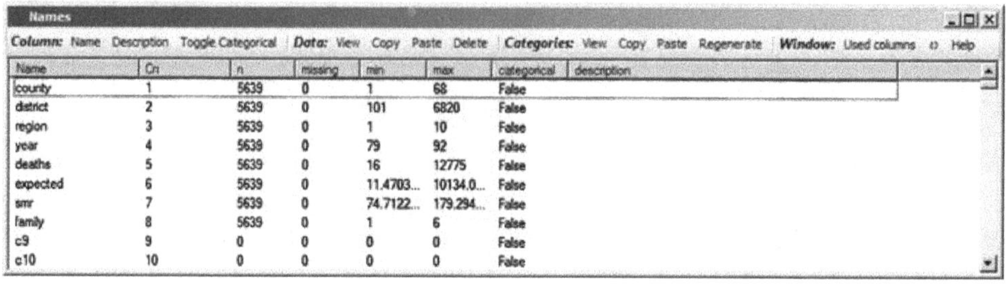

Name	Cn	n	missing	min	max	categorical	description
county	1	5639	0	1	68	False	
district	2	5639	0	101	6820	False	
region	3	5639	0	1	10	False	
year	4	5639	0	79	92	False	
deaths	5	5639	0	16	12775	False	
expected	6	5639	0	11.4703...	10134.0...	False	
smr	7	5639	0	74.7122...	179.294...	False	
family	8	5639	0	1	6	False	
c9	9	0	0	0	0	False	
c10	10	0	0	0	0	False	

Data Window

The data may be viewed and edited in a spreadsheet format.

Go to the **Data manipulation** menu
Select **View or edit data**
Alternatively, the **Data** window may be accessed from the **Names** window:
In the **Names** window, highlight columns 1–8 (use the shift or control keys to highlight multiple columns)
Click the **View** button in the **Data** section at the top of the **Names** window

The **view** button at the top of the **Data** window can be used to change or extend the selection of variables shown; simply select the desired variables from the drop-down list.

All windows can be re-sized by clicking on the borders and dragging; also the scroll bars at the bottom and on the right-hand side can be used to view more of the selected data.

Data

goto line 1 | View | Show value labels | Font | Help

	county(5639)	district(5639)	region(5639)	year(5639)	deaths(5639)	expected(5639)	smr(5639)	family(5639)
1	1.000	101.000	3.000	79.000	50.000	36.072	138.611	1.000
2	1.000	101.000	3.000	81.000	28.000	28.159	99.435	1.000
3	1.000	101.000	3.000	82.000	53.000	37.721	140.506	1.000
4	1.000	101.000	3.000	83.000	43.000	38.468	111.780	1.000
5	1.000	101.000	3.000	84.000	41.000	39.181	104.642	1.000
6	1.000	101.000	3.000	85.000	34.000	32.200	105.592	1.000
7	1.000	101.000	3.000	86.000	32.000	38.185	83.803	1.000
8	1.000	101.000	3.000	87.000	38.000	37.363	101.706	1.000
9	1.000	101.000	3.000	88.000	28.000	37.477	74.712	1.000
10	1.000	101.000	3.000	89.000	30.000	36.463	82.275	1.000
11	1.000	101.000	3.000	90.000	38.000	35.658	106.569	1.000
12	1.000	101.000	3.000	91.000	43.000	32.528	132.193	1.000
13	1.000	101.000	3.000	92.000	32.000	37.279	85.840	1.000
14	1.000	111.000	3.000	79.000	2160.000	1533.833	140.824	6.000
15	1.000	111.000	3.000	80.000	2094.000	1526.076	137.215	6.000
16	1.000	111.000	3.000	81.000	2081.000	1568.919	132.639	6.000
17	1.000	111.000	3.000	82.000	2041.000	1585.704	128.713	6.000
18	1.000	111.000	3.000	83.000	2011.000	1582.598	127.070	6.000
19	1.000	111.000	3.000	84.000	1854.000	1595.079	116.233	6.000
20	1.000	111.000	3.000	85.000	1997.000	1604.626	124.453	6.000
21	1.000	111.000	3.000	86.000	1971.000	1604.318	122.856	6.000
22	1.000	111.000	3.000	87.000	1868.000	1610.334	116.001	6.000
23	1.000	111.000	3.000	88.000	1864.000	1609.627	115.803	6.000
24	1.000	111.000	3.000	89.000	1760.000	1604.886	109.665	6.000

The first 13 observations are made on DISTRICT 101, COUNTY 1, REGION 3. The 13 observations on this DISTRICT can be seen to correspond to 13 YEARs of data; there is no observation for 1980. The estimated SMR in this district ranges from 75 in 1988 to 141 in 1982. The district classification (FAMILY) was group 1—Inner London.

Graph Window

Before starting to model the data, we may wish to examine them in a graph.

> Go to the **Graphs** menu
> Select **Customised Graphs**

The graphical output in MLwiN is separated into three components. A *display* is what can be displayed on the computer screen at any one time and up to ten different displays may be specified. The pull-down menu at the top left-hand corner of the customised graph window corresponds to the display function—this currently shows **D1** denoting display 1. Each display can contain a number of *graphs*. A graph is a frame with x and y (horizontal and vertical) axes showing lines, points or bars, and each display can show an array of up to 5 × 5 graphs. The **position** tab towards the top right of the customised graph window is used to specify the layout—the position of the graphs in the display. Finally, each graph can plot one or more *datasets*, each one consisting of a set of x and y coordinates selected from the worksheet columns. Different datasets may be specified by clicking on different rows in the table under the **ds#** heading shown at the left-hand side of the customised graph display.

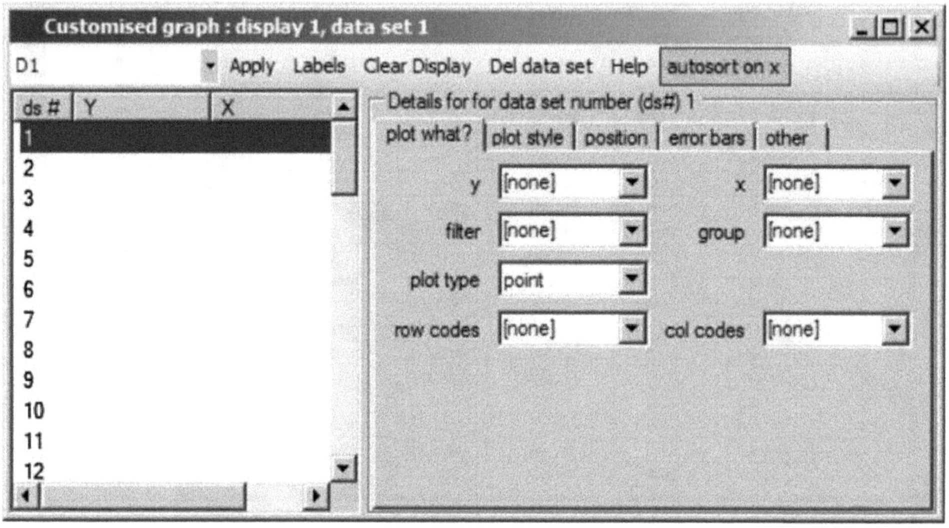

To obtain a scatter plot of SMRs by year, ensure that the **plot what?** tab is selected and

Select the **y** variable to be SMR from the drop-down list
Select the **x** variable to be YEAR from the drop-down list
Click the **Apply** button

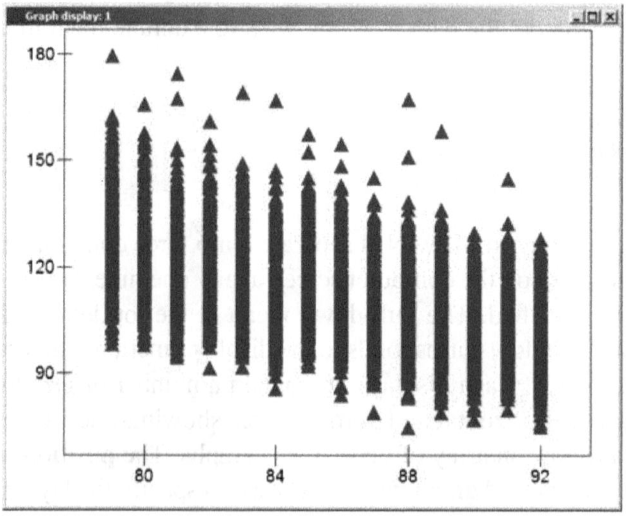

It is clear that there have been considerable reductions in SMR over these 14 years; nearly every district had an SMR greater than 100 in 1979. (The fact that standardisation was to 1992 means that the overall SMR—for the whole of England and Wales—was 100 for that year.)

To change this graph to a line plot with a line for each district:

In the **Customised Graph** window, select **group** to be DISTRICT
Change **plot type** to **line**
Select the **plot style** tab
Change **colour** to **rotate**
Click the **Apply** button

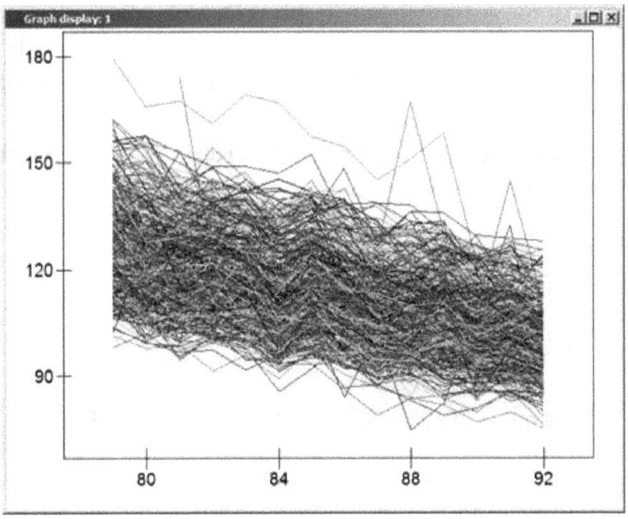

It is possible to identify points on the graph: point and click anywhere on the graph and the **Graph options** window will appear with details of the closest data point. Also included in the **Graph options** window are facilities for adding titles to the graph and axes, and for making other changes to the display including the scales.

Closing Windows

At any time you may wish to close or minimise windows to prevent your screen from becoming too cluttered. You may do this, as with any other Windows package, by clicking on the X or _ buttons respectively in the top right corner of each window. Alternatively, you may go to the **Window** menu and select **close all windows**.

This section has covered data exploration using:
Names window—data summaries

(continued)

Data window—spreadsheet
Graph—scatter plot
Graph—line graph

Model Specification

Creating New Variables

A number of functions are available in MLwiN that allow the creation of new variables or amendments to existing variables. In order to include a constant or intercept term in a model using MLwiN, we need to create a column of 1's that spans the entire data set. This variable will also be used to model the variance at each level in a multilevel model. We use the **Generate vector** window to create a column containing 5639 occurrences of the value 1.

Go to **Data manipulation** menu
Select **Generate vector**
Select **Type of vector** to be **Constant vector**
Select C9 to be the **Output column**
Enter 5639 (the number of data points) beside **Number of copies**
Enter 1 beside **Value**
Click the **Generate** button

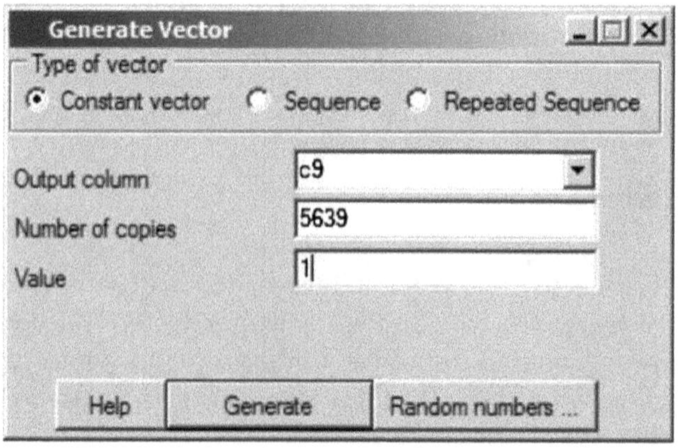

Returning to the **Names** window, column C9 now contains 5639 data points each with the value of 1. We can give this new variable a name:

Click on C9 in the **Names** window
Click on the **Name** button in the Column section at the top of the window
Type CONS and press <return>

We can also use the **Generate vector** window to create a unique identifier for every data point or observation.

In the **Generate vector** window:
Select **Type of vector** to be **Sequence**
Select C10 to be the **Output column**
Enter 1 beside **Start number**
Enter 5639 (the number of data points) beside **End number**
Enter 1 beside **Step value**
Click the **Generate** button

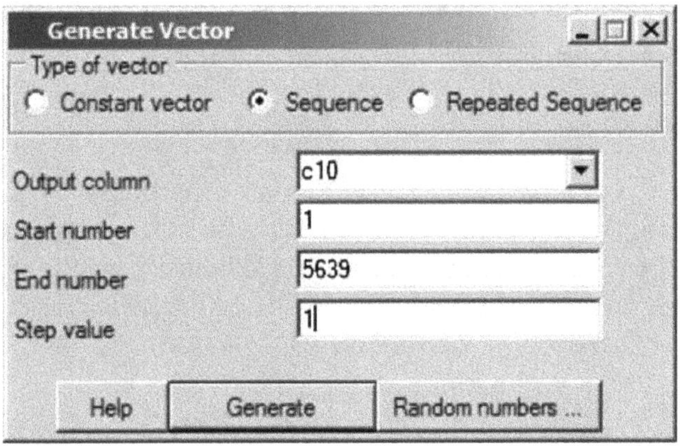

In the **Names** window, column C10 should now contain 5639 data points with a minimum of 1 and a maximum of 5639. We will name this variable:

Click on C10 in the **Names** window
Click on **Name** at the top of the window
Type ID and press <return>

Equations Window

Specifying models in MLwiN is done mainly via the **Equations** window.

Go to **Models** menu
Select **Equations**

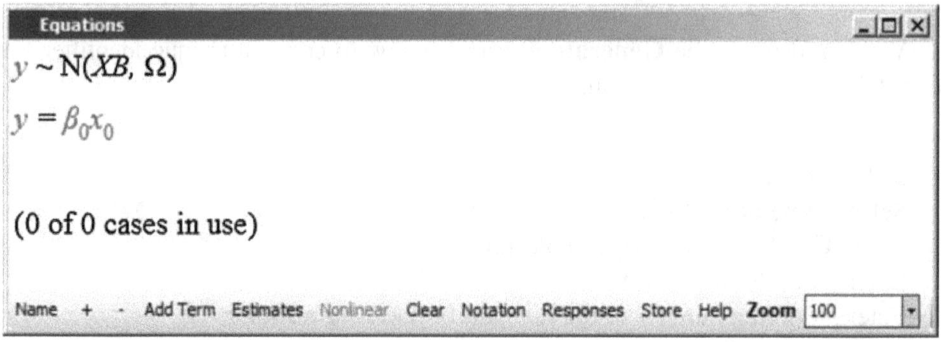

The terms in red are those which must be defined before a model can be fitted to the data. We begin by specifying our outcome:

Click on either of the ***y*** terms
Select SMR as the dependent variable

The structure of the hierarchical model is also specified at this stage, first by stating the number of levels the model will have and then by specifying what the levels of the hierarchy are using the appropriate identifier variables. We will start by fitting a single-level (Ordinary Least Squares—OLS) model. The level 1 units, our observations, are identified by the variable ID.

Select 1 – i for **N levels**
Select ID for **level 1(i)**
Click on **Done**

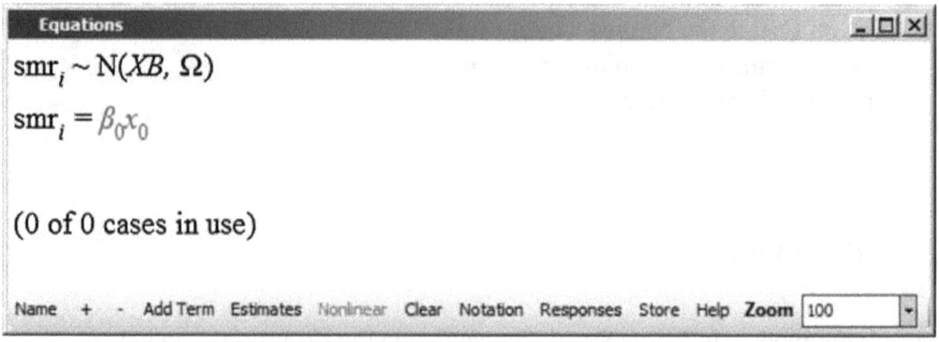

The red response variable ***y*** has been replaced by the term $\boldsymbol{smr_i}$, the black colour indicating that this term has been defined; moreover, the addition of a subscript

i indicates that this is a single-level model. In a similar manner, we can define CONS—the column of 1's that we just created—to be an independent variable.

> Click on the $\boldsymbol{\beta}_0\boldsymbol{x}_0$ term
> Select CONS from the drop-down list

The check boxes indicate in what part of the model each variable is to be included; by default, CONS has been added to the fixed part of the model and its coefficient will provide an estimate of the intercept. The other option in this window relates to the random part of the model. We allow for random error at level 1 by setting the CONStant term to be random at this level.

> Click on the check box by **i(ID)**
> Click on **Done**

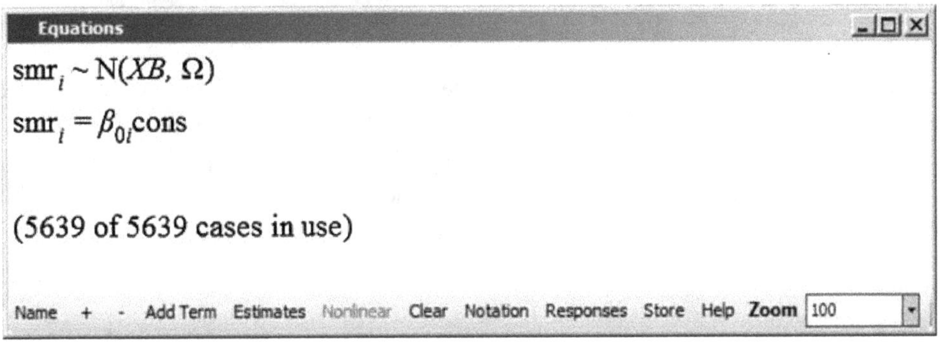

Note that the term $\boldsymbol{\beta}_0$ changes to $\boldsymbol{\beta}_{0i}$, denoting the fact that it is random at level 1 (between occasions).

To expand this model to see the distributional assumptions and error structure, click twice on the '+' at the bottom of the **Equations** window.

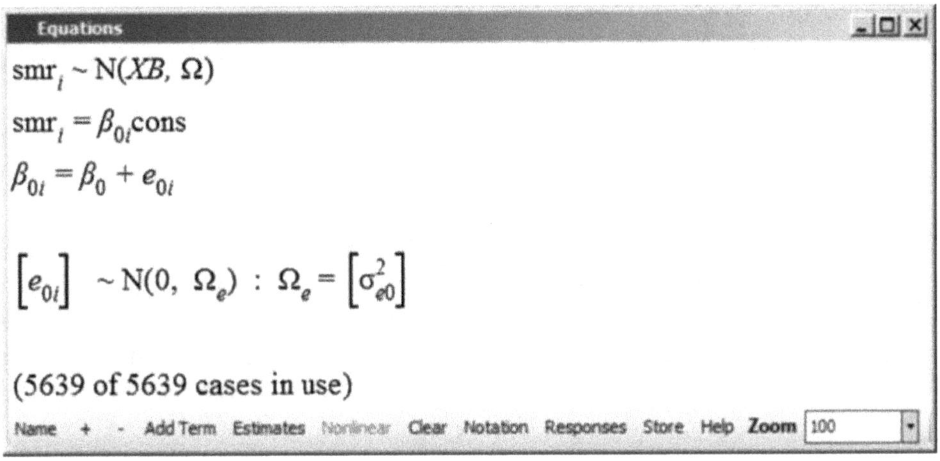

This shows our assumption of a normal distribution for the residuals $e_{0i} \sim N(0, \sigma_{e0}^2)$. At any time we can toggle between the representation of the model that includes the names of all of the variables and a purely algebraic representation; simply click on the **Name** button at the bottom of the **Equation** window.

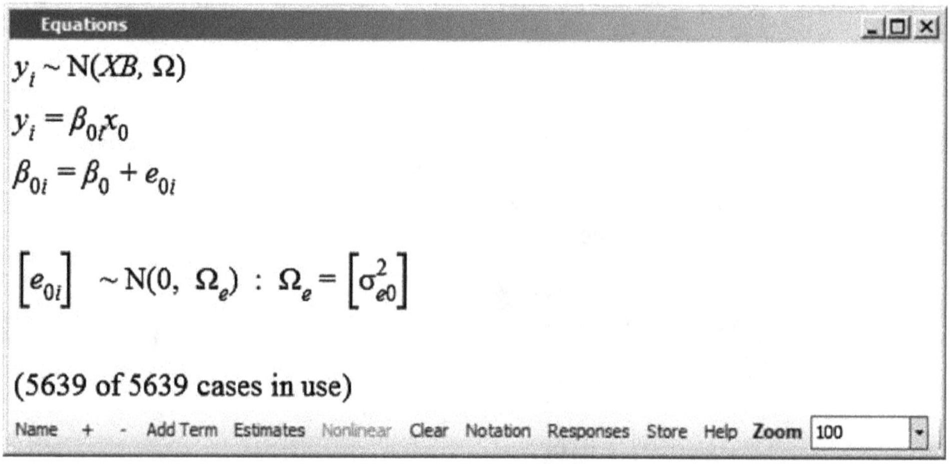

Note that the names of the specified dependent and independent variables, SMR and CONS, have been replaced by $\boldsymbol{y}$ and $\boldsymbol{x}$. If you click on the **Estimates** button, you can see that two terms in the model are blue: the grand intercept $\boldsymbol{\beta}_0$ and the level 1 variance $\boldsymbol{\sigma}_{e0}^2$. The fact that they are blue indicates that these terms are to be estimated; when the model converges, the blue will change to green.

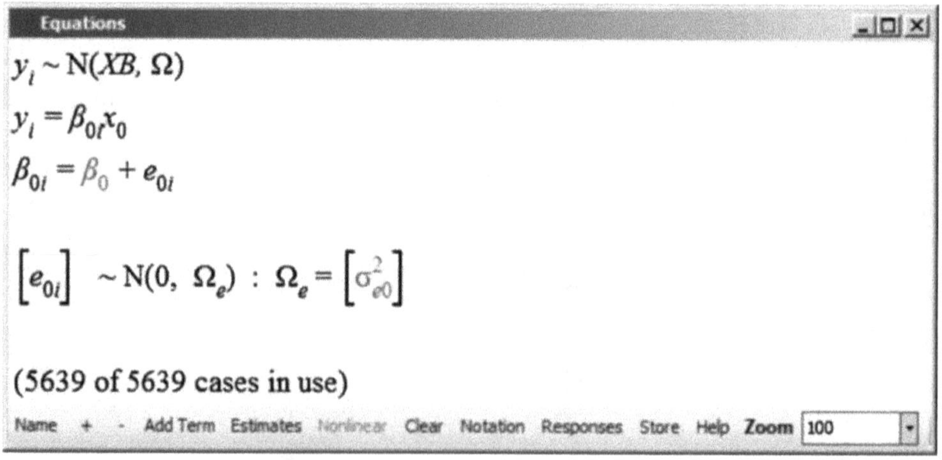

Clicking on the **Estimates** button again will replace these two terms with their current estimates (both the default value of 0.000 because no model has yet been estimated). Since our variable CONS is just a column of 1's, the above equation is just fitting the SMR of the *i*th observation using a mean $\boldsymbol{\beta}_0$ and a residual or error term $\boldsymbol{e}_{0i}$. We are going to begin by assuming that these $\boldsymbol{e}_{0i}$ are independent and identically distributed. This means that if the SMR in a particular DISTRICT is higher than the mean one YEAR, we believe that the SMR in another YEAR is just as likely to be below the mean as above. In other words, we are fitting a model that assumes that there will not be certain DISTRICTs with persistently high SMRs and others where mortality is consistently below the mean.

In addition to the mean, we will add year as an independent variable in the fixed part of the model in order to answer our first research question.

Click on the **Add Term** button
Select YEAR from the drop-down list under **variable** in the **Specify term** window
Click **Done**

The third term to be estimated, β_1, is the regression coefficient (slope) associated with YEAR and this will estimate the trend in SMRs during the study period.

Fitting the Model

The model is now ready to be estimated.

Click the **Start** button on the tool bar at the top left-hand corner of the MLwiN screen

After two iterations (the iteration number is given at the bottom of the MLwiN screen), the model converges; the blue estimates in the equation window turn green, indicating that they have converged.

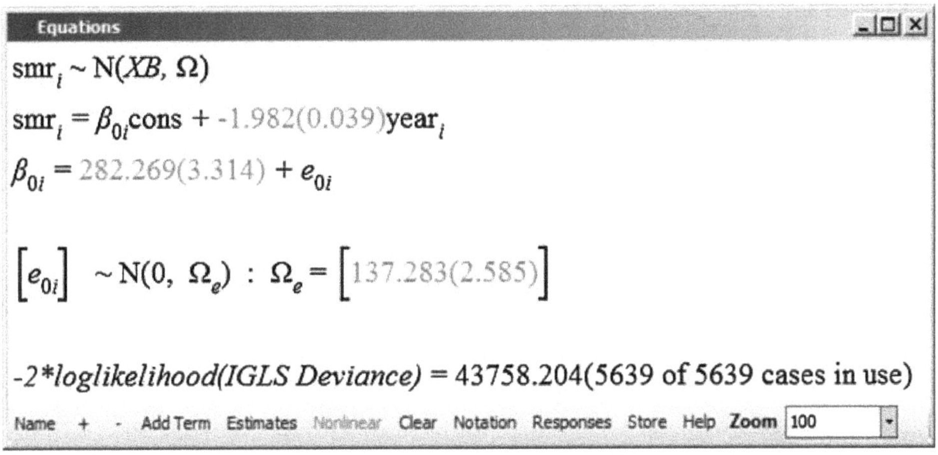

The parameter estimates are shown with their estimated standard errors in brackets. Our intercept is about 282, and the SMR has been decreasing at 1.982 per year. This decrease is highly significant in comparison with its standard error; a 95% confidence interval around this decrease would range from $1.982 \pm 1.96 * 0.039 = (1.906, 2.058)$. The variance of all of the observations around this fitted trend is 137. This means that the standard deviation is $\sqrt{137.283} = 11.717$ and so 95% of observations lie within ± 22.965 of the mean in any given year. The current model has a single term to describe the variation around the mean and is therefore just an ordinary least squares (OLS) regression model, but it is a starting point for our multilevel analysis. The value $-2{*}$*loglikelihood* is provided as an aid to model comparison and selection.

Before continuing, consider the interpretation of the intercept term. This is the predicted value of the SMR in all districts when the variable YEAR takes the value 0: in other words, in 1900. Since the data do not cover this period, it is not sensible to make any inference about the SMR at this time, and we can change the origin to something more meaningful. Explanatory variables are frequently centred around an average value; in this case, however, we will set the origin at the first year for which we have data (1979). We can use the **Equations** window to change this to a new variable which takes the value 0 in 1979 and 13 in 1982.

> In the **Equation** window, click on the term $\boldsymbol{year_i}$ in the equation
> Select **Modify term** in the X variable window
> In the **centring** section of the **Specify term** window, check **around value** and
> type **79** in the corresponding box
> Click **Done**

You will notice in the **Equations** window that the term $\boldsymbol{year_i}$ has been replaced by $(\boldsymbol{year} - 79)_i$. As the model has changed the estimates have changed from green to blue, indicating that we need to re-estimate this model. Note also that the new

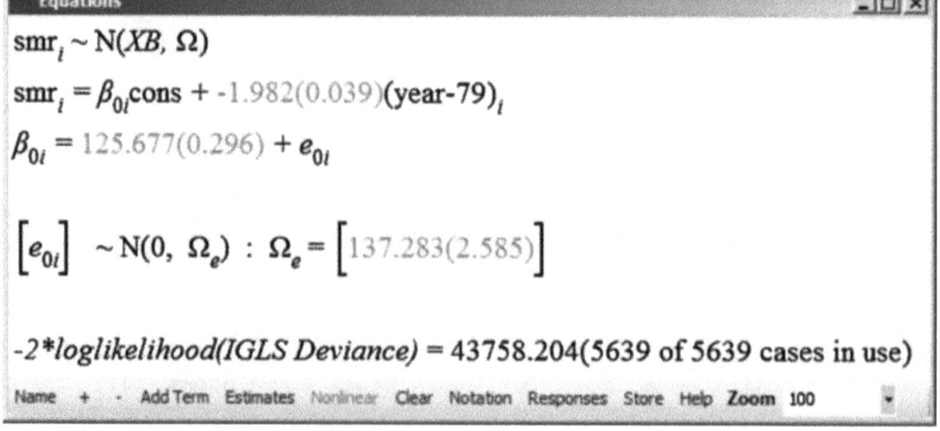

variable appears in column 11 in the **Names** window. Rather than click on the **Start** button again to estimate this model, click on the **More** button in the top left-hand corner of the MLwiN screen to continue estimation from the current values.

The estimated slope has not changed and nor has the variance. There is, however, a big change in the intercept. In 1979, the average SMR was therefore about 126.

We can store the results of successive models to allow easy comparison.

Click on the **Store** button at the bottom of the **Equations** window
Enter a suitable name in the box in the **Model name** window, e.g. Trend 1-level
Click **OK**

This section has covered data manipulation using:
Generate vector window—creating a constant
Generate vector window—creating a sequence
Name window—naming variables
This section has also covered model set-up using:
Equations window—defining the response (dependent variable)
Equations window—adding an intercept (CONS)
Equations window—adding an explanatory (independent) variable
Equations window—modelling random error at level 1
Estimating a model—the **Start** and **More** buttons
Equations window—modifying a term in the regression model
Centring the data to assist model interpretation
Equations window—storing results

Variance Components

All of the variance in the current model is at the lowest level of observation; this is just an ordinary least squares (OLS) regression equation. This model may be expanded by including the level of DISTRICT in the model, enabling us to partition the variance into that which is attributable to random variation between DISTRICTs and that which arises due to fluctuations between observations (YEARs) within DISTRICTs.

A 2-Level Variance Components Model

In the **Equations** window, we want to specify that our model has two levels, identified by DISTRICT (at level 2) and ID (at level 1).

Click on either ***smr$_i$*** term
Change **N levels** to *2 – ij*
Select DISTRICT from the drop-down list by **level 2(j)**
Click **Done**

We now need to fit a random intercept across DISTRICTs. We do this by allowing the coefficient of the CONStant to vary randomly across DISTRICTs as well as at level 1.

Click on β_{0i}
Check the box by **j(DISTRICT)**
Click **Done**

The intercept term now has an additional subscript (j), indicating that it varies across DISTRICTs as well as across YEARs. The intercept now has three parts: the overall fixed part intercept for 1979, the error term e_{0ij} and a term u_{0j} which is specific to DISTRICT *j*. The u_{0j} are random effects at level 2 and are assumed to be normally distributed. The intercept for the *j*th district in 1979 will be given by $\beta_0 + u_{0j}$. The parameter estimates have again changed from green to blue, indicating that the model has changed and must be estimated again.

Equations

$$\text{smr}_{ij} \sim \text{N}(XB, \Omega)$$

$$\text{smr}_{ij} = \beta_{0ij}\text{cons} + -1.982(0.039)(\text{year-79})_{ij}$$

$$\beta_{0ij} = 125.677(0.296) + u_{0j} + e_{0ij}$$

$$\left[u_{0j}\right] \sim \text{N}(0,\ \Omega_u) \ :\ \Omega_u = \left[0.000(0.000)\right]$$

$$\left[e_{0ij}\right] \sim \text{N}(0,\ \Omega_e) \ :\ \Omega_e = \left[137.283(2.585)\right]$$

*-2*loglikelihood(IGLS Deviance)* = 43758.204(5639 of 5639 cases in use)

UNITS:

district: 403 (of 403) in use

Name + - Add Term Estimates Nonlinear Clear Notation Responses Store Help **Zoom** 100

Sorting the Data

Before fitting a multilevel model, the data need to be sorted within their hierarchy (in this example by DISTRICTs and then by ID within DISTRICT). If your data are not sorted, then MLwiN will produce estimates but these will not be correct. *Failure to sort your data when using MLwiN is a common reason for getting 'strange' results!*

Go to **Data manipulation** menu
Select **Sort**
Increase the **Number of keys to sort on** to 2
Select DISTRICT as the first **Key code column** and ID as the second
Select all named variables, from COUNTY to (YEAR-79), under the heading **Input columns**
Press **Same as input** button to overwrite current columns with sorted data
Press **Add to action list** and then **Execute**

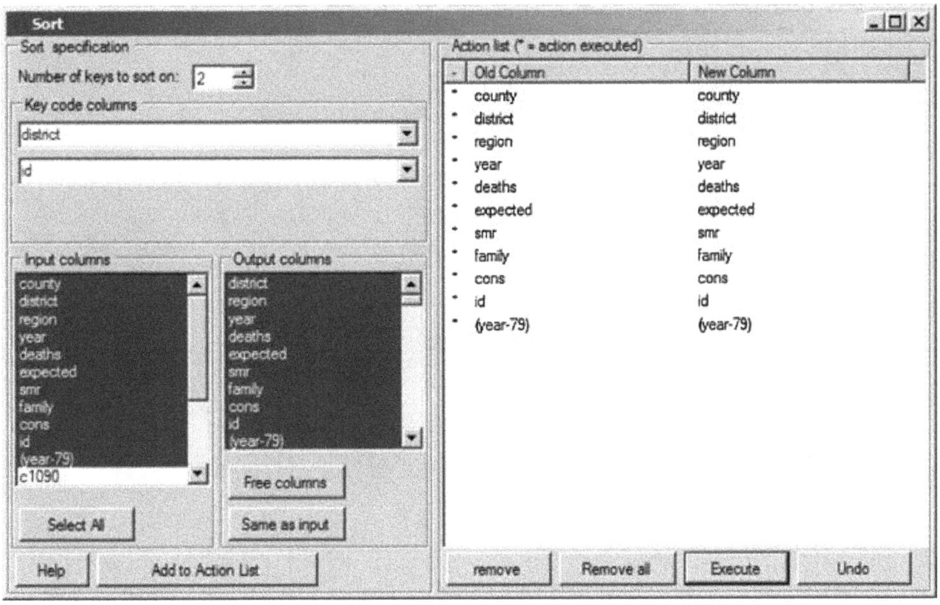

This model may now be fitted by clicking **More**.

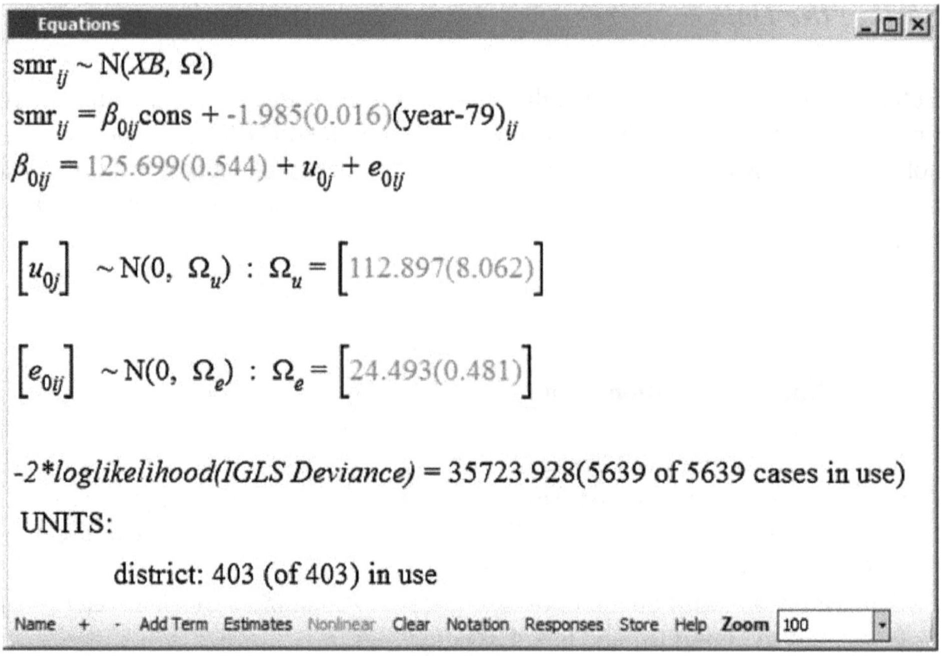

If we store these results, we can then make a comparison with the OLS estimates previously obtained.

Click on the **Store** button at the bottom of the **Equations** window
Enter a suitable name in the box in the **Model name** window, e.g. Trend 2-level
Click **OK**
Go to the **Model** menu
Select **Compare stored models**

Results Table

Copy

	Trend 1-level	S.E.	Trend 2-level	S.E.
Response	smr		smr	
Fixed Part				
cons	125.677	0.296	125.699	0.544
(year-79)	-1.982	0.039	-1.985	0.016
Random Part				
Level: cons				
Level: id				
Var(cons)	137.283	2.585	24.493	0.481
Level: district				
Var(cons)			112.897	8.062
Units: cons	1			
Units: id	5639		5639	
Units: district			403	
Estimation:	IGLS		IGLS	
-2*loglikelihood:	43758.204		35723.928	

There is little change in the estimates of the intercept and slope between the two models. However, in the random part most of the variation has moved up to level 2, indicating that there is substantial variation between DISTRICTs rather than year-on-year variation within DISTRICTs. The total variance in our second model is obtained by summing the variances between and within DISTRICTs ($\sigma_{u0}^2 + \sigma_{e0}^2$); the label 'CONS/CONS' in the first column indicates that these terms are the variances of the intercepts (remembering that we created and used the variable CONS to model the variance at each level). The total variance in our 'Trend 2-level' model is 137.390, very close to the estimate of 137.283 obtained for σ_{e0}^2 in our 'Trend 1-level' model. The proportion of the total variance which arises due to differences between DISTRICTs is 112.897/(112.897 + 24.493) or 82.2%. This figure is known as the *intra-unit* or *intraclass correlation*, and indicates that the correlation between two observations made in different years on the same DISTRICT is 0.822. The level 1 variance may be interpreted as the variation between years within DISTRICTs. So, in answer to the second research question, it would appear that the majority of the variation in mortality is due to between-district differences rather than year-on-year fluctuations.

Note that the addition of a single variance term has produced a substantial reduction in the value of $-2*\log(\text{likelihood})$ from 43758 to 35724. This reduction has been brought about by the addition of a single parameter—the variance σ^2_{u0}—to our single-level model. Changes in the value of $-2*\log(\text{likelihood})$ for nested models (that is, for models that differ only by having terms added) are assessed using a chi-squared distribution with the number of degrees of freedom equivalent to the number of additional parameters. Since the reduction in $-2*\log(\text{likelihood})$ is of the order of 8000, we can dispense with the formal hypothesis testing (which will be covered later in this chapter) and conclude that the full model—that including the level of DISTRICT—is a significant improvement on the single-level model.

Predictions and confidence envelopes
At this stage, you may wish to look at the section Predictions and confidence envelopes at the end of this chapter. This compares the precision of estimates from the 2-level model with those from a single-level model. The work is in a section at the end of this chapter because it covers predictions, a subject which is given more attention later in this tutorial. You may read through this section or work through the example, in which case you will be prompted to save your worksheet at the current point. Alternatively, you can save the worksheet now as, for example, lmdpapp1.wsz and return to this section later.

The Hierarchy Viewer

We can view the data structure using the **Hierarchy viewer**. This will tell us how many lower-level units are in each high level unit.

Go to **Model** menu
Select **Hierarchy Viewer**

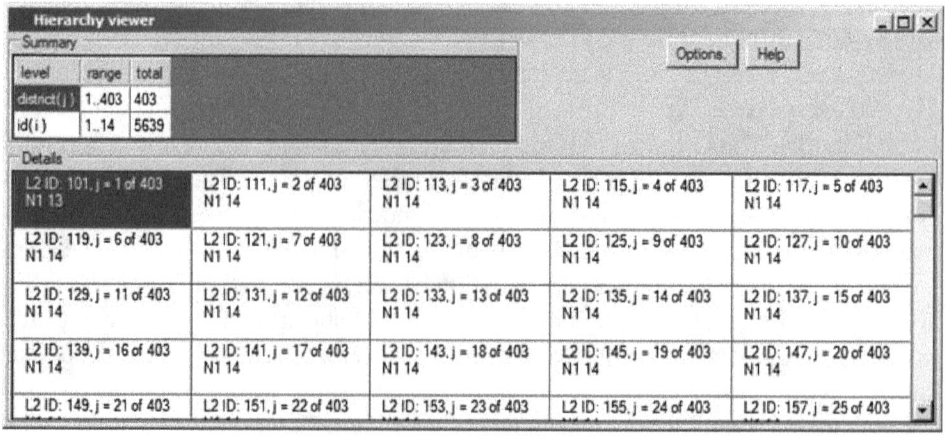

The box in the top left corner provides a summary of the data hierarchy: there are 403 DISTRICTs at level 2 and up to 14 observations at level 1 (defined by ID) within each DISTRICT, with a total of 5639 observations. Every level 2 unit (DISTRICT) has a box in the grid in the main part of the **Hierarchy viewer** screen; the first level 2 unit has identifying code 101 and has 13 level 1 units (observations). The second DISTRICT has identifying code 111 and so on. (These identifying codes are those found in the column DISTRICT.) The **Hierarchy viewer** is a useful tool to check that your data structure is correctly specified; failure to sort the data, for example, may lead to a data structure containing too many high level units.

Adding a Further Level

We can add COUNTY as a third level to the model and examine the relative importance of these large areas compared to the smaller DISTRICTs. First sort the data again according to this new hierarchy of COUNTY then DISTRICT then ID.

Go to **Data manipulation** menu
Select **Sort**
Increase the **Number of keys to sort on** to 3
Select COUNTY as the first **Key code column,** DISTRICT as the second and ID as the third
Select all named variables under the heading **Input columns**
Press **Same as input** button to overwrite current columns with sorted data
Press **Add to action list** and then **Execute**

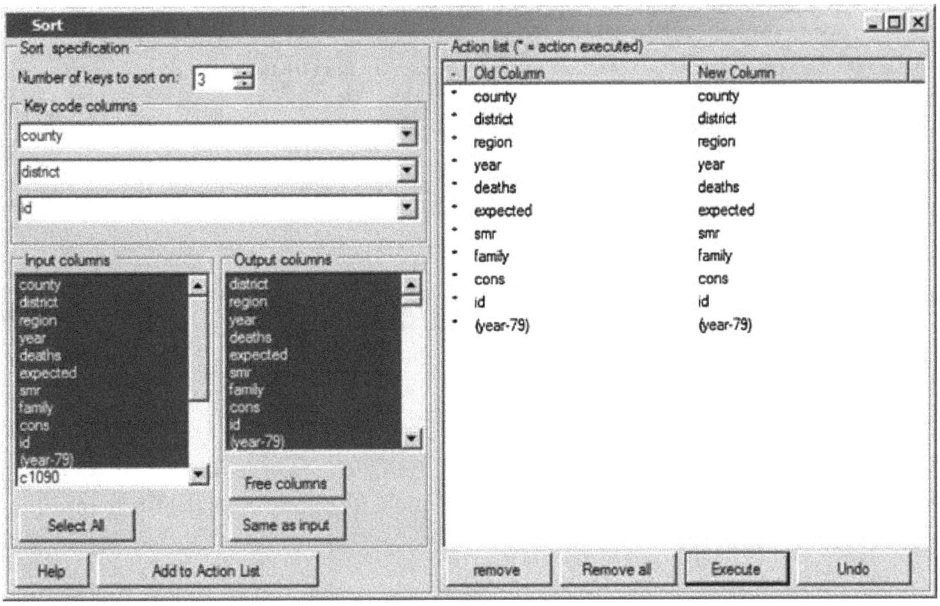

Now return to the **Equations** window. We are going to add COUNTY in at level 3 and make the coefficient of CONS, the intercept, random across COUNTY (as well as DISTRICT and ID).

Click on either smr_{ij} term
Change **N levels** to **3 – ijk**
Select COUNTY from the drop-down list by **level 3(k)**
Click **Done**
Click on β_{0ij}
Check the box by **k(COUNTY)**
Click **Done**

The intercept term now has an additional subscript to indicate that it varies across COUNTY as well as across DISTRICTs and ID. The terms v_{0k} are level 3 random effects and are again assumed to arise from a normal distribution. We can check the data structure using the **Hierarchy viewer**:

Go to **Model** menu
Select **Hierarchy Viewer**

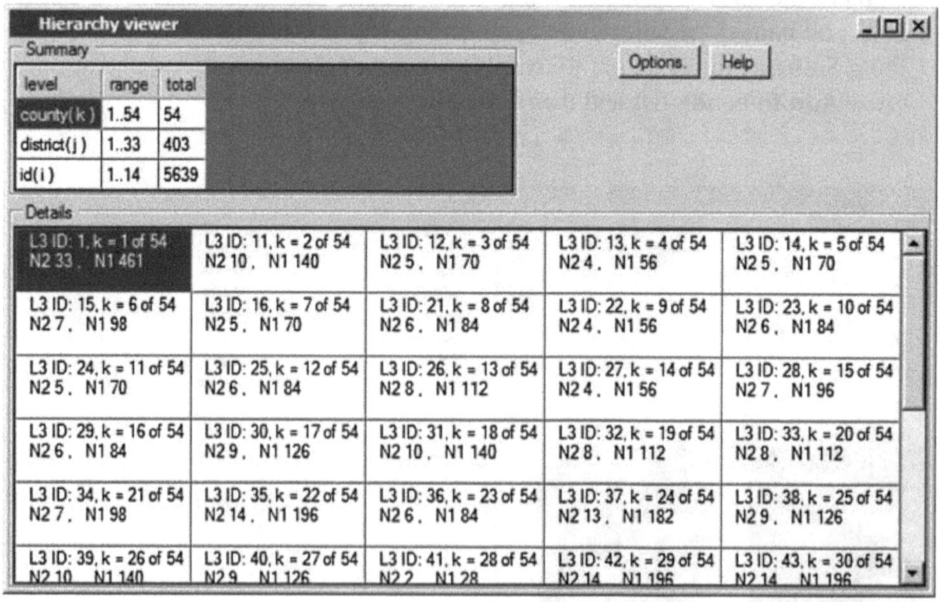

We still see 5639 observations and 403 DISTRICTs, but these are nested in 54 COUNTYs. The first COUNTY has 33 DISTRICTs and a total of 461 observations at level 1.

Click **More** to estimate the new model

Equations

$$\text{smr}_{ijk} \sim \text{N}(XB, \Omega)$$

$$\text{smr}_{ijk} = \beta_{0ijk}\text{cons} + -1.984(0.016)(\text{year-79})_{ijk}$$

$$\beta_{0ijk} = 126.191(1.245) + v_{0k} + u_{0jk} + e_{0ijk}$$

$$\left[v_{0k}\right] \sim \text{N}(0,\ \Omega_v) : \Omega_v = \left[75.800(15.949)\right]$$

$$\left[u_{0jk}\right] \sim \text{N}(0,\ \Omega_u) : \Omega_u = \left[42.851(3.378)\right]$$

$$\left[e_{0ijk}\right] \sim \text{N}(0,\ \Omega_e) : \Omega_e = \left[24.494(0.479)\right]$$

*-2*loglikelihood(IGLS Deviance)* = 35479.459(5639 of 5639 cases in use)

UNITS:

county: 54 (of 54) in use

district: 403 (of 403) in use

Name + - Add Term Estimates Nonlinear Clear Notation Responses Store Help **Zoom** 100

Click on the **Store** button at the bottom of the **Equations** window
Enter a suitable name in the box in the **Model name** window, e.g. Trend 3-level
Click **OK**
Go to the **Model** menu
Select **Compare stored models**

Results Table

Copy

	Trend 1-level	S.E.	Trend 2-level	S.E.	Trend 3-level	S.E.
Response	smr		smr		smr	
Fixed Part						
cons	125.677	0.296	125.699	0.544	126.191	1.245
(year-79)	-1.982	0.039	-1.985	0.016	-1.984	0.016
Random Part						
Level: cons						
Level: id						
Var(cons)	137.283	2.585	24.493	0.481	24.494	0.479
Level: district						
Var(cons)			112.897	8.062	42.851	3.378
Level: county						
Var(cons)					75.800	15.949
Units: cons	1					
Units: id	5639		5639		5639	
Units: district			403		403	
Units: county					54	
Estimation:	IGLS		IGLS		IGLS	
-2*loglikelihood:	43758.204		35723.928		35479.459	

The fixed part is more or less unchanged as is the level 1 (between years within DISTRICTs) variance. However, the higher-level variance has been partitioned further into that attributable to COUNTYs and that due to differences between DISTRICTs within COUNTYs. About 53% (75.800/[75.800 + 42.851 + 24.494]) of the total variation can be seen to be between COUNTYs with 30% between DISTRICTs and just 17% due to year-on-year fluctuations.

This section has covered multilevel model set-up using:
Equations window—adding additional levels
Equations window—random intercepts (CONS) at different levels
Sort window—sorting the data by the hierarchy
Hierarchy viewer window—viewing the data structure
Results table window—comparing a series of models

Interpreting the Model

Residuals

In an ordinary least squares (OLS) regression equation, the residual or error term is the difference between the observed and fitted values. In the above model, the equation may be written as

$$y_{ijk} = (\beta_0 x_0 + \beta_1 x_{1ijk}) + (v_{0k} x_0 + u_{0jk} x_0 + e_{0ijk} x_0)$$

The terms inside the first set of brackets comprise the fixed part of the model, i.e. the fitted values for all data points. The terms inside the second set of brackets comprise the random part of the model and describe the departures from the fitted values at each level of the hierarchy. Thus, the difference between the observed and fitted values is comprised of residuals at three levels—the v_{0k}, u_{0jk} and e_{0ijk} in the regression equation. (Remember that x_0 is the variable CONS, i.e. it takes the value 1 for every observation.) Each set of residuals is assumed to follow a normal distribution and this assumption may be checked using similar residual diagnostics as those that would be appropriate if using OLS. First we will consider the residuals at level 1.

Go to the **Models** menu
Select **Residuals**

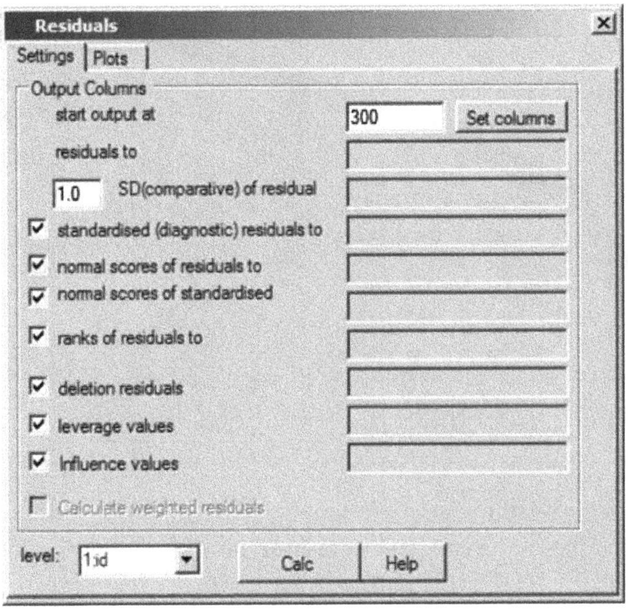

There is a variety of options which allow a range of standard diagnostic checks to be carried out—for example, to check the normality of the data or to look for outliers. By default all nine functions are calculated and the results are stored in columns c300–c308; this can be changed by entering a different number in the box by **start output at**. The drop-down box in the bottom left corner specifies the level at which the residuals are calculated; the default is level 1. We will calculate the residuals at level 1—the e_{0ijk}—and plot the standardised residuals against their normal scores.

In the **Residuals** window, click on the **Set columns** button
Click **Calc**
Select the **Plots** tab at the top of the **Residuals** window
Select the first option **standardised residual x normal scores**
Click **Apply**

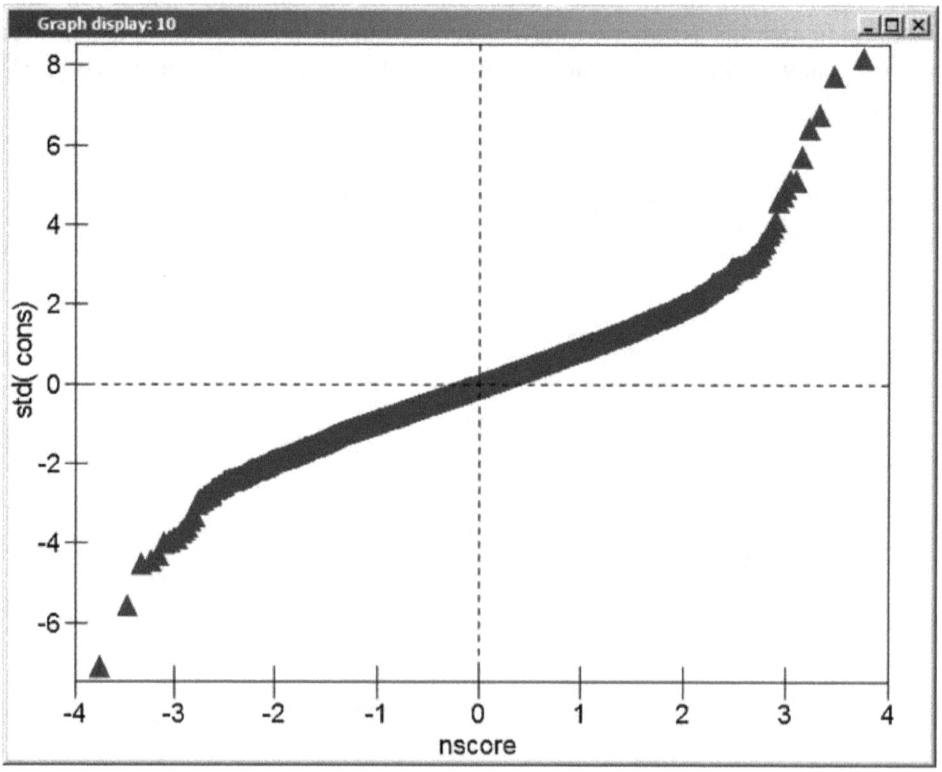

The points in the resulting graph should lie on a straight line; the fact that they do not suggests that there is some departure from normality. For the moment we will ignore this and look at the residuals at level 2 (DISTRICT), calculating these and 1.96 times their standard deviation (so that we can examine 95% confidence intervals).

Click on the **Settings** tab in the **Residuals** window
Select **2:DISTRICT** to be the **level** at which the residuals are calculated
Change the multiplier in the box by **SD(comparative) of residual** to 1.96
Click on **Set columns**
Click **Calc**

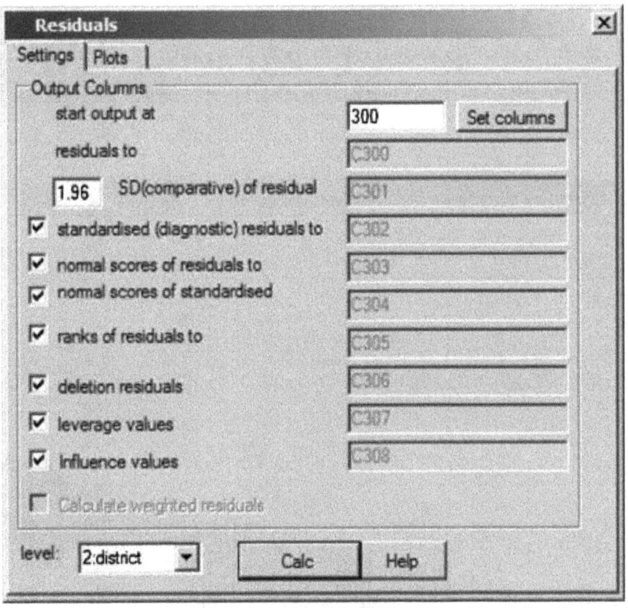

Select the **Plots** tab
Choose a plot of **residual +/-1.96 sd x rank**
Click on **Apply**

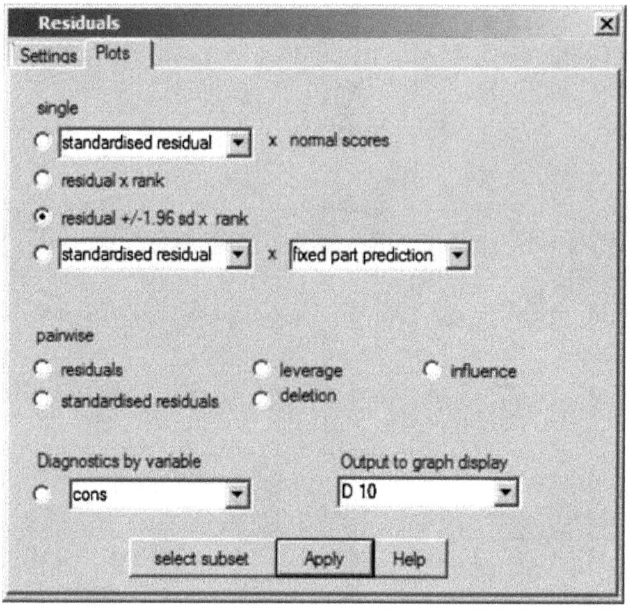
Residuals
Settings
Plots
single
standardised residual
x normal scores
residual x rank
residual +/-1.96 sd x rank
standardised residual
x
fixed part prediction
pairwise
residuals
leverage
influence
standardised residuals
deletion
Diagnostics by variable
cons
Output to graph display
D 10
select subset
Apply
Help

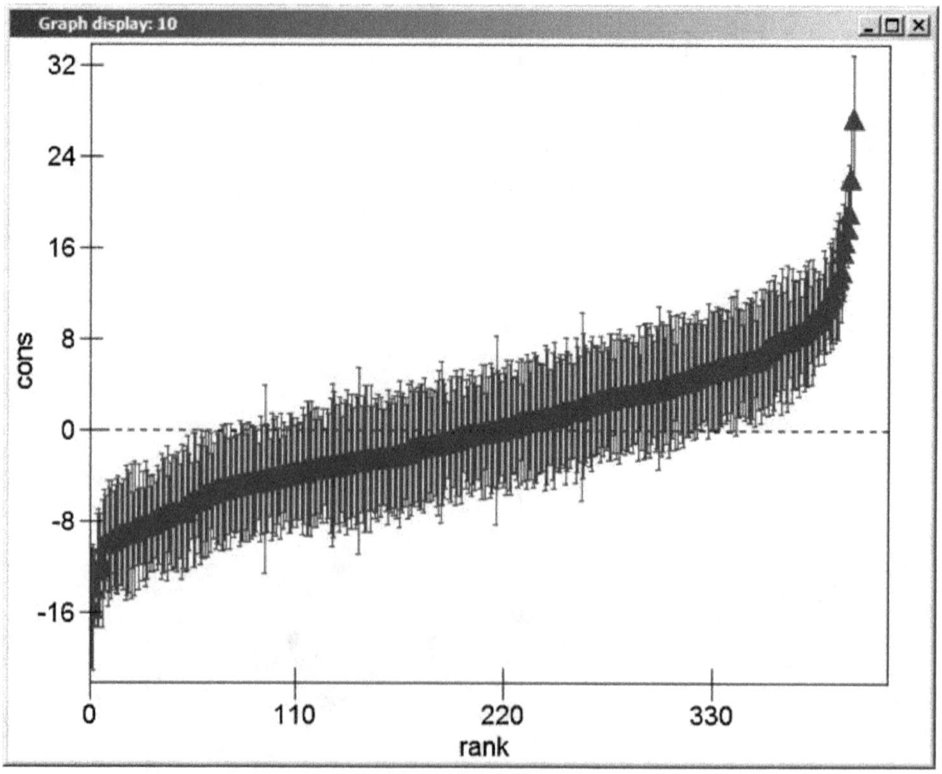
Graph display: 10
32
24
16
8
0
-8
-16
cons
0
110
220
330
rank

This plot shows the residuals or random effects for each of the 403 DISTRICTs, ordered from those with the smallest residuals on the left to those DISTRICTs with the largest residuals on the right. The range of values is from a reduction in the SMR of 16 points to an increase of 27 points. Since there is another level above DISTRICT, that of COUNTY, the residuals do not represent differences from the national average but from the COUNTY average. (We could add the residual for each DISTRICT to that of the appropriate COUNTY and plot these composite residuals $v_{0k} + u_{0jk}$.) The residuals are accompanied by error bars of half-width 1.96 S.D.; a DISTRICT whose error bar does not cross the horizontal line through zero has an SMR which is significantly different from the COUNTY average.

Finally, consider the residuals at level 3 (COUNTY).

Click on the **Settings** tab in the **Residuals** window
Select **3:COUNTY** to be the **level** at which the residuals are calculated
Ensure the multiplier in the box by **SD(comparative) of residual** is set to 1.96
Click on **Set columns**
Click **Calc**
Select the **Plots** tab
Choose a plot of **residual +/-1.96 sd x rank**
Click on **Apply**

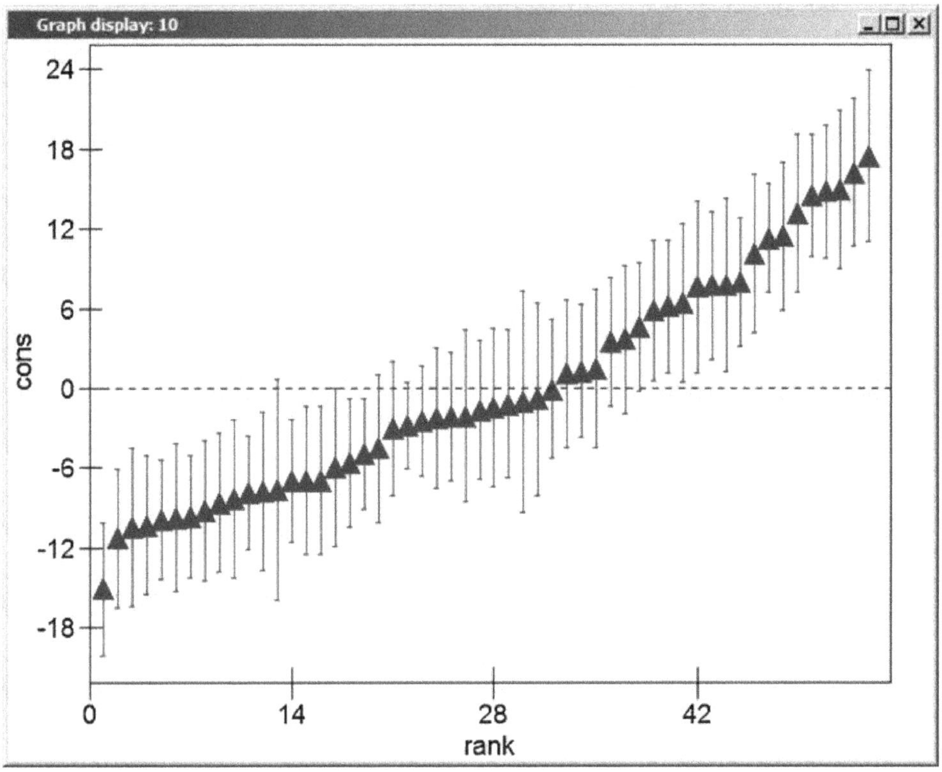

The range of values of the COUNTY residuals is from a reduction in SMR of 15 points to an increase of 17 points. Although this is not as great as the range that is apparent among the DISTRICTs, bear in mind that there are considerably fewer COUNTYs than DISTRICTs (54 as opposed to 403). Thirty-three of the COUNTYs have residuals which are significantly different from zero. Note that not all DISTRICTs within these COUNTYs need to have SMRs which are significantly different from 100; a COUNTY with a positive residual may contain DISTRICTs with negative residuals because the components of the composite random part—$\boldsymbol{u}_{0jk}$ and $\boldsymbol{v}_{0k}$—are assumed to be independent.

Predictions Window

A number of different predictions may be made from a multilevel model depending on whether one includes fixed effects only or a combination of fixed and random effects. For example, prediction lines for COUNTYs are derived from the fixed part of the model together with the residuals from the COUNTY level (the $\boldsymbol{v}_{0k}$).

> Go to the **Model** menu
> Select **Predictions**

The elements of the model are arranged in two columns in the bottom half of the **Predictions** window, one for each explanatory variable. Initially, all the terms are in grey indicating that none has been selected and that they are not included in the prediction equation at the top of the **Predictions** window. The prediction equation is built by selecting the appropriate terms; clicking on the variable name at the head of the column (***cons*** or $(\boldsymbol{year} - 79)_{ijk}$) selects all the terms in that column (turning them black), whilst clicking on individual terms (such as $\boldsymbol{\beta}_0$ or $\boldsymbol{v}_{0k}$) toggles that term in or out of the prediction equation. To make predictions for the 54 COUNTYs at level 3, we need to include the fixed part and the level 3 residuals.

> Click on ***cons*** and $(\boldsymbol{year} - 79)_{ijk}$
> Click on $\boldsymbol{u}_{0jk}$ and $\boldsymbol{e}_{0ijk}$ to remove these terms from the prediction
> In the drop-down list by **output from prediction to** select C12
> Click on **Calc**

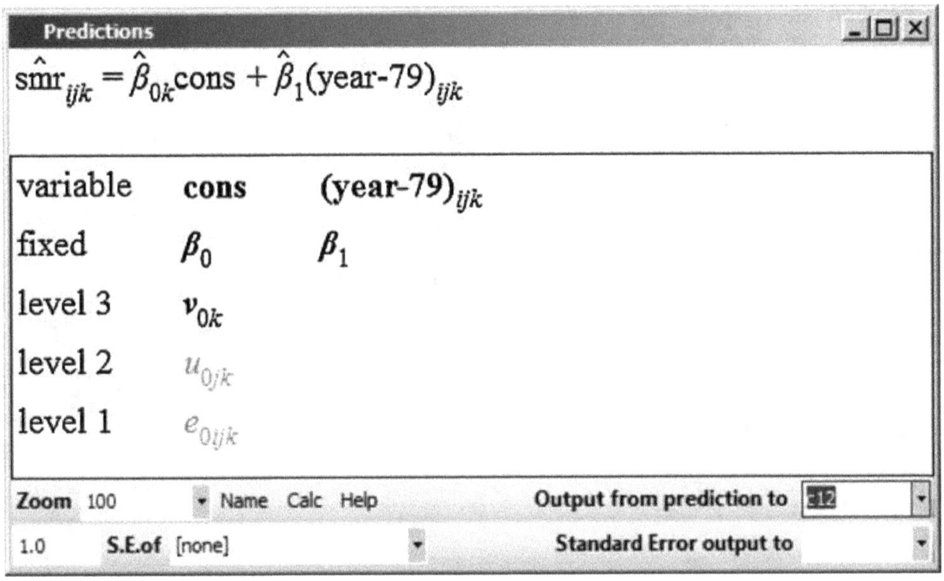

The results from this prediction are now in C12. (You may need to click on the **Refresh** button in the **Window** section at the top right-hand corner of the **Names** window to see the values that have been put in this column.) The COUNTY level predictions range from 85.3 to 143.6. Use the **Names** window to name this variable PRED3 to indicate that it is a prediction including the level 3 (COUNTY) random effects. Then plot the predicted values for each COUNTY against YEAR.

In the **Names** window, click on C12
Click on **Name** in the Column section at the top of the **Names** window
Type PRED3 and press <return>
Go to the **Graph** menu
Select **Customised Graph**

Note that details of earlier graphs are still held. D1 contains plots of the crude data whilst D10 contains the plot of residuals carried out in the previous section. To create a new graph

Select **D2** from the drop-down box in the top left-hand corner
Select the **y** variable to be PRED3
Select the **x** variable to be YEAR
Select **group** to be COUNTY
Select **plot type** to be **line**
Click the **Apply** button

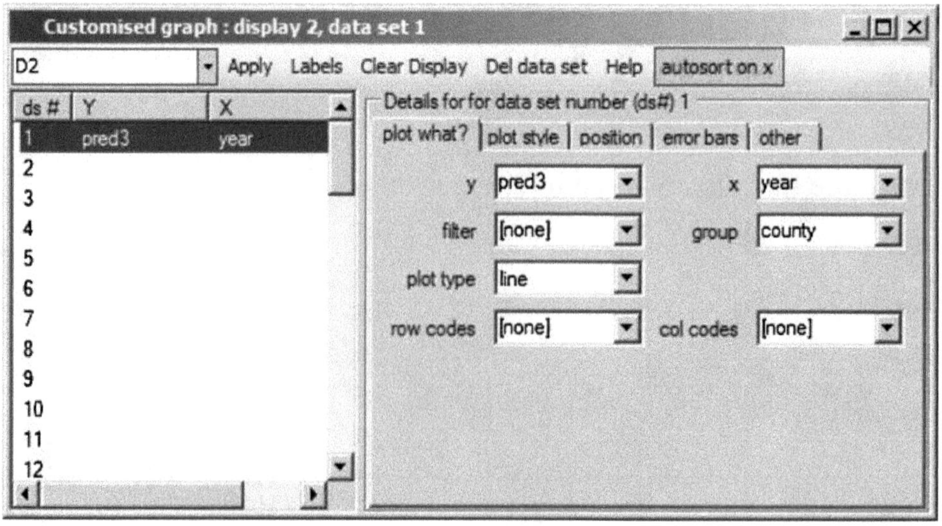
Customised graph : display 2, data set 1
D2
Apply
Labels
Clear Display
Del data set
Help
autosort on x
ds #
Y
X
1
pred3
year
2
3
4
5
6
7
8
9
10
11
12
Details for for data set number (ds#) 1
plot what?
plot style
position
error bars
other
y
pred3
x
year
filter
[none]
group
county
plot type
line
row codes
[none]
col codes
[none]

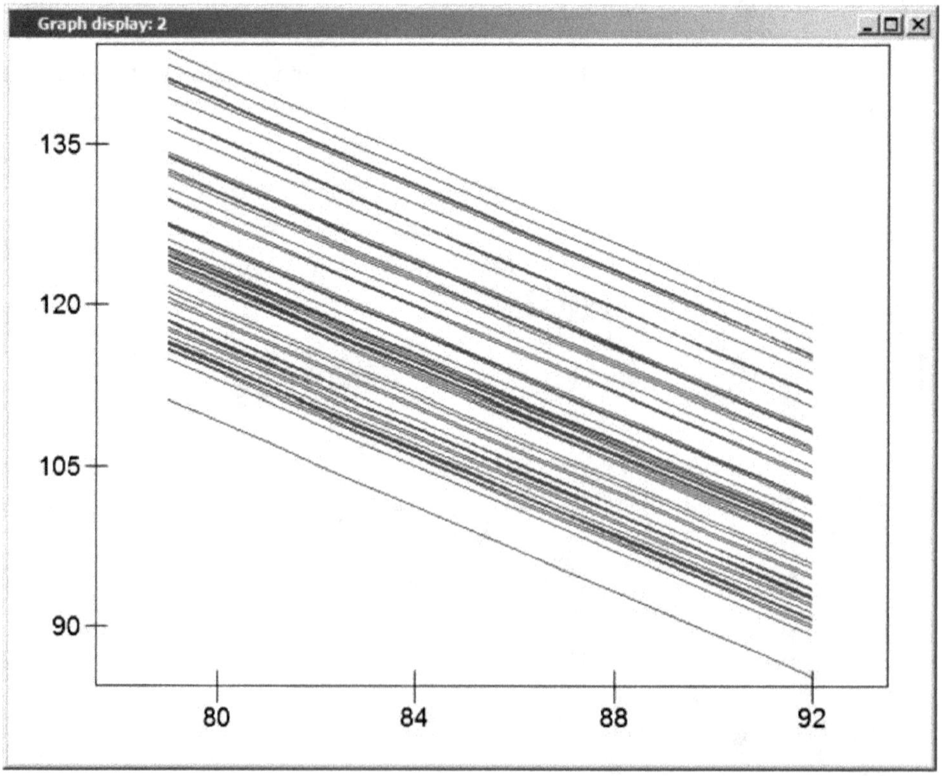
Graph display: 2
135
120
105
90
80
84
88
92

This produces a plot of 54 parallel lines, one for each COUNTY. We will superimpose on this graph the prediction of the fixed part of the model, the mean line given by

$$\hat{y}_{ijk} = \hat{\beta}_0 x_0 + \hat{\beta}_1 x_{1ijk}$$

This means that we only wish to include the fixed part of the model—all of the residual terms in the equation window should be grey.

Return to the **Predictions** window
Click on v_{0k} to remove it from the prediction equation
In the drop-down list by **output from prediction to** select C13
Click on **Calc**

In the **Names** window, change the name of C13 to PREDFP to indicate that it is a prediction from the fixed part only. We will plot the predicted values from the fixed part as dataset number 2 in display 2, plotting the mean over the prediction for each COUNTY.

Open the **Customised Graph** window
Ensure **D2** is selected
Under **ds #** (dataset number) click on number **2**
Select the **y** variable to be PREDFP
Select the **x** variable to be YEAR
Select **plot type** to be **line**
Click the **plot style** tab
Change the **colour** to **green**
Change the **line thickness** to **3**
Click the **Apply** button

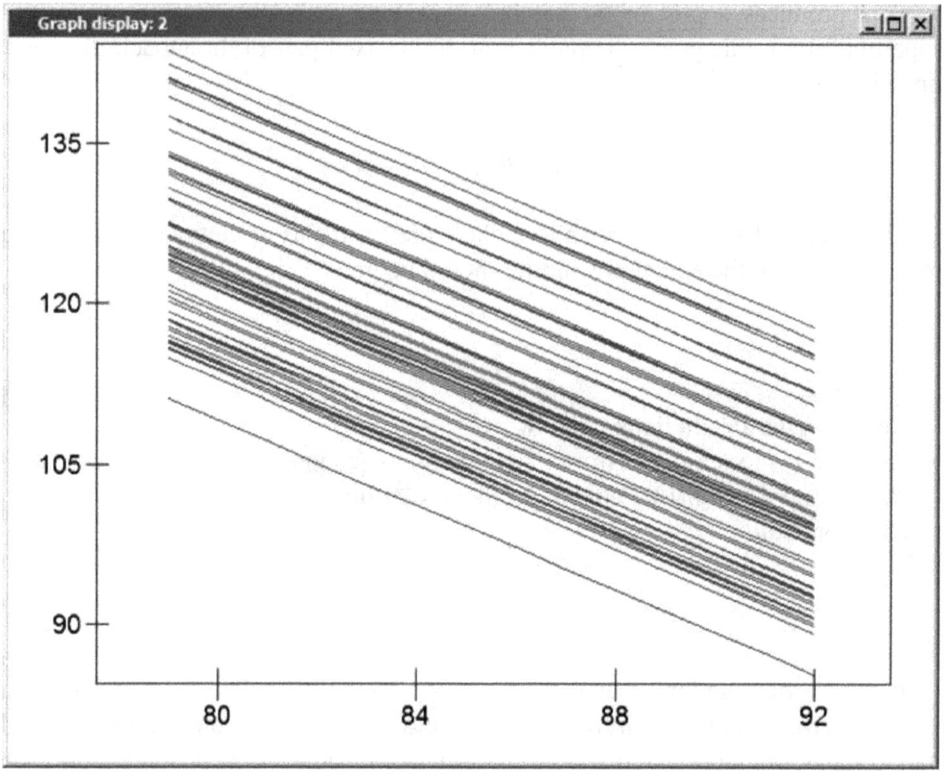

The national mean SMR is highlighted in green with the predicted mean for each COUNTY shown around it. The lines are all parallel since the effect of each COUNTY, v_{0k}, is assumed to be the same throughout the study period. This residual is the horizontal distance between the national intercept and the COUNTY-specific intercept; a positive value of v_{0k} indicates the COUNTY mean SMR is greater than the national mean.

Now look at the predicted means for DISTRICTs within a specific COUNTY. First we need to generate the predicted values for each DISTRICT by including all terms apart from the level 1 residuals e_{0ijk}:

$$\widehat{y}_{ijk} = \widehat{\beta}_{0jk}x_0 + \widehat{\beta}_1 x_{1ijk}$$

Return to the **Predictions** window
Click on v_{0k} and u_{0jk} to add them to the prediction equation
In the drop-down list by **output from prediction to** select C14
Click on **Calc**

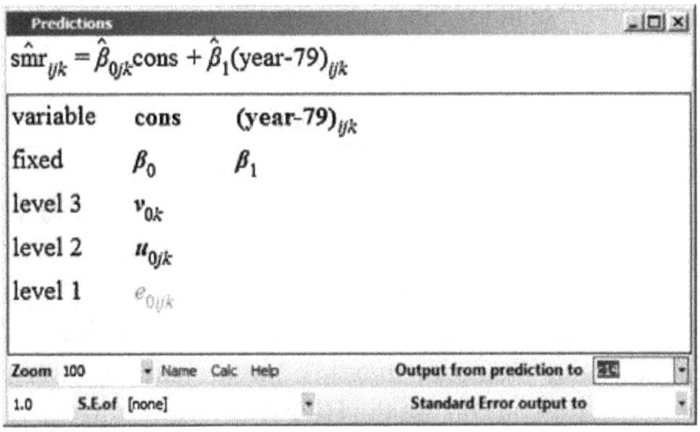

In the **Names** window, change the name C14 to PRED2 to indicate that these predicted values include the level 2 (DISTRICT) random effects.

We can look at these three sets of predictions using the **View or edit data** window.

Go to the **Data Manipulation** menu
Select **View or edit data**
Click on **view** to see a choice of variables
Select COUNTY, DISTRICT, YEAR, SMR, PRED3, PREDFP and PRED2 (multiple columns can be selected using the Control key)
Click on **OK**

Data

goto line 1 view Show value labels Font Help

	county(5639)	district(5639)	year(5639)	smr(5639)	pred3(5639)	predfp(5639)	pred2(5639)
1	1.000	101.000	79.000	138.611	123.371	126.191	119.130
2	1.000	101.000	81.000	99.435	119.402	122.222	115.161
3	1.000	101.000	82.000	140.506	117.418	120.238	113.177
4	1.000	101.000	83.000	111.780	115.434	118.253	111.192
5	1.000	101.000	84.000	104.642	113.449	116.269	109.208
6	1.000	101.000	85.000	105.592	111.465	114.284	107.223
7	1.000	101.000	86.000	83.803	109.480	112.300	105.239
8	1.000	101.000	87.000	101.706	107.496	110.315	103.254
9	1.000	101.000	88.000	74.712	105.511	108.331	101.270
10	1.000	101.000	89.000	82.275	103.527	106.347	99.285
11	1.000	101.000	90.000	106.569	101.542	104.362	97.301
12	1.000	101.000	91.000	132.193	99.558	102.378	95.316
13	1.000	101.000	92.000	85.840	97.573	100.393	93.332
14	1.000	111.000	79.000	140.824	123.371	126.191	133.459
15	1.000	111.000	80.000	137.215	121.387	124.207	131.474
16	1.000	111.000	81.000	132.639	119.402	122.222	129.490
17	1.000	111.000	82.000	128.713	117.418	120.238	127.506
18	1.000	111.000	83.000	127.070	115.434	118.253	125.521
19	1.000	111.000	84.000	116.233	113.449	116.269	123.537
20	1.000	111.000	85.000	124.453	111.465	114.284	121.552

The variable PREDFP contains just the values from the fixed part of the model—the intercept and slope. These values change across YEAR—the slope—but are constant (in the same YEAR) across DISTRICTs and COUNTYs. PRED3 contains the predicted mean for each COUNTY and although they vary from one YEAR to another they are the same for all DISTRICTs in the same COUNTY. PRED2 contains predictions for each DISTRICT within each COUNTY. The slope is constant across time and does not vary between DISTRICTs or COUNTYs; for any of our three predictions, the difference between the predictions in neighbouring years is 1.984 (the coefficient of YEAR in our current **Equations** window).

To illustrate the different prediction lines in a single chart, select a single COUNTY, e.g. COUNTY number 1. (You can use the **Hierarchy viewer** to see which COUNTY codes exist; for example, there is no COUNTY with code between 2 and 10 inclusive.) To create an indicator for COUNTY number 1, for example, we use the logical function == (two equals signs) meaning 'is equal to' in the **Calculate** window:

Go to **Data manipulation** menu
Select **Calculate**
Select the empty column C15 from the list of variables and press the right arrow button near the top of the **Calculate** window
Click on the = button on the window's keypad
Select COUNTY from the list of variables and press the right arrow button
Use the window's keypad to enter **==1**
Press **Calculate**

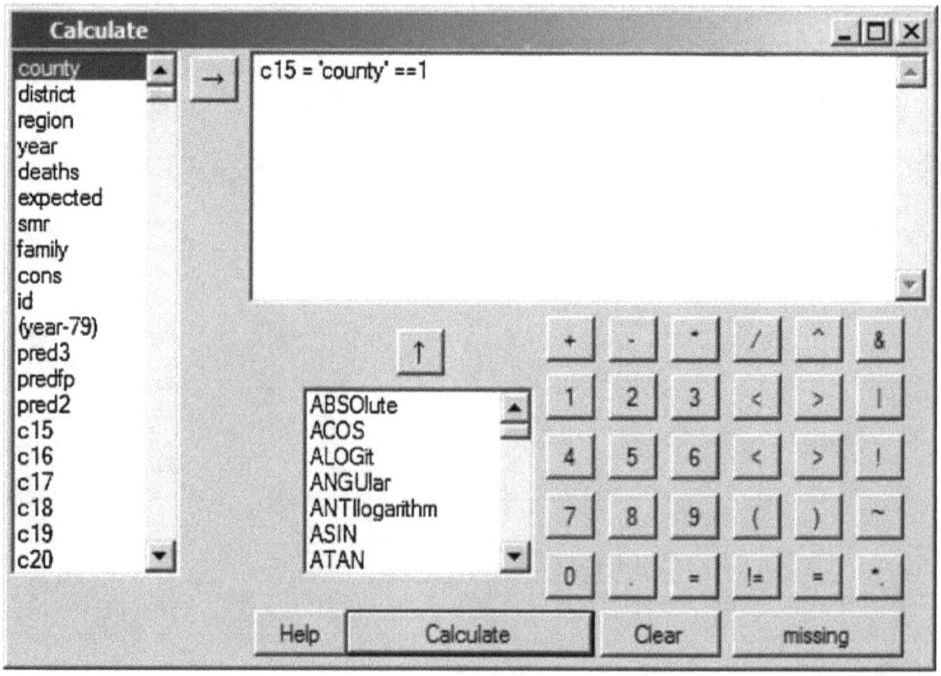

This will create a dummy variable with the value 1 if the data are from COUNTY number 1, 0 otherwise.

Go to the **Names** window and change the name of C15 to COUNTY1. Then, in the **Customised Graph** window we can filter out all COUNTYs apart from the one that we have chosen.

Return to the **Customised Graph** window
Ensure **D2** is selected
Highlight data set number **1** under **ds #**
Select the **filter** to be COUNTY1 under the **plot what?** tab
Click on the **plot style** tab
Change the **line thickness** to **3**
Click the **Apply** button

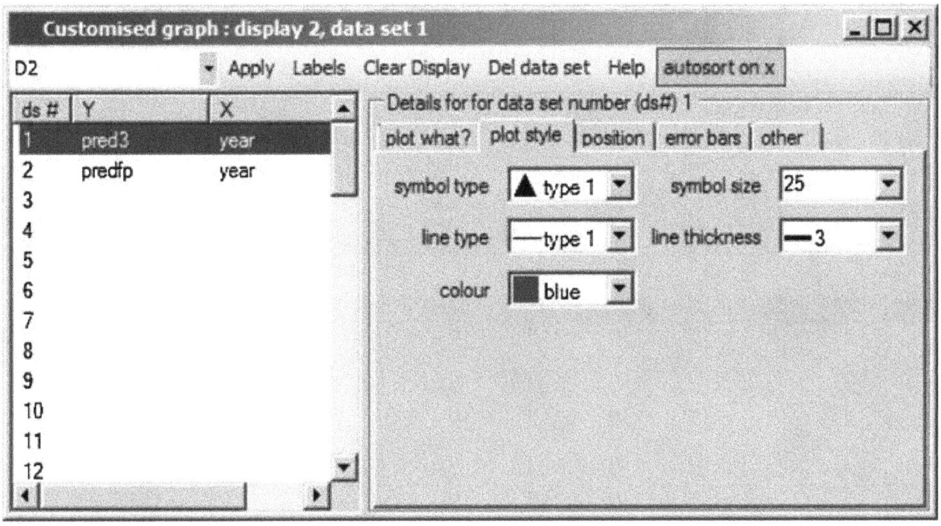

The resulting graph now has just two lines—one for the national mean and one for the selected COUNTY. To plot the predicted lines for the DISTRICTS in COUNTY number 1, we again need to use the filter; we can plot the DISTRICT predictions in red.

Return to the **Customised Graph** window
Select **ds # 2**
Select the **filter** to be COUNTY1
Click the **Apply** button
Under **ds #** click on number **3**
Select the **y** variable to be PRED2
Select the **x** variable to be YEAR
Select the **filter** to be COUNTY1

(continued)

Select **group** to be DISTRICT
Select the **plot type** to be **line**
Click the **plot style** tab
Change the **colour** to **red**
Click the **Apply** button

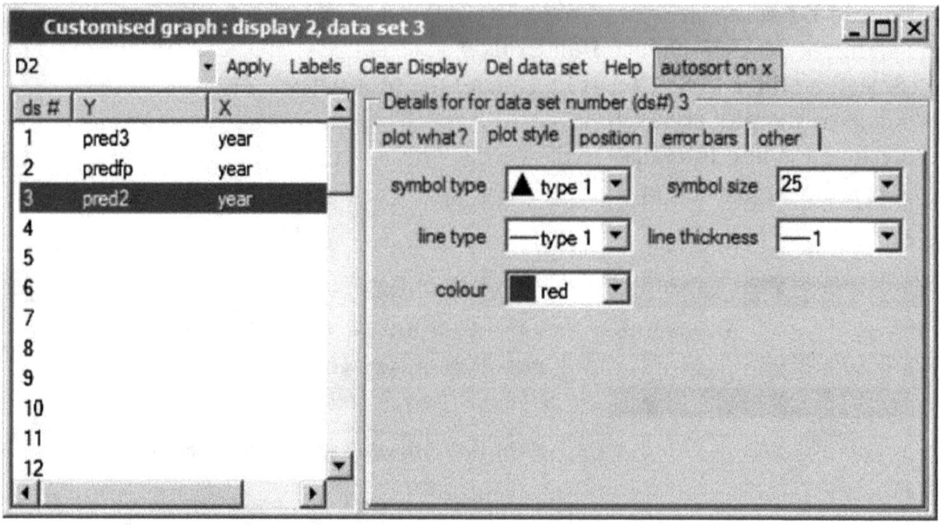

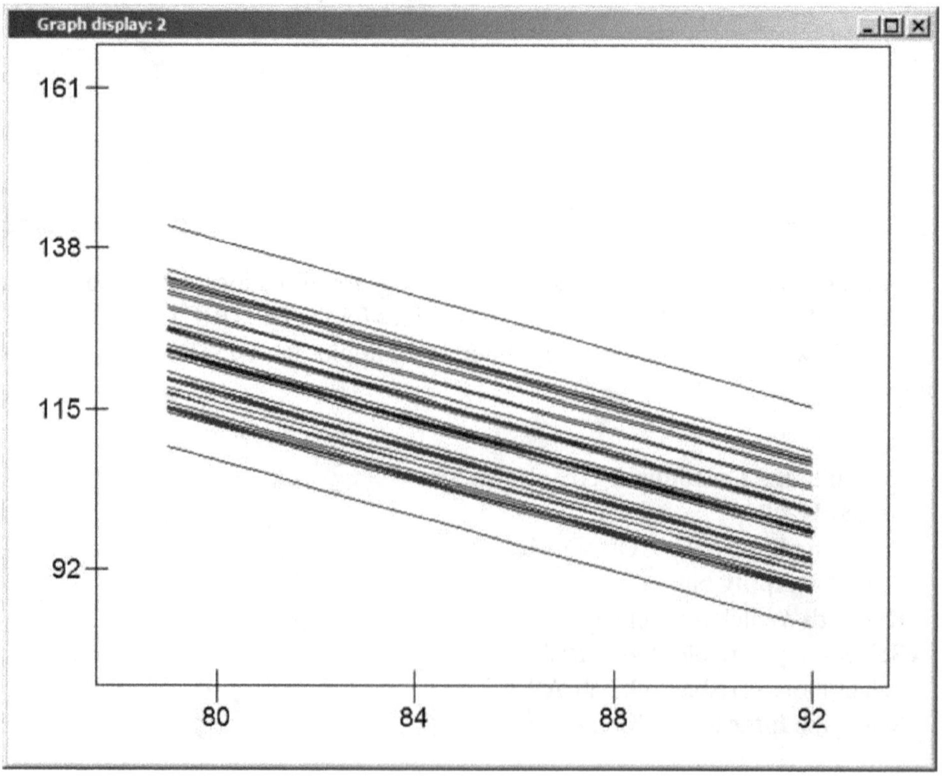

In addition to the national mean (green) and COUNTY mean (blue), the graph now displays the DISTRICT predictions for the selected COUNTY. The vertical distance between the green and blue lines is the level 3 (COUNTY) residual v_{01} (the subscript k is replaced by the number of the COUNTY). The fact that the COUNTY mean is below the national mean indicates that this residual is negative. The vertical distance between each DISTRICT mean and the COUNTY mean is the level 2 (DISTRICT) residual u_{0j1}. The vertical distance between each DISTRICT mean and the national mean is then the composite residual $v_{01} + u_{0j1}$. You may note that, despite the average for this COUNTY being below the national average, some of the DISTRICT means still lie above the national average (the green line) because the composite residual $v_{01} + u_{0j1}$ is greater than zero.

This section has covered model diagnostics and interpretation using:
Residuals window—checking normality at level 1
Residuals window—higher-level residuals with confidence intervals
Predictions window—predictions from the fixed part of the model
Predictions window—predictions including residuals
Graph—plotting predicted values
Graph—overlaying (multiple) graphs
Calculate window—creating a new variable

Model Building

Adding More Fixed Effects

The models fitted so far include only an intercept term (CONS) and a trend coefficient (YEAR) in the fixed part. Now consider the addition of further variables. Firstly, we add a quadratic term in year since the assumption of a linear trend may be too simplistic. We can use the ^ (to the power of) function in the **Calculate** window to raise our trend variable (YEAR-79) to the power of 2.

Go to **Data manipulation** menu
Select **Calculate**
Select the empty column C16 from the list of variables and press the right arrow button
Click on the = button on the window's keypad
Select (YEAR-79) from the list of variables and press the right arrow button
Use the window's keypad to enter **^2**
Press **Calculate**

In the **Names** window, change the name of C16 to (YEAR-79)^2. We can add this term in the **Equations** window and re-estimate the model:

Return to the **Equations** window
Click on **Add Term**
Select (YEAR-79)^2 from the drop-down list under **variable** in the **Specify term** window
Click **Done**
Click on the **More** button to re-estimate the model

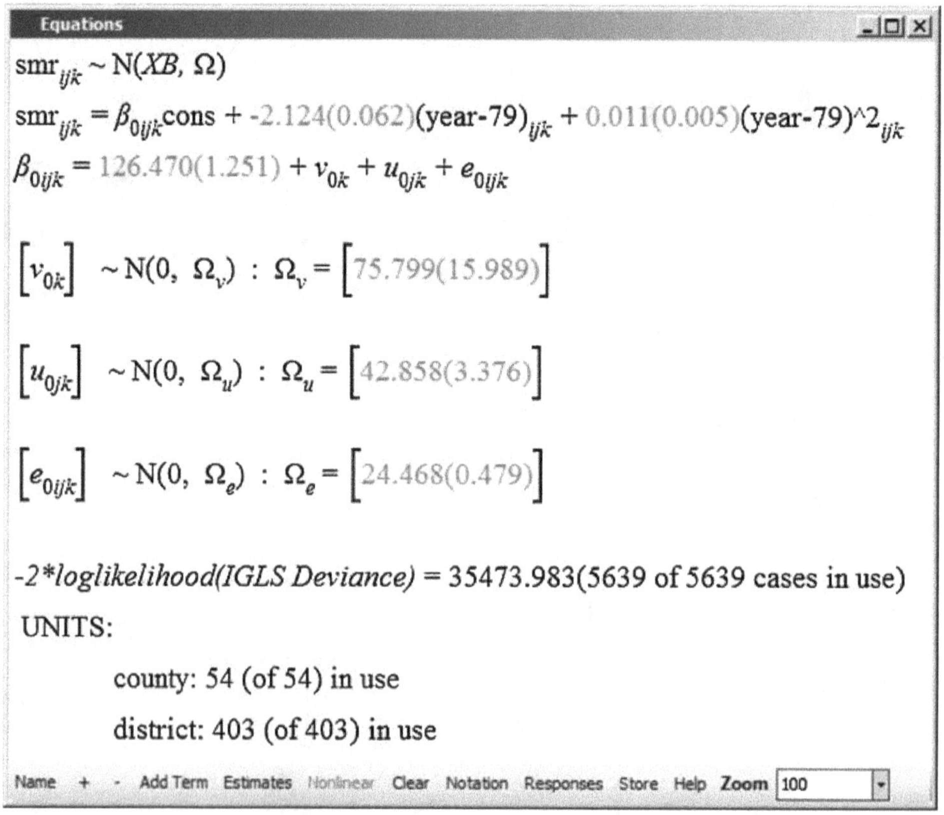

Click on the **Store** button at the bottom of the **Equations** window
Enter a suitable name in the box in the **Model name** window, e.g. M4
Click **OK**
Go to the **Model** menu
Select **Compare stored models**

Results Table

Copy

	Trend 1-level	S.E.	Trend 2-level	S.E.	Trend 3-level	S.E.	M4	S.E.
Response	smr		smr		smr		smr	
Fixed Part								
cons	125.677	0.296	125.699	0.544	126.191	1.245	126.470	1.251
(year-79)	-1.982	0.039	-1.985	0.016	-1.984	0.016	-2.124	0.062
(year-79)^2							0.011	0.005
Random Part								
Level: cons								
Level: id								
Var(cons)	137.283	2.585	24.493	0.481	24.494	0.479	24.468	0.479
Level: district								
Var(cons)			112.897	8.062	42.851	3.378	42.858	3.376
Level: county								
Var(cons)					75.800	15.949	75.799	15.989
Units: cons	1							
Units: id	5639		5639		5639		5639	
Units: district			403		403		403	
Units: county					54		54	
Estimation:	IGLS		IGLS		IGLS		IGLS	
-2*loglikelihood:	43758.204		35723.928		35479.459		35473.983	

The reduction in $-2*\log(\text{likelihood})$ is 5.476 from 1 degree of freedom—comfortably greater than the critical value of 3.84—so this term has significantly improved the fit of the model. The addition of this term has, however, done nothing to reduce the variance at any of the three levels in the model.

The next covariate we can consider adding to the fixed part of the model is the variable FAMILY, a classification of the DISTRICTs into different types. Before adding this to the model, we can see how mean SMRs differ across the categories of family. We do this using the **Tabulate** window:

Go to **Basic statistics** menu
Select **Tabulate**
In the **Output mode** section at the top right of the **Tabulate** window, select **Means**
From the drop-down list next to **Variate column,** select SMR
From the drop-down list next to **Columns,** select FAMILY
Click **Tabulate**

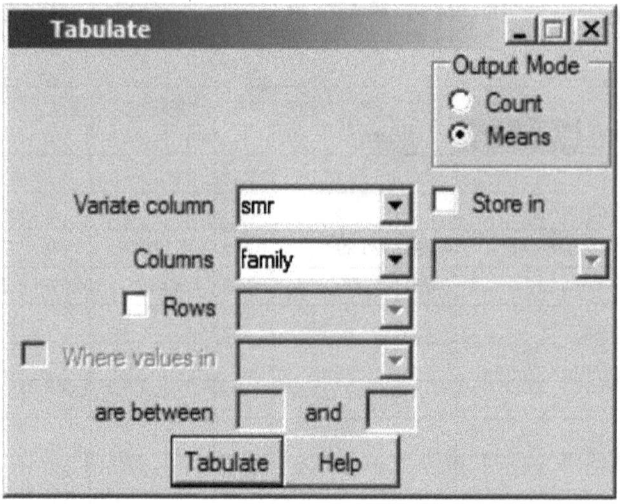

The output window opens containing the table of means and SDs:

```
Output
->TABUlate  'smr'    'family'


Variable tabulated is smr

              1          2          3          4          5          6       TOTALS

      N     251       1594       1554        588        840        812        5639
  MEANS   115.081    110.660    107.089    104.642    118.687    126.950    112.787
   SD'S    10.674     13.224     11.669     10.308     12.982     12.241     14.182

Zoom 100   Copy as table  Clear  Include output from system generated commands
```

This shows lower mean SMRs in categories 3 and 4 (prospering and maturer areas) and higher SMRs in mining areas (category 6). To add a categorical variable such as this to our model, we first need to specify that it is categorical; we do this using the **Names** window.

In the **Names** window, click on the variable FAMILY
Click on the **Toggle Categorical** button in the **Column** section at the top of the **Names** window
Click on the **View** button in the **Categories** section
With family_1 highlighted, click **Edit** and type LONDON
Highlight family_2, click **Edit** and type RURAL
Highlight family_3, click **Edit** and type PROSPER
Highlight family_4, click **Edit** and type MATURE
Highlight family_5, click **Edit** and type URBAN
Highlight family_6, click **Edit** and type MINING
Click on **OK**

We can now add the variable FAMILY to the model. As with any categorical variable, we fit one fewer dummy variable than the number of categories; for this reason, we need a reference category against which all comparisons will be made. We will use LONDON as the reference category.

In the **Equations** window, click on the **Add term** button
Select FAMILY from the drop-down list under **variable** in the **Specify term** window
Check that LONDON is selected as the **Reference category**
Click **Done**
Click on the **More** button to re-estimate the model

We have created five dummy variables named RURAL, PROSPER, etc., which take the value 1 for a DISTRICT if it is of that type, 0 otherwise. These variables can be seen in the **Names** window in columns 17–21.

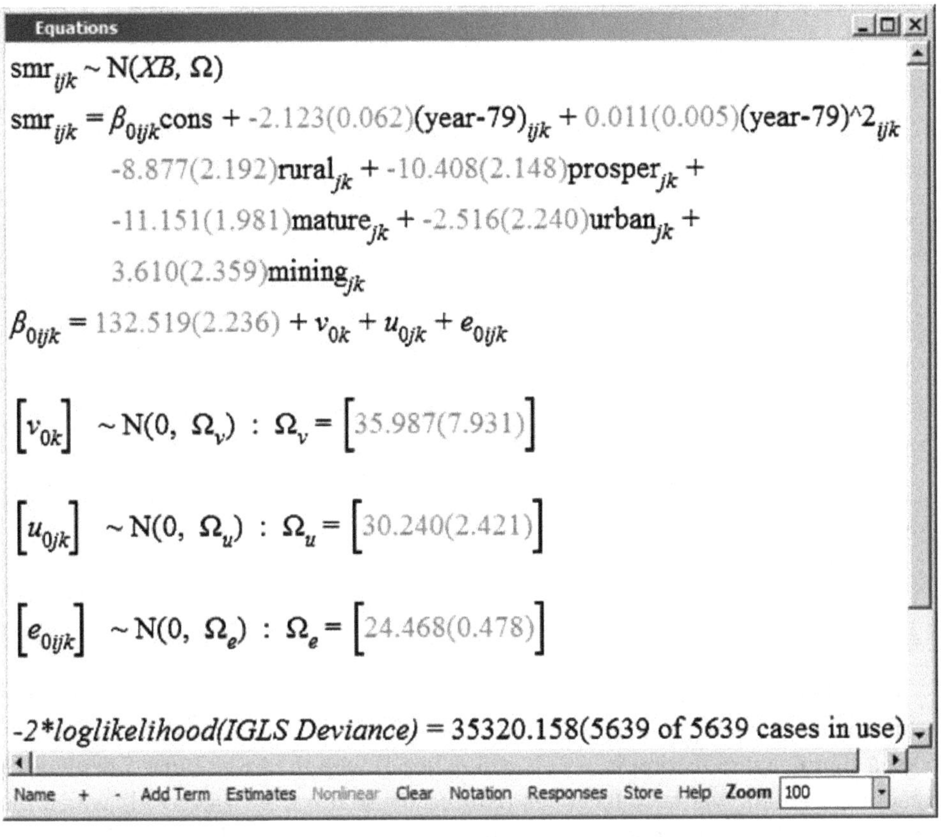

In the **Equations** window, note that the dummy variables representing the categories of FAMILY have subscripts **jk** as opposed to the variables (YEAR-79) and (YEAR-79)^2 which have subscripts **ijk**. This is because the FAMILY variable is measured at the DISTRICT level—it remains constant for each DISTRICT from one year to another.

Click on the **Store** button at the bottom of the **Equations** window
Enter a suitable name in the box in the **Model name** window, e.g. M5
Click **OK**
Go to the **Model** menu
Select **Compare stored models**

Results Table

Copy

	Trend 1-level	S.E.	Trend 2-level	S.E.	Trend 3-level	S.E.	M4	S.E.	M5	S.E.
Fixed Part										
cons	125.677	0.296	125.699	0.544	126.191	1.245	126.470	1.251	132.519	2.236
(year-79)	-1.982	0.039	-1.985	0.016	-1.984	0.016	-2.124	0.062	-2.123	0.062
(year-79)^2							0.011	0.005	0.011	0.005
rural									-8.877	2.192
prosper									-10.408	2.148
mature									-11.151	1.981
urban									-2.516	2.240
mining									3.610	2.359
Random Part										
Level: cons										
Level: id										
Var(cons)	137.283	2.585	24.493	0.481	24.494	0.479	24.468	0.479	24.468	0.478
Level: district										
Var(cons)			112.897	8.062	42.851	3.378	42.858	3.376	30.240	2.421
Level: county										
Var(cons)					75.800	15.949	75.799	15.989	35.987	7.931
Units: cons	1									
Units: id	5639		5639		5639		5639		5639	
Units: district			403		403		403		403	
Units: county					54		54		54	
Estimation:	IGLS		IGLS		IGLS		IGLS		IGLS	
-2*loglikelihood:	43758.204		35723.928		35479.459		35473.983		35320.158	

The intercept or coefficient of the CONS term has changed as this is now the estimated mean in 1979 for areas in Inner London (the reference category). There has been a significant reduction in $-2*\log(\text{likelihood})$ with the loss of just 5 degrees of freedom. The total variance has been reduced by 36.6% from 143 to 91; whilst the year-on-year (level 1) variation has changed little, the between DISTRICT (level 2) variance has been reduced by 29% and the between COUNTY (level 3) variance by 53%. The addition of a level 2 variable has then had the greatest effect on the apparent variation between level 3 units, indicating that to a large extent there is homogeneity of the type of DISTRICT found within each COUNTY. (This is not surprising; as an example, consider the fact that all of the DISTRICTs classified as being Inner London must lie within the same COUNTY, i.e. London.)

We can calculate the explained variance ($\boldsymbol{R}^2 = 1 - \widehat{\boldsymbol{\sigma}}^2/s_y^2$) at any time by making a comparison of the variance in our current model, $\widehat{\boldsymbol{\sigma}}^2$, and the variance in the original data, s_y^2. (See, for example, Gelman and Hill 2007.) From M5 in the table above, we have $\widehat{\boldsymbol{\sigma}}^2 = 90.695$. To obtain s_y^2 we could refit the first model—labelled 'Trend 1-level' above—excluding the trend variable (YEAR-79) from the fixed part. Alternatively, we can use the **Averages and Correlation** window to obtain the SD of the dependent variable SMR.

> Go to the **Basic Statistics** menu
> Select **Averages and Correlations**
> Ensure that **Averages** is selected in the **Operation** section
> Select SMR from the drop-down list
> Click **Calculate**

In the output window, we can see that the variable SMR has a mean of 112.79 and a standard deviation of 14.182, giving a variance of 201.129. So the $\boldsymbol{R}^2$ for M5 is 0.550.

Intervals and Tests Window

So far the change in likelihood has been used to assess improvement in the fit of the model to the data. It is also possible to carry out hypotheses tests for either fixed or random parameters using the **Intervals and tests** window. To illustrate how tests are formulated, consider the following two hypotheses. Firstly, if we are interested in testing whether SMRs in urban DISTRICTs are the same as those in Inner London then, since Inner London is the baseline category, this is equivalent to testing whether the coefficient for URBAN is significantly different from 0, i.e.

$$\textit{Hypothesis}\,1: \quad \beta_6 = 0$$

We are not limited to single parameter tests but can also formulate significance tests involving a function of two or more parameters, as well as joint significant tests involving two or more functions of the model parameters. For example, consider a test of the hypothesis that SMRs in rural, prospering and mature DISTRICTs are the same, i.e.

$$
\begin{aligned}
\textit{Hypothesis 2}: \quad & \boldsymbol{\beta}_3 = \boldsymbol{\beta}_4 = \boldsymbol{\beta}_5 \textit{ or equivalently} \\
& (\boldsymbol{\beta}_3 - \boldsymbol{\beta}_4 = 0) \textit{ and } (\boldsymbol{\beta}_3 - \boldsymbol{\beta}_5 = 0) \textit{ implying } (\boldsymbol{\beta}_4 - \boldsymbol{\beta}_5 = 0)
\end{aligned}
$$

The **Intervals and tests** window gives us a choice of testing contrasts among the fixed or random parameters; in this case, we want to test the fixed parameters.

Go to the **Model** menu
Select **Intervals and tests**
Select **fixed** at the bottom of the window

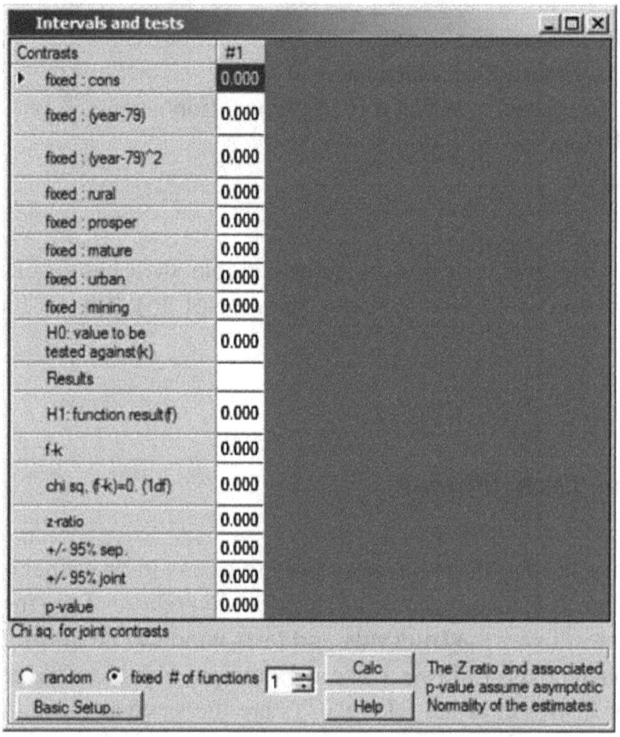

The **# of functions** relates to the number of functions or contrasts of the parameter estimates being tested under a single hypothesis; for hypothesis 1 only one function is necessary whilst two functions are required for hypothesis 2. The boxes beside each fixed parameter are used to enter the function of the parameters to be tested, whilst the constant (k) contains the value to which the function is compared which, in both of the following cases, is the default value zero. So for hypothesis 1:

Select the box beside **fixed : urban**
Type 1
Press **Calc**

Note that the function **f** is a single multiple of the URBAN parameter and so equals $\boldsymbol{\beta}_6$, and because $k = 0$, $(f - k)$ also equals the parameter $\boldsymbol{\beta}_6$. The test statistic, based on Wald's Test, appears at the bottom of the window, **joint chi sq test(1df) = 1.261**, and this may be compared to a chi-squared distribution to either accept or reject the hypothesis that $\boldsymbol{\beta}_6 = 0$. In this instance we can see that the p-value of 0.261 is greater than the conventional threshold of 0.05 and, as such, we do not reject the hypothesis that the mean SMR is the same in Inner London and urban DISTRICTs.

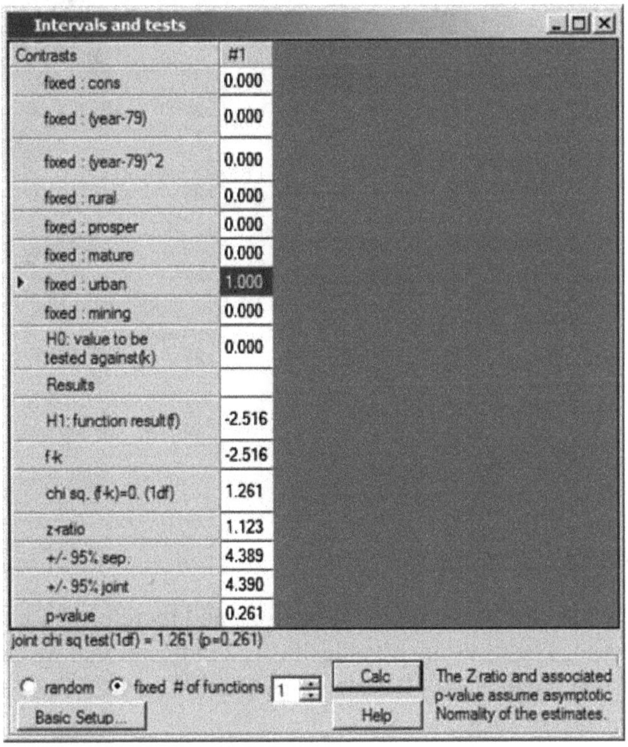

Now to formulate a test for *Hypothesis 2* (if the **Intervals and tests** window is still open, close it down and open it again to erase details of the previous test), we need to set up the two tests corresponding to RURAL – PROSPER = 0 and RURAL – MATURE = 0. (The third test, corresponding to PROSPER – MATURE = 0, is implied by the other two tests.)

Ensure **fixed** is selected at the bottom of the **Intervals and tests** window
Change the **# of functions** to **2**
In the first column, enter a **1** beside **fixed:rural** and a **–1** beside **fixed:prosper**
In the second column, enter a **1** beside **fixed:rural** and a **–1** beside **fixed: mature**
Press **Calc**

Each column specifies a function of the parameters which is compared to **constant (*k*)** equal to zero; for example, in column 1, the function is $(1 \times \beta_3) - (1 \times \beta_4) = 0$ (i.e. $\beta_3 = \beta_4$).

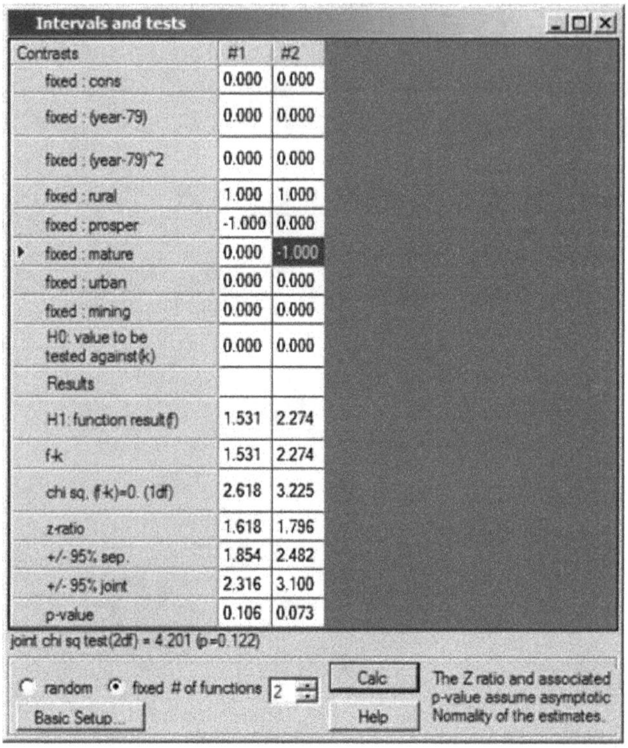

Contrasts	#1	#2
fixed : cons	0.000	0.000
fixed : (year-79)	0.000	0.000
fixed : (year-79)^2	0.000	0.000
fixed : rural	1.000	1.000
fixed : prosper	-1.000	0.000
fixed : mature	0.000	-1.000
fixed : urban	0.000	0.000
fixed : mining	0.000	0.000
H0: value to be tested against(k)	0.000	0.000
Results		
H1: function result(f)	1.531	2.274
f-k	1.531	2.274
chi sq, (f-k)=0. (1df)	2.618	3.225
z-ratio	1.618	1.796
+/- 95% sep.	1.854	2.482
+/- 95% joint	2.316	3.100
p-value	0.106	0.073

joint chi sq test(2df) = 4.201 (p=0.122)

This time we are jointly testing two functions and therefore base the test on two degrees of freedom. The resulting p-value of 0.122 indicates that we cannot reject the hypothesis that the mean SMRs of categories RURAL, PROSPER and MATURE are the same.

In practice at this stage we might want to collapse the variable FAMILY into just three categories: a baseline category comprising Inner LONDON and URBAN areas and a combination of RURAL, PROSPERing and MATUREr areas, which would involve creating a new variable using the **Calculate** window and replacing the variables RURAL, PROSPER and MATURE in the model with this new variable. However, we will continue for now with all six categories.

This section has covered model building using:

Equations window—adding an explanatory (independent) variable

Tabulate window—tabulating variable means across categories

Names window—declaring categories for a variable

Averages and correlation window—obtaining the mean and standard deviation of a variable

Intervals and tests window—testing hypotheses involving single and multiple parameters

Random Coefficients

We now consider another important class of multilevel model: random coefficients (also known as random slopes). In variance components models only the intercept is considered random; however, in the following model we will also allow the slope to vary across higher levels.

Random Slopes

The following section considers the possibility that the rate at which the SMRs have been decreasing may vary from one COUNTY to another. The models fitted so far have contained random intercepts for both COUNTY and DISTRICT; however, the following model will also consider random slopes across the level 3 units (COUNTYs). This is achieved in the **Equations** window by specifying that we want the coefficient of (YEAR-79) to vary randomly across COUNTYs.

> Return to the **Equations** window
> Click on $(\textit{year} - 79)_{ijk}$ and check the box by **k(COUNTY)**
> Then click **Done**

Equations

$$\text{smr}_{ijk} \sim \text{N}(XB, \Omega)$$

$$\text{smr}_{ijk} = \beta_{0ijk}\text{cons} + \beta_{1k}(\text{year-79})_{ijk} + 0.011(0.005)(\text{year-79})\text{\^{}}2_{ijk} + -8.877(2.192)\text{rural}_{jk} + -10.408(2.148)\text{prosper}_{jk} + -11.151(1.981)\text{mature}_{jk} + -2.516(2.240)\text{urban}_{jk} + 3.610(2.359)\text{mining}_{jk}$$

$$\beta_{0ijk} = 132.519(2.236) + v_{0k} + u_{0jk} + e_{0ijk}$$

$$\beta_{1k} = -2.123(0.062) + v_{1k}$$

$$\begin{bmatrix} v_{0k} \\ v_{1k} \end{bmatrix} \sim \text{N}(0, \Omega_v) : \Omega_v = \begin{bmatrix} 35.987(7.931) & \\ 0.000(0.000) & 0.000(0.000) \end{bmatrix}$$

$$\begin{bmatrix} u_{0jk} \end{bmatrix} \sim \text{N}(0, \Omega_u) : \Omega_u = \begin{bmatrix} 30.240(2.421) \end{bmatrix}$$

$$\begin{bmatrix} e_{0ijk} \end{bmatrix} \sim \text{N}(0, \Omega_e) : \Omega_e = \begin{bmatrix} 24.468(0.478) \end{bmatrix}$$

Name + - Add Term Estimates Nonlinear Clear Notation Responses Store Help Zoom 100

The coefficient of $(\boldsymbol{year} - \boldsymbol{79})_{ijk}$ has changed from $\boldsymbol{\beta}_1$ to $\boldsymbol{\beta}_{1k}$ indicating that this parameter now varies randomly across COUNTYs. The estimate of $\boldsymbol{\beta}_{1k}$ is now given as a mean $\boldsymbol{\beta}_1$, common to all COUNTYs, plus a level 3 residual $\boldsymbol{v}_{1k}$, unique to the kth COUNTY. The level 3 residuals $\boldsymbol{v}_{0k}$ and $\boldsymbol{v}_{1k}$ now have a joint multivariate normal distribution with variances $\boldsymbol{\sigma}^2_{v0}$ and $\boldsymbol{\sigma}^2_{v1}$ respectively and covariance $\boldsymbol{\sigma}_{v01}$. Click on **More** to estimate this model.

Equations

$$\text{smr}_{ijk} \sim \text{N}(XB, \Omega)$$

$$\begin{aligned}\text{smr}_{ijk} = {} & \beta_{0ijk}\text{cons} + \beta_{1k}(\text{year-79})_{ijk} + 0.011(0.004)(\text{year-79})\text{^}2_{ijk} + \\ & -9.703(2.135)\text{rural}_{jk} + -10.742(2.096)\text{prosper}_{jk} + \\ & -11.276(1.954)\text{mature}_{jk} + -2.901(2.187)\text{urban}_{jk} + \\ & 2.526(2.279)\text{mining}_{jk}\end{aligned}$$

$$\beta_{0ijk} = 133.288(2.276) + v_{0k} + u_{0jk} + e_{0ijk}$$

$$\beta_{1k} = -2.143(0.070) + v_{1k}$$

$$\begin{bmatrix} v_{0k} \\ v_{1k} \end{bmatrix} \sim \text{N}(0,\ \Omega_v)\ :\ \Omega_v = \begin{bmatrix} 57.202(12.160) & \\ -1.709(0.401) & 0.070(0.016) \end{bmatrix}$$

$$\begin{bmatrix} u_{0jk} \end{bmatrix} \sim \text{N}(0,\ \Omega_u)\ :\ \Omega_u = \begin{bmatrix} 30.254(2.416) \end{bmatrix}$$

$$\begin{bmatrix} e_{0ijk} \end{bmatrix} \sim \text{N}(0,\ \Omega_e)\ :\ \Omega_e = \begin{bmatrix} 23.346(0.459) \end{bmatrix}$$

Name + - Add Term Estimates Nonlinear Clear Notation Responses Store Help **Zoom** 100

Click on the **Store** button at the bottom of the **Equations** window
Enter a suitable name in the box in the **Model name** window, e.g. M6
Click **OK**
Go to the **Model** menu
Select **Compare stored models**

Results Table

Copy

	Trend 1-level	S.E.	Trend 2-level	S.E.	Trend 3-level	S.E.	M4	S.E.	M5	S.E.	M6	S.E.
cons	125.677	0.296	125.699	0.544	126.191	1.245	126.470	1.251	132.519	2.236	133.288	2.276
(year-79)	-1.982	0.039	-1.985	0.016	-1.984	0.016	-2.124	0.062	-2.123	0.062	-2.143	0.070
(year-79)^2							0.011	0.005	0.011	0.005	0.011	0.004
rural									-8.877	2.192	-9.703	2.135
prosper									-10.408	2.148	-10.742	2.096
mature									-11.151	1.981	-11.276	1.954
urban									-2.516	2.240	-2.901	2.187
mining									3.610	2.359	2.526	2.279
Random Part												
Level: cons												
Level: id												
Var(cons)	137.283	2.585	24.493	0.481	24.494	0.479	24.468	0.479	24.468	0.478	23.346	0.459
Level: district												
Var(cons)			112.897	8.062	42.851	3.378	42.858	3.376	30.240	2.421	30.254	2.416
Level: county												
Var(cons)					75.800	15.949	75.799	15.989	35.987	7.931	57.202	12.160
Covar((year-79)/cons)											-1.709	0.401
Var((year-79))											0.070	0.016
Units: cons	1											
Units: id	5639		5639		5639		5639		5639		5639	
Units: district			403		403		403		403		403	
Units: county					54		54		54		54	
Estimation:	IGLS		IGLS		IGLS		IGLS		IGLS		IGLS	
-2*loglikelihood:	43758.204		35723.928		35479.459		35473.983		35320.158		35138.778	

Note that should you want you can select a subset of stored models to compare by going to the **Manage stored models** window in the **Model** menu.

There is little change in the fixed part of the model, nor in the level 1 or level 2 variances. There has, however, been a large reduction in the value of $-2*\log$ (likelihood). Therefore, the addition of random slopes has improved the overall fit of the model. (If the covariance between the intercept and slope at the COUNTY level does not show up in the results table then go to **Manage stored models** in the **Model** menu, ensure that the box by covariance in the **Metric** section is checked, and click on the **Compare** button.) The three random terms at level 3 now refer to the variance of the intercept (CONS) for COUNTYs—$\boldsymbol{\sigma}_{v0}^2$, the variance of the slope (YEAR79) for COUNTYs—$\boldsymbol{\sigma}_{v1}^2$, and the covariance between the two, $\boldsymbol{\sigma}_{v01}$. Whilst the two additional random terms appear large compared to their standard error, it is possible to test this formally using the **Intervals and tests** window. This time we are testing contrasts on two random parameters.

Go to **Model** menu
Select **Intervals and tests**
Select **random** at the bottom of the window
In the box beside **# of functions** type 2

There are two functions to test; our hypothesis is

$$\textit{Hypothesis } 3: \quad \sigma_{v1}^2 = \sigma_{v01} = 0 \ \textit{or}$$
$$\sigma_{v1}^2 = 0 \ \textit{and} \ \sigma_{v01} = 0$$

In the first column, enter a **1** beside **county:year79/cons**
In the second column, enter a **1** beside **county:year79/year79**
Press **Calc**

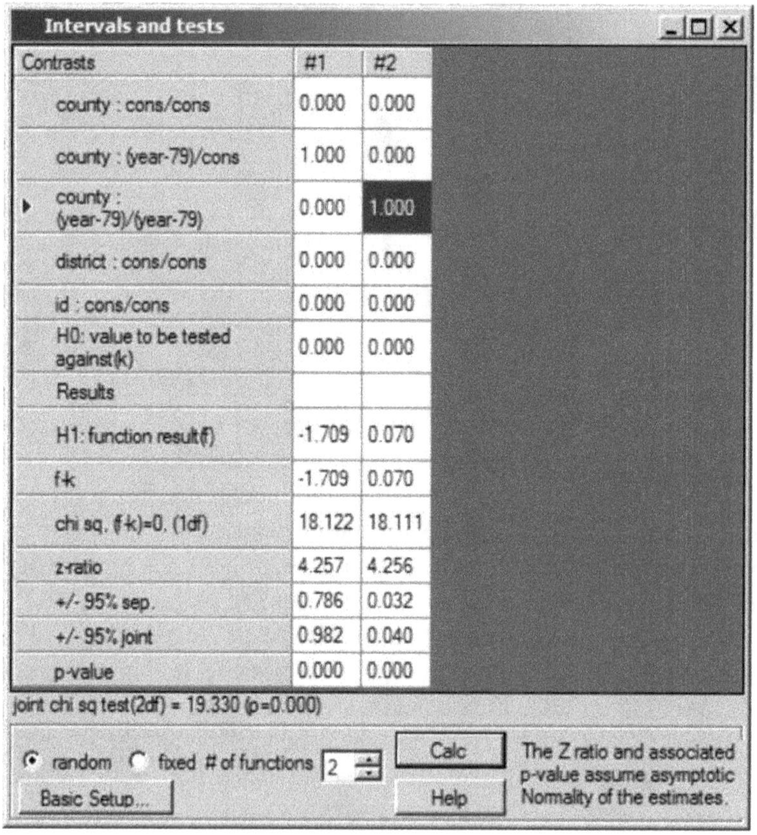

The value of 19.330 is highly significant when compared with a chi-squared distribution with two degrees of freedom ($p < 0.001$); we therefore reject the hypothesis that the two random terms are not significantly different from 0. In general, when testing the significance of random parameters (variances and covariances), using either the likelihood ratio test (comparing values of $-2*\log(\text{likelihood}))$ or the Wald test (using the **Intervals and tests** window), we need to halve the p-value. This is essentially because variances are non-negative and the alternative hypothesis is therefore one-sided. For a more detailed explanation of this issue, the reader is referred to Snijders and Bosker (2012).

The level 3 variance is now more complex and more difficult to interpret; however, the **Variance function** window can be used as an aid.

Variance Function Window

Go to **Model** menu
Select **Variance function**

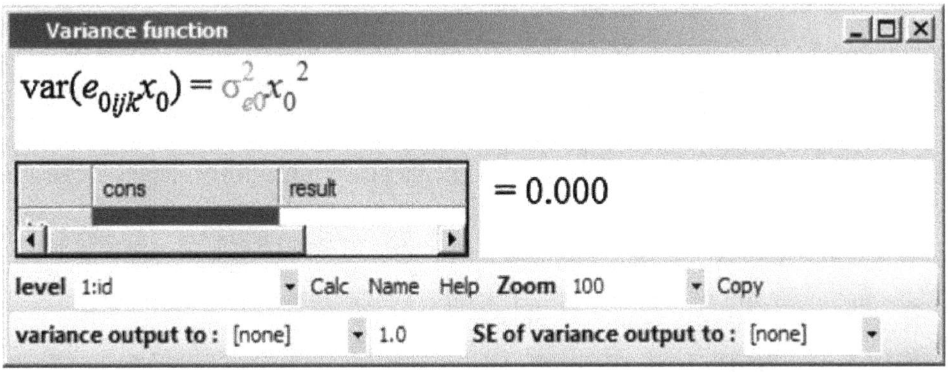

The purpose of this window is to display and calculate the variance function at any level of the current model. The variance function for level 1 is shown by default; this only involves one term because the current model assumes that the level 1 variance is constant for all observations. (Remember that $\boldsymbol{x}_0$ is our CONStant and takes the value 1 for all observations.) To view the level 3 variance function:

In the drop-down list by **level** in the bottom left-hand corner, select **3: COUNTY**

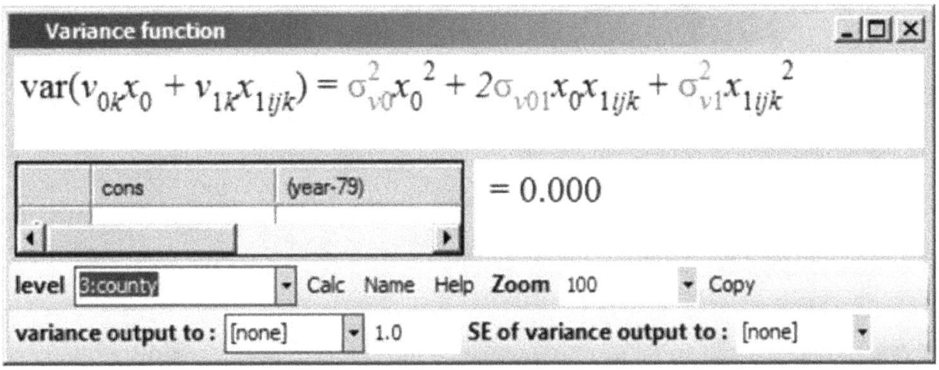

The current model has two terms random at level 3, the intercept and the slope, so the level 3 variance is a function of two random variables. The function shown is the variance of the sum of the two random terms $v_{0k}x_0$ and $v_{1k}x_{1ijk}$. Since x_0 is just the CONStant term, taking the value 1, the level 3 variance is a quadratic in x_{1ijk} (YEAR-79). We can use the **Variance function** window to calculate this function and use the **Graph** window to plot it. This will tell us how the variance between COUNTYs has been changing over time.

Note that the columns in the table in the **Variance function** window named **cons, (year-79), result** and **result se** allow us to estimate the variance function at specific values of (YEAR-79). However, rather than enter the values from 0 to 13 it is simpler to estimate the function for all data points.

In the drop-down menu by **variance output to**, select C22
Click **calc**

In the **Names** window name C22 VARF3. To plot the level-3 variance across the observed values of YEAR79:

From the **Graph** menu, select the **Customised Graph** window
Select a new display **D3**
Highlight **ds # 1**
Select **y** to be VARF3
Select **x** to be YEAR
Click **Apply**

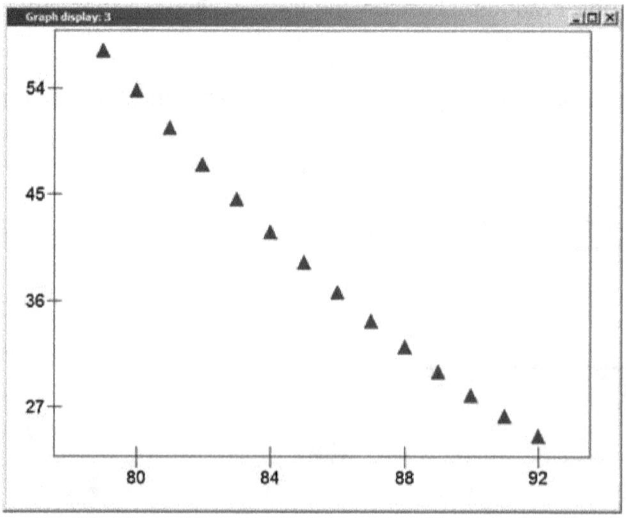

The level 3 (between COUNTY) variance has steadily decreased from a high of 57.2 in 1979 to a low of 24.6 in 1992. It therefore appears that absolute differentials between COUNTYs have been decreasing over time. Another way of examining this change is by looking at the prediction graphs. First calculate the predicted values using the random intercepts and slopes at COUNTY level:

Choose the **Predictions** window from the **Model** menu
Click on **cons**, $(year - 79)_{ijk}$ and $(year - 79)\hat{}2_{ijk}$ to ensure that they are included
Click on u_{0jk} and e_{0ijk} to remove them from the prediction but ensure that v_{0k} and v_{1k} are included
Select PRED3 for **output from prediction to**
Click **Calc**

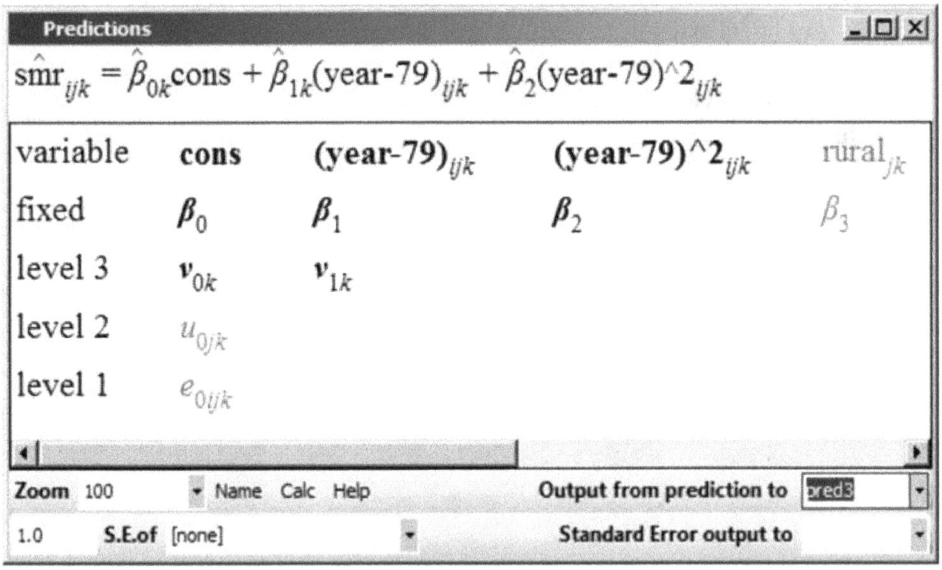

Next re-calculate the predicted values using the fixed part of the model only:

Click on v_{0k} and v_{1k} to remove these terms from the prediction
Select PREDFP for **output from prediction to**
Click **Calc**

We have ignored the categories of the FAMILY variable indicating the type of each DISTRICT. This is because we are only interested at the moment in seeing how mortality has changed over time in each COUNTY, and not how mortality varies according to FAMILY. (The inclusion of the categories of FAMILY would give us up to six lines for each COUNTY, corresponding to the different DISTRICT types within each COUNTY.) We can plot these new level 3 predictions using the

Customised graph window, overlaying the national mean in green on top of the COUNTY-specific slopes.

Return to the **Customised Graph** window
Select a new display **D4**
Highlight **ds # 1**
Select **y** to be PRED3
Select **x** to be YEAR
Select COUNTY as the **group**
Change **plot type** to **line**
Click **Apply**
Highlight **ds # 2**
Select **y** to be PREDFP
Select **x** to be YEAR
Change **plot type** to **line**
Under the **plot style** tab, set **colour** to **green**
Set **line thickness** to **3**
Click **Apply**

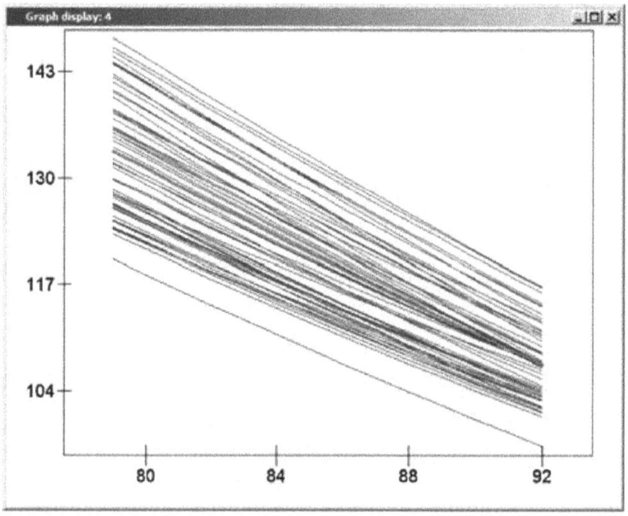

The plot shows the individual predicted trends for each COUNTY plotted around the mean trend line shown in green. The fact that the COUNTY lines are converging towards the mean line over time demonstrates the decrease in level 3 variation over time.

Higher-Level Residuals

There are now two sets of residuals at the COUNTY level; we can look at these using the **Residuals** window.

Under the **Model** menu, open the **Residuals** window
Click on the **Settings** tab
Select the **level** to be **3:COUNTY**
Change the multiplier to 1.96 for the **SD (comparative) of residual**
Click on **Set columns**

Each of the output items now requires two columns: the first column relates to the intercept CONS and the second to the slope YEAR79. For example, C300 will store the residual for CONS and C301 the residual for YEAR79. We can plot both sets of residuals, together with 95% confidence intervals:

Click **Calc**
Select the **Plots** tab
Select **residual +/- 1.96 sd x rank**
Click **Apply**

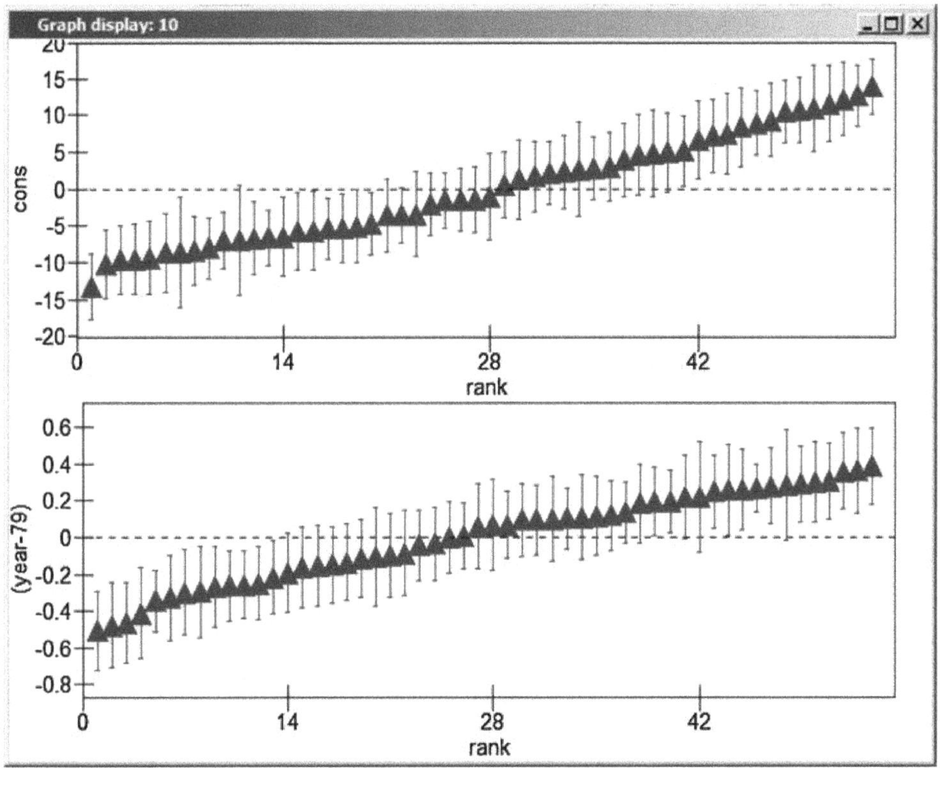

These plots can be used to examine how many COUNTYs have slopes which differ from the average as well as how many have intercepts which differ from the average. Note that a COUNTY's rank for the intercept residual will not necessarily be the same as its rank for the slope residual. To see how the intercept and slope residuals are correlated between COUNTYs:

Return to the **Plots** tab in the **Residuals** window
Under the **pairwise** heading, select a **residuals** plot
Click **Apply**

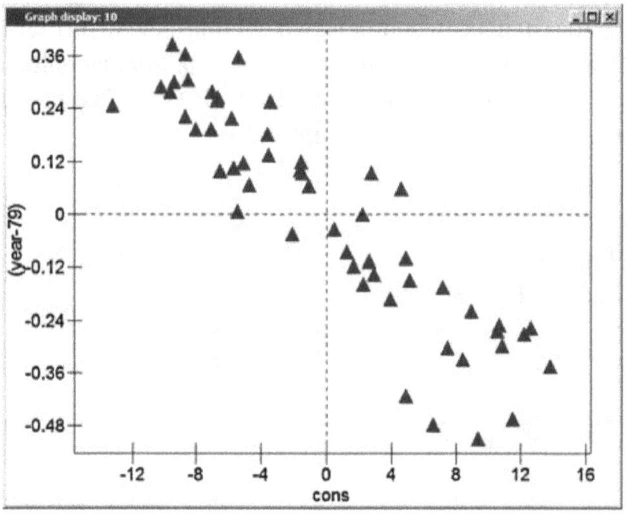

This shows the strong negative correlation between the two sets of residuals. Those in the top left quadrant refer to those COUNTYs with negative intercept (CONS) residuals and positive slope (YEAR-79) residuals. This suggests that those COUNTYs which had lower than average SMRs in 1979 experienced a more gradual decrease in SMR over the 14 YEARs. Similarly, the COUNTYs featured in the bottom right quadrant are those which had above average SMRs in 1979 (positive CONS residual) but which experienced mortality decreasing at a faster than average rate (negative (YEAR-79) residual).

Complex Level 1 Variation

The multilevel framework allows variables to be random at any level so, for example, we may wish to extend the previous model such that trends in SMR not only vary across COUNTYs but also vary across DISTRICTs at level 2. However, random variables at level 1 have a slightly different interpretation; this concerns the effects of heterogeneity (i.e. non-constant variance). In this example, we may consider whether the variation between observations is constant throughout the 14 years or whether it changes. We do this by making the coefficient of the variable YEAR79 random across observations (ID—our level 1 identifier).

Return to the **Equations** window
Click on $(\textit{year} - 79)_{ijk}$
Check the box at **i(id)**
Click **Done**

Now estimate this model by clicking on the **More** button.

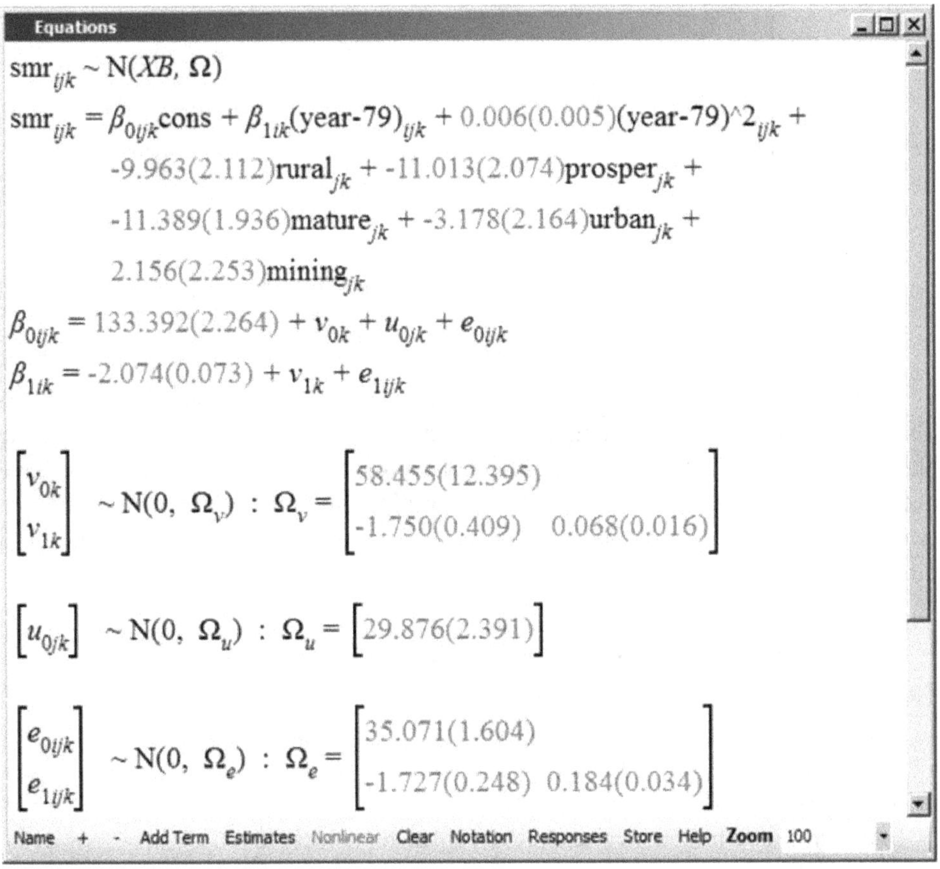

Click on the **Store** button at the bottom of the **Equations** window
Enter a suitable name in the box in the **Model name** window, e.g. M7
Click **OK**
Go to the **Model** menu
Select **Compare stored models**

Results Table

Copy

	M6	S.E.	M7	S.E.
Level: county				
Var(cons)	57.202	12.160	58.455	12.395
Covar((year-79)/cons)	-1.709	0.401	-1.750	0.409
Var((year-79))	0.070	0.016	0.068	0.016
Level: district				
Var(cons)	30.254	2.416	29.876	2.391
Level: id				
Var(cons)	23.346	0.459	35.071	1.604
Covar((year-79)/cons)			-1.727	0.248
Var((year-79))			0.184	0.034
Units: county	54		54	
Units: district	403		403	
Units: id	5639		5639	
Estimation:	IGLS		IGLS	
-2*loglikelihood:	35138.778		35032.992	

There is evidence of heterogeneity with a substantial reduction in −2∗log(likelihood). This means that the degree of scatter of individual observations about the predicted DISTRICT (level 2) means is not constant over time; it appears to have been decreasing. We can use the **Variance function** window to estimate the variance at each level, creating two new variables VARF2 and VARF1 and plotting these three variables against YEAR in the **Graph** window.

Open the **Variance function** window under the **Model** menu
Ensure that **1:ID** is selected to be the **level**
In the drop-down menu by **variance output to**, select C23
Click **Calc**
Select **2:DISTRICT** to be the **level**
In the drop-down menu by **variance output to**, select C24
Click **Calc**
Select **3:COUNTY** to be the **level**
In the drop-down menu by **variance output to**, select VARF3
Click **Calc**

In the **Names window** name C23 VARF1 and C24 VARF2. We can plot all of these variance functions on the same scale across the observed values of YEAR; this will show us how the variance at COUNTY, DISTRICT and YEAR level have been changing over time.

Go to the **Customised Graph** window
Select display **D3**
Highlight **ds#1**
Select **y** to be VARF3
Select **x** to be YEAR
Select the **plot type** to be **line**
Under the **plot style** tab, select the **line thickness** to be **3**
Click **Apply**
Under the **plot what?** tab, select **ds#2** with VARF2 as the **y** variable, YEAR as the **x** variable, and the **plot type** to be **line**
Under the **plot style** tab, select the **colour** to be **red** and the **line thickness** to be **3**
Click **Apply**
Under the **plot what?** tab, select **ds#3** with VARF1 as the **y** variable, YEAR as the **x** variable, and the **plot type** to be **line**
Under the **plot style** tab, select the **colour** to be **light magenta** and the **line thickness** to be **3**
Click **Apply**

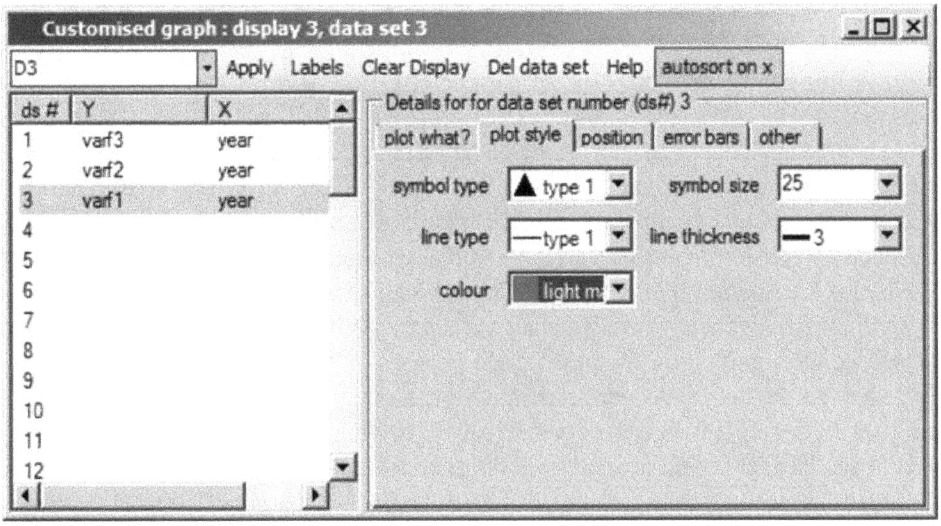

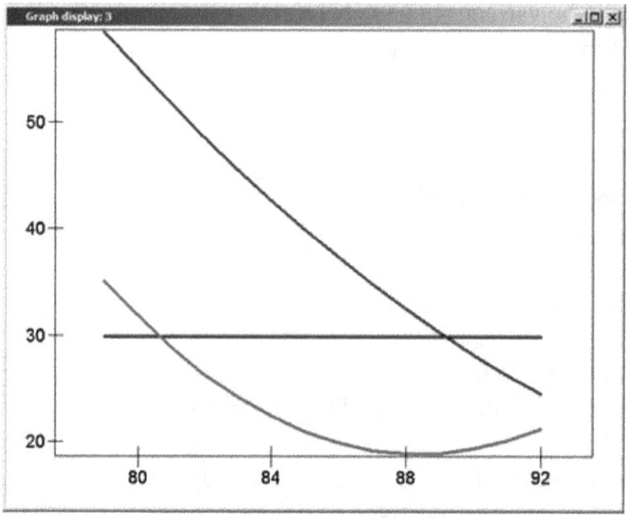

We have not fitted any random effects at level 2, so the variation between DISTRICTs within COUNTYs is assumed to be constant. The variation between COUNTYs decreased steadily between 1979 and 1992; however, the level 1 variance decreased from 1979 to 1988 but may have increased slightly since then. (This may also be an 'edge effect'.) The total variation has decreased from 123 in 1979 to just 76 in 1992. In a similar manner it is possible to explore the extent to which the level 2 variation (between DISTRICTs) has also been changing over time.

By this stage the user has become familiar with the basics of model fitting for continuous (normally distributed) responses. The fixed part of the model can be built up as with an ordinary least squares (OLS) regression model, including any combination of continuous and categorical variables and interactions between them. The significance and effect of variables can be examined through changes in the likelihood or through comparisons of the parameter estimates with their estimated standard errors.

The difference between such models and OLS regression is the ability to separate the variance into the different levels in the model—COUNTY, DISTRICT and the yearly observations within DISTRICTs in this example—and then to model this variance by considering other variables to be random at any of the levels. At higher levels this has the interpretation of fitting random slopes; at the lowest level this is modelling heterogeneity (non-constant variance) within the data. We are again able to test for the significance of any of these random terms.

The example used has been illustrative of the methods employed when fitting a multilevel model; it is not, however, the way in which we would normally model such data. The following section goes on to consider a generalised linear model for these data; however, before proceeding to the more complex modelling it is important to have a good understanding of the basics covered up to this point.

This section has covered random coefficients using:
Equations window—making a variable random at different levels
Intervals and tests window—testing hypotheses about random parameters, e.g. the significance of a random slope
Variance function window—calculating a non-constant variance
Graph window—plotting random slopes
Predictions window—predictions including random intercepts and random slopes
Residuals window—plotting intercept and slope residuals with confidence intervals
Residuals window—pairwise comparisons of intercept and slope residuals
Equations window—modelling heterogeneity at level 1

A Poisson Model: Introduction

The model that we have fitted assumes that the standardised mortality ratio follows a normal distribution. We found that the variance decreased over the period 1979–1992; over this time the standardised mortality ratio also fell. This suggests that there may be a link between the variance in a particular year and the average mortality rate in that year. We have also attached equal importance to every area and in every year; this is probably not sensible since the size of areas in terms of their populations and the number of deaths observed varies considerably both across areas and over time. One possibility would be to weight each observation according to the population of the district in that year; this requires weighting at each level of analysis and would ensure that areas from which we have the most information—the largest areas in terms of their populations—are afforded the most weight. In this section, we adopt an alternative approach.

The local mortality datapack is based on *counts* of deaths. Instead of modelling a transformation of this response—the SMR—we can consider modelling the actual counts of deaths. Such data are discrete rather than continuous—you cannot observe fractions of deaths—and they also tend to be extremely skewed (see histogram below). Therefore, the assumption of a normal distribution is usually not appropriate.

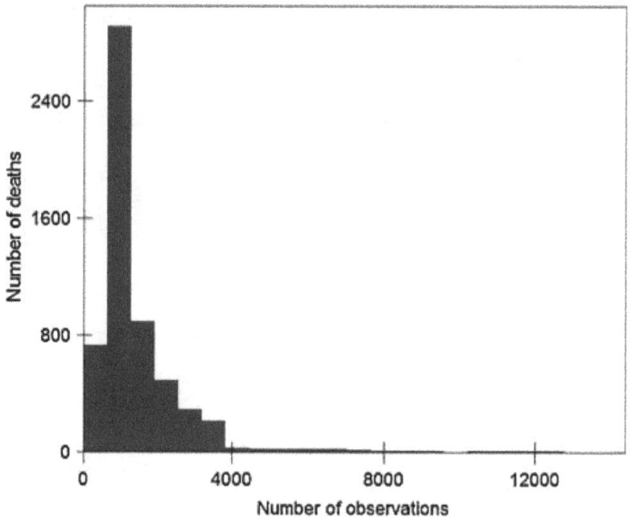

Instead we can fit a generalised linear model and approximate a Poisson distribution for the data. This is the basis of the analysis conducted by Leyland (2004) on data including these.

Setting Up a Generalised Linear Model in MLwiN

First open the original worksheet lmdp.ws again.

Go to the **File** menu
Select **Open worksheet**
Navigate to and open the worksheet called **lmdp.ws**

We use the **Generate vector** window to create a constant and a unique identifier for every data point or observation.

Select the **Generate vector** window from the **Data Manipulation** menu
Select **Generate vector**
Select **Type of vector** to be **Constant vector**
Select C9 to be the **Output column**
Enter 5639 (the number of data points) beside **Number of copies**
Enter 1 beside **Value**
Click the **Generate** button
Select **Type of vector** to be **Sequence**

(continued)

Select C10 to be the **Output column**
Enter 1 beside **Start number**
Enter 5639 (the number of data points) beside **End number**
Enter 1 beside **Step value**
Click the **Generate** button

In the **Names** window name C9 CONS and C10 ID. Then go to the **Equations** window. We will set DEATHS to be the response variable in a 3-level model: ID (observations) in DISTRICTs in COUNTYs.

Click on either of the **y** terms
Select DEATHS as the dependent variable
Select 3 – ijk for **N levels**
Select COUNTY for **level 3(k)**
Select DISTRICT for **level 2(j)**
Select ID for **level 1(i)**
Click on **Done**

So far we have simply repeated the steps for the 3-level model in the introductory tutorial with the response variable being DEATHS rather than SMR. We now have to amend the default distribution for the response. In the **Equations** window, we will specify a **Poisson** distribution with a **log** link.

Click on the **N** that defines the normal distribution
Check the box marked **Poisson**
Click on **Done**

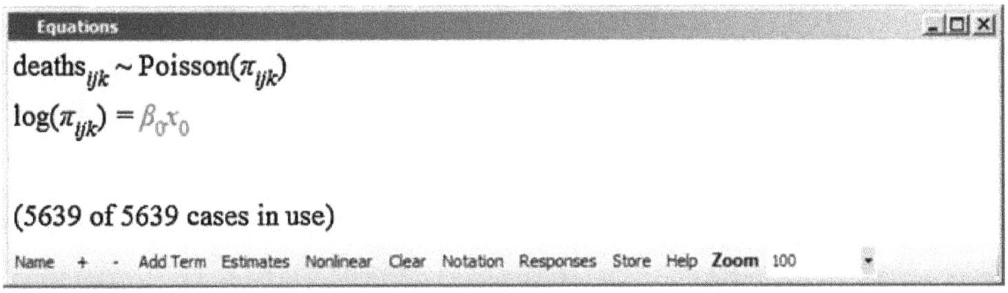

These steps have specified the response to be a Poisson random variable, which defines the lowest level variance function, and the linearising function of the response (the relationship between the response variable, DEATHS, and any of our explanatory variables) is taken to be the natural logarithm.

Now return to the **Equations** window and add CONS to the fixed part of the model only.

Click on $\beta_0 x_0$
Select CONS from the drop-down list
Click on **Done**

This time you may notice that there was no possibility to make the CONStant random at the lowest level (ID). This is because we have already defined the error structure at the lowest level when we specified that the data had a Poisson distribution. MLwiN automatically generated a new variable—which it called BCONS.1—which it will use in the estimation. This new variable can be seen in the **Names** window.

We are using the CONStant in the fixed part of the model to estimate the intercept or mean. We are going to fit a single-level Poisson model to start with, ignoring any variation between DISTRICTs and COUNTYs. As in the introductory tutorial, we will fit a quadratic in YEAR centred around 1979.

Go to **Data manipulation** menu
Select **Calculate**
Select the empty column C12 and press the right arrow button
Click the '=' button on the keypad
Select YEAR from the list of variables and press the right arrow button
Use the window's keypad to enter **–79**
Press **Calculate**
Clear this calculation using the backspace or delete buttons on your keyboard or by pressing the **Clear** button in the **Calculate** window
Next, select the empty column C13 and press the right arrow button
Click the '=' button on the keypad
Select C12 from the list of variables and press the right arrow button
Use the window's keypad to enter **^2**
Press **Calculate**

Use the **Names** window to name C12 and C13 YEAR79 and YEAR79^2, respectively. Next, return to the **Equations** window to add both terms to the fixed part of the model only.

Click on the **Add term** button
Select the **variable** YEAR79 from the drop-down list
Click on **Done**

(continued)

Click on the **Add term** button
Select the **variable** YEAR79^2 from the drop-down list
Click on **Done**

The **Equations** window should now look like this (remember you can use the **Name**, **Estimates** and **+** buttons to display more information about the current model in the **Equations** window):

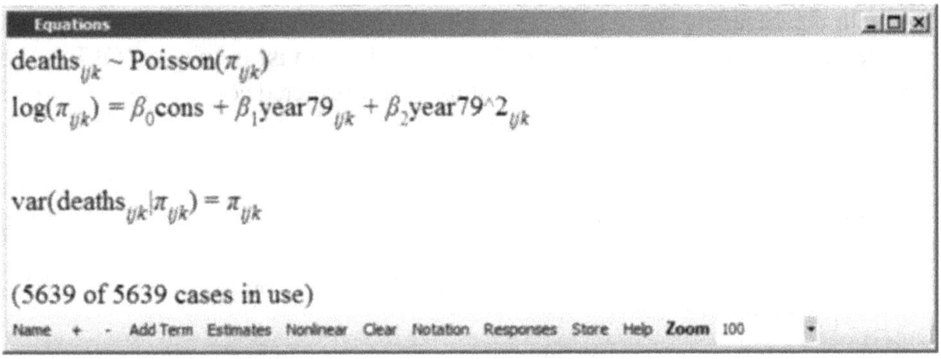

The response, DEATHs, is assumed to follow a Poisson distribution with parameter π_{ijk}. The predicted number of deaths is then estimated by taking the log of π_{ijk} (i.e. linearising the response) and setting this equal to the linear predictor on the right-hand side. This linear predictor is estimated as a quadratic function of time and the intercept in the predictor, β_0, does not vary across COUNTYs or DISTRICTs since we have included no random effects at these levels. This model will provide estimates of how the average number of deaths has changed over time (the fixed part) allowing just for random fluctuations from one year to the next (the random part).

The Offset

The model described above will fit the observed number of DEATHS in an area using just a mean and a linear and quadratic term in YEAR. However, unlike the SMR this response variable has not been scaled. That is, the SMR of an average DISTRICT in 1992 should be 100; the number of DEATHS in that DISTRICT may be 10 or 10,000 depending on the size of the population. All that an SMR of 100 tells us is that the observed number of DEATHS is the same as the EXPECTED number; we are now trying to fit that observed number and so need to account for the EXPECTED number in our model. We will do this by including it as an *offset* term. We can think of this as modelling the log of the ratio of the predicted deaths π_{ijk} to the EXPECTED deaths E_{ijk} as

$$\log\left({}^{\pi_{ijk}}/_{E_{ijk}}\right) = \beta_0 x_0 + \beta_1 x_{1ijk} + \beta_2 x_{2ijk}$$

In terms of the predicted number of deaths, this can be rewritten as

$$\log\left(\pi_{ijk}\right) = \log\left(E_{ijk}\right) + \beta_0 x_0 + \beta_1 x_{1ijk} + \beta_2 x_{2ijk}$$

In other words, the logarithm of the EXPECTED number of deaths in each area, based on population size and age-sex composition, is entered into the regression equation but its coefficient is fixed at 1 rather than being estimated freely, as is the case with the covariate coefficients for CONS, YEAR79 and YEAR79^2. MLwiN provides a facility to do this; **the variable to be offset must be named OFFS**. We can create a variable containing the logarithm of the expected count using the LOGE function in the **Calculate** window.

Go to **Data manipulation** menu
Select **Calculate**
Select the empty column C14 and press the right arrow button
Click the '=' button on the keypad
Select LOGE from the list of functions and press the up arrow button
Click the '(' button on the keypad
Select EXPECTED from the list of variables and press the right arrow button
Click the ')' button on the keypad
Click the **Calculate** button

In the **Names** window, name C14 OFFS. This variable is now included in all subsequent Poisson models unless it is renamed.

Non-linear Estimation

As mentioned above, generalised linear models are approximated in MLwiN using a linearising function based upon an expansion of the Taylor series. Specialist knowledge of this approximation is not necessary; however, users should be aware of the following options which are available when using non-linear estimation.

Click the **Nonlinear** button at the bottom of the **Equations** window

A window appears and provides details of the options for three settings:

- **Distributional assumptions** give us the options of **Poisson** or **extra Poisson** variation at level 1. A **Poisson** distribution has an equal mean and variance such that $E(y_{ijk}) = Var(y_{ijk}) = \pi_{ijk}$. However, it may be that such a distribution does not fit the data well; the most common situation is one in which the tail of the observed distribution is too heavy. We can sometimes obtain a better approximation to the data by allowing **extra Poisson** variation; the mean remains unchanged but we fit the variance as $Var(y_{ijk}) = \pi_{ijk}\sigma_e^2$. **Poisson** (distributional) variation can then be seen to be a special case of this in which $\sigma_e^2 = 1$.

- **Linearisation** gives us the choice of using a **first order** or **second order** approximation to the Taylor series.
- **Estimation type** gives us the option of using marginal quasi-likelihood (**MQL**) or penalised quasi-likelihood (**PQL**).

The latter two options affect the way in which coefficients are estimated. Bias in parameter estimates tends to be lower when using **second order** approximations and **PQL** estimation; however, there is an associated cost in as much as estimation may take longer. The **PQL** estimation procedure is also somewhat less robust and you may experience problems with convergence. A guideline is often to use **first order, MQL** when exploring the data and to use **second order, PQL** to test the model and obtain final estimates.

We will begin by using the default settings, assuming **Poisson** variation and a **first order, MQL** estimation procedure. These options may be set by clicking the **Use Defaults** button in the **Nonlinear Estimation** window and then clicking **Done**.

This section has covered setting up a GLM using:
Equations window—changing the distributional assumptions
Calculate window—using arithmetical functions
Adding an OFFSet to a Poisson model
Equations window—non-linear estimation options

Model Interpretation

Press the **Start** button to estimate the model.

To view the estimates, it will be helpful to change the precision of the display.

Go to the **Options** menu
Select **Numbers**
Increase the **# digits after decimal point** to 4
Click **Apply** and then **Done**

By clicking on the **Estimates** button in the **Equations** window, the following should appear:

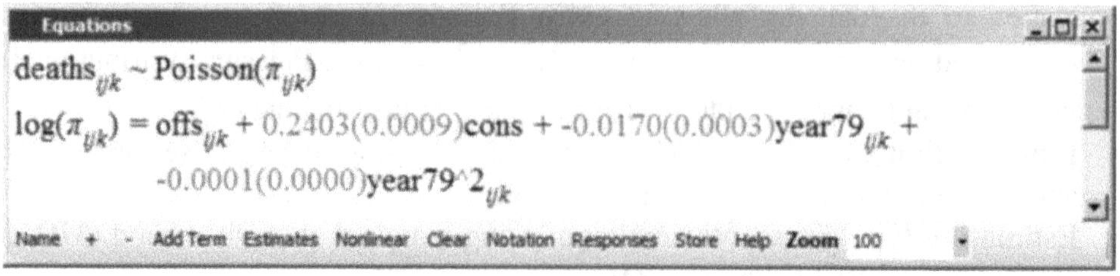

The parameter estimates are now on the log scale and should be treated as such with the OFFSet term included; for example, the predicted number of deaths in 1979 (when both YEAR79 and YEAR79^2 equal 0) has been fitted as 1.272 (=$e^{0.2403}$) times the expected number of deaths. Since the expected number of deaths varies from DISTRICT to DISTRICT, so will the predicted number of deaths. Note that MLwiN does not give values of $-2{*}loglikelihood$ for generalised linear models.

We can now consider the effects of COUNTY and DISTRICT by letting the intercept or mean CONS vary at random across these two levels.

Return to the **Equations** window
Click on CONS
Click on the check box by **j(DISTRICT)**
Click on the check box by **k(COUNTY)**
Click on **Done**
Click on the **More** button to re-estimate the model

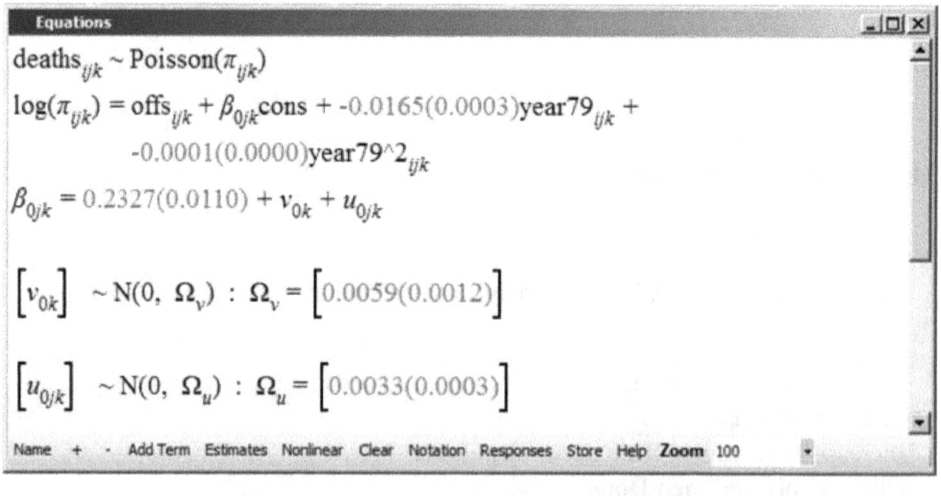

The parameter estimates in the fixed part are little changed; what is clear, however, is that there is variation over and above the Poisson variation in the counts that we might expect from one year to the next. Of the higher-level variation, about

64% (0.0059/[0.0059 + 0.0033]) is at the COUNTY (as opposed to the DISTRICT) level; this figure is very similar to that obtained from the 3-level variance components model of the SMR.

We can see what is going on more clearly using the **Graph** window. First of all we will get **Predictions** by DISTRICT and output these to C15.

> Go to **Model** menu
> Select **Predictions**
> Click on ***cons***, ***year79***$_{ijk}$ and ***year79^2***$_{ijk}$ to include all terms in the **Predictions** equation
> Select C15 for **output from prediction to**
> Click **Calc**

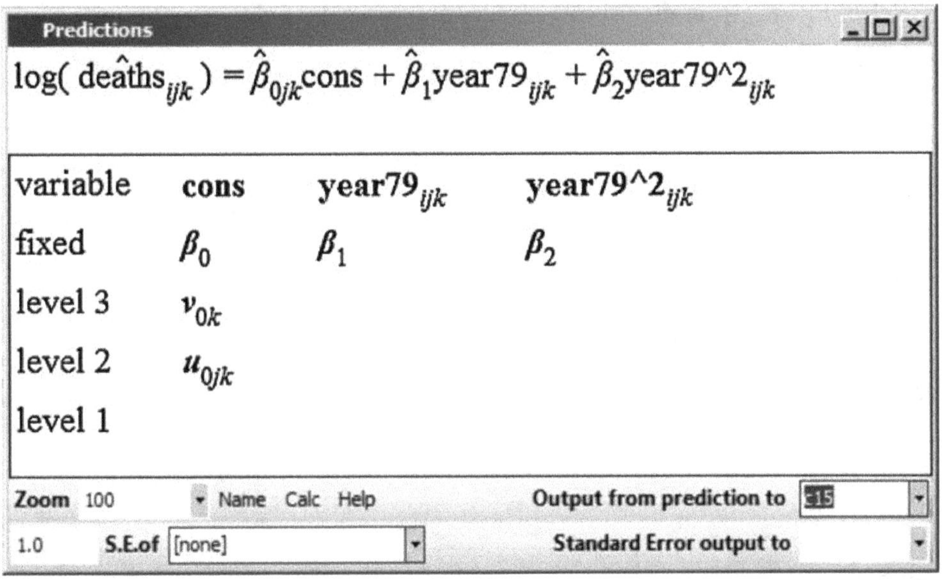

In the **Names** window, change the name of C15 to PRED2. In a similar manner we can put the predicted values for the fixed part in c16 and the level 3 predictions in c17.

> Return to the **Predictions** window
> Click on v_{0k} and u_{0jk} to remove them from the **Predictions** equation
> Select C16 for **output from prediction to**
> Click **Calc**
> Click on v_{0k} to include it in the **Predictions** equation
> Select C17 for **output from prediction to**
> Click **Calc**

Name the variables C16 and C17 PREDFP and PRED3, respectively. You will note from the summary statistics in the **Names** window that these prediction equations are on the log scale; they also do not include our OFFSet term. As such, we really have the predicted values $\log\left(\widehat{y/E_{ijk}}\right)$.

We can very easily convert these to predicted SMRs by taking the EXPOnents in the **Calculate** window:

Go to **Data manipulation** menu
Select **Calculate**
Select the PRED2 and press the right arrow button
Type =100* using the keypad
Select the function EXPOnential from the list and press the up arrow button
Click the '(' button on the keypad
Select PRED2 from the list of variables and press the right arrow button
Click the ')' button on the keypad
Click the **Calculate** button

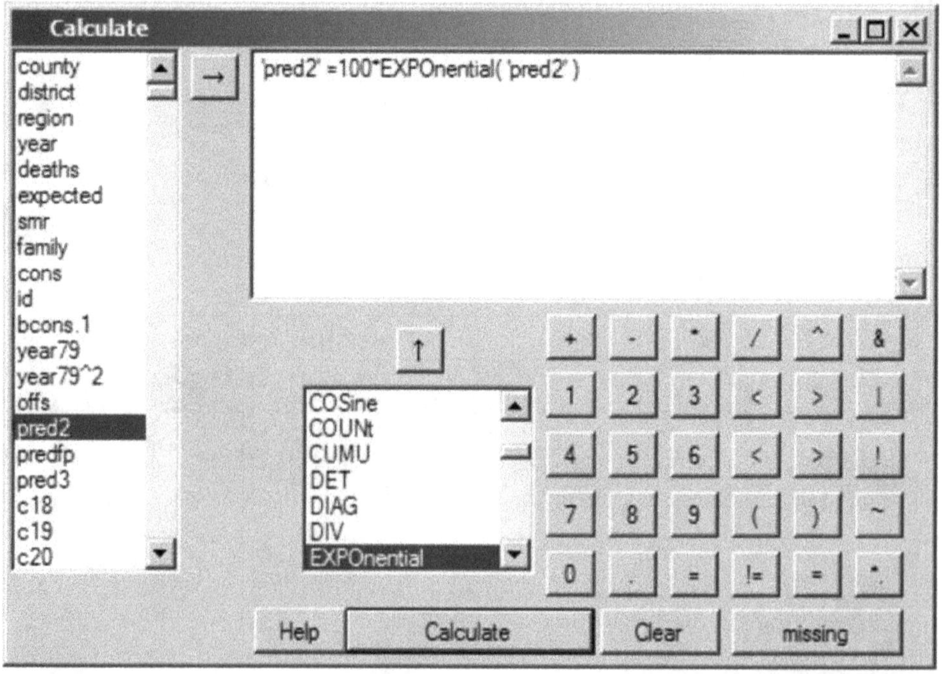

Repeat this process for the variables PREDFP and PRED3. We can now plot the predicted SMR against the observed values; PRED2 includes DISTRICT and COUNTY effects but assumes that the year-on-year fluctuations are part of a Poisson process.

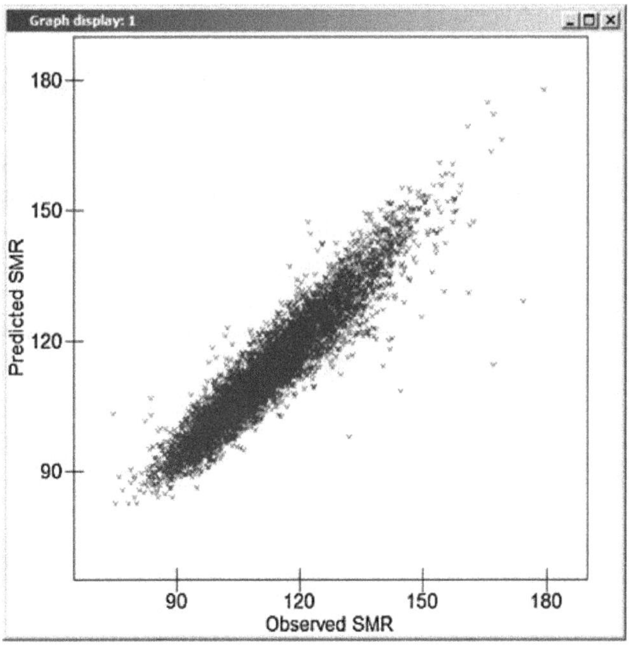

The variability in the predicted SMRs (range 82–178) is slightly less than in the observed SMRs (range 75–179). However, some of the points on this graph are a long way from the diagonal (if a point lies on the diagonal, then the observed and predicted SMRs are equal). We can identify some of the points that lie further from the diagonal by clicking on those points in the graph. Some of those in the lower right-hand quadrant—where observed SMRs are considerably larger than the predicted—can be

Data

goto line 1 view Show value labels Font Help

	county(5639)	district(5639)	year(5639)	deaths(5639)	expected(5639)	smr(5639)	pred2(5639)	predfp(5639)	pred3(5639)
1586	28.0000	2830.0000	83.0000	1034.0000	899.8230	114.9115	115.2132	118.0290	113.7186
1587	28.0000	2830.0000	84.0000	1042.0000	924.8376	112.6684	113.2637	116.0318	111.7943
1588	28.0000	2830.0000	85.0000	1103.0000	950.5851	116.0338	111.3322	114.0531	109.8879
1589	28.0000	2830.0000	86.0000	1062.0000	970.8724	109.3862	109.4191	112.0932	107.9996
1590	28.0000	2830.0000	87.0000	1036.0000	1005.3714	103.0465	107.5245	110.1523	106.1296
1591	28.0000	2830.0000	88.0000	1084.0000	1034.8282	104.7517	105.6485	108.2305	104.2780
1592	28.0000	2830.0000	89.0000	1075.0000	1060.7599	101.3424	103.7915	106.3281	102.4450
1593	28.0000	2830.0000	90.0000	1056.0000	1091.5106	96.7467	101.9534	104.4451	100.6308
1594	28.0000	2830.0000	91.0000	1140.0000	1112.5481	102.4675	100.1346	102.5818	98.8355
1595	28.0000	2830.0000	92.0000	1080.0000	1123.5365	96.1250	98.3350	100.7383	97.0593
1596	28.0000	2835.0000	81.0000	20.0000	11.4703	174.3632	128.8103	122.0782	117.6199
1597	28.0000	2835.0000	82.0000	18.0000	14.7798	121.7880	126.6645	120.0445	115.6605
1598	28.0000	2835.0000	83.0000	17.0000	13.4120	126.7520	124.5378	118.0290	113.7186
1599	28.0000	2835.0000	84.0000	22.0000	15.8785	138.5518	122.4305	116.0318	111.7943
1600	28.0000	2835.0000	85.0000	17.0000	11.9065	142.7790	120.3427	114.0531	109.8879
1601	28.0000	2835.0000	86.0000	16.0000	16.2276	98.5976	118.2747	112.0932	107.9996
1602	28.0000	2835.0000	87.0000	25.0000	20.0699	124.5646	116.2268	110.1523	106.1296
1603	28.0000	2835.0000	88.0000	27.0000	16.1551	167.1298	114.1990	108.2305	104.2780
1604	28.0000	2835.0000	89.0000	19.0000	14.5950	130.1811	112.1917	106.3281	102.4450
1605	28.0000	2835.0000	90.0000	20.0000	18.5083	108.0595	110.2049	104.4451	100.6308
1606	28.0000	2835.0000	91.0000	29.0000	20.0285	144.7934	108.2388	102.5818	98.8355
1607	28.0000	2835.0000	92.0000	20.0000	18.1693	110.0757	106.2936	100.7383	97.0593
1608	29.0000	2905.0000	79.0000	1231.0000	902.8111	136.3519	136.5076	126.1988	135.1608

identified as belonging to district 2835 in county 28. It may be worth examining some of these points in more detail using the **View or edit data** window, clicking the **view** button to select the required variables and resizing the window if necessary:

For most years in district 2835 there were more deaths than expected; however, the expected number of deaths (and therefore the population) was rather small (range 16–29). The observed SMRs for this district show considerable disparity, ranging from 174 in 1981 to 99 in 1986. The values in PRED3 suggest that county 28 as a whole has an SMR which is slightly below average, the value of 97 in 1992 being lower than the fitted average in PREDFP of 101. PRED2 contains the predicted SMRs based on the fixed part of the model—containing just an intercept and a linear and quadratic term in YEAR—and the residuals at levels 2 (DISTRICT) and 3 (COUNTY). Since both sets of residuals have been shrunk towards zero, the predicted SMRs are also known as shrunken estimates. (This name may seem confusing, since the estimates for individual years are not always closer to the average in PREDFP. For example, in 1982 the observed SMR of 122 is nearer to the average of 120 than the shrunken estimate of 127. This is because the shrunken estimate for any one year is derived from data for all years in that district—and, indeed, for all districts and all counties—and in this sense is thought to be a closer approximation to a 'true', underlying relative risk of mortality.) Note that the values of the predicted SMR are much closer to the observed values for the previous DISTRICT, 2830, reflecting the larger number of expected deaths and the consequent increase in confidence that the observed rate is close to the 'true' mortality rate.

We can also plot the predicted values at national and COUNTY level by YEAR:

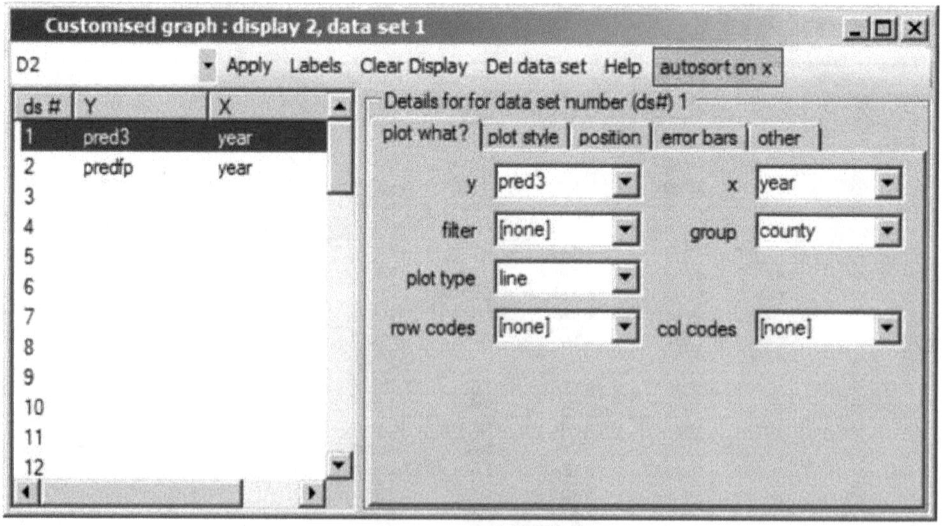

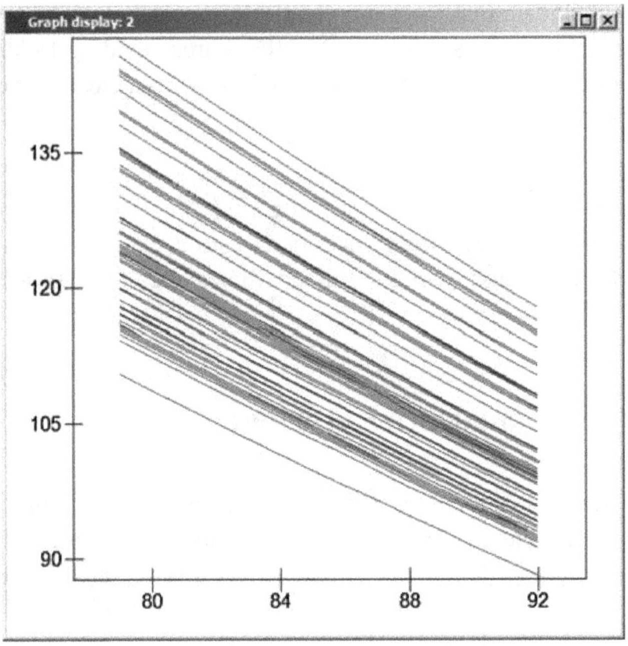

This graph illustrates the convergence of SMRs that we noted in the previous analysis even though we have not included a random slope; this is to be expected since the assumption of Poisson variation means that we can expect the variance to decrease as the number of DEATHS decreases.

You can continue to build up the model as before, entering random effects where appropriate. The plots of predicted SMRs can be broken down into the three area groupings—urban areas and inner London (URBANL), rural, prospering and maturer areas (RUPRMA) and MINING using the layout option of the Graph window. These might look as follows.

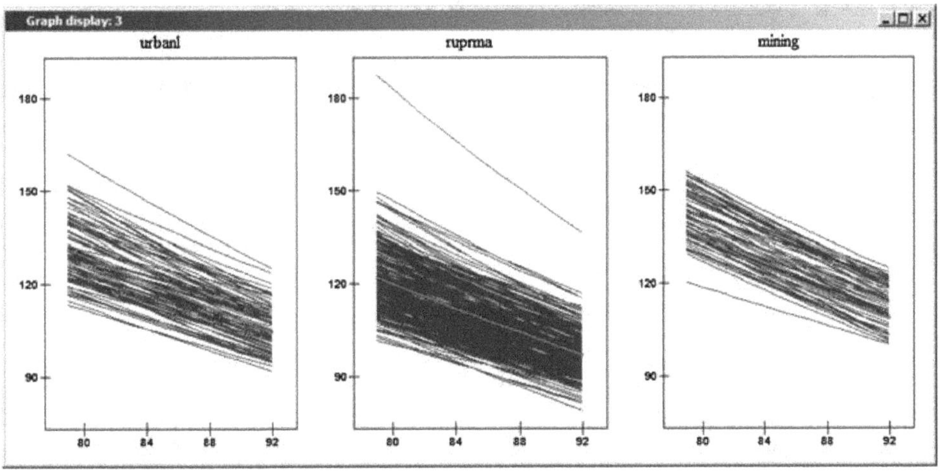

These graphs indicate that there are clear differences between the three types of area in terms of their mean SMR, with MINING areas tending to have the highest SMRs. One of the RURAL districts—DISTRICT 4820—appears to be outlying with the highest predicted SMR over the period.

This section has GLM interpretation using:
Equations window—interpreting parameter estimates
Calculate window—converting predicted values back to SMRs

Predictions and Confidence Envelopes

Compare the parameter estimates obtained from the basic 1-level and 2-level models with YEAR79 as the sole covariate. Note particularly the standard errors in the fixed part of the two models; whilst the standard error associated with the intercept (CONStant) has increased with the addition of another level, as we might expect, that associated with the slope (YEAR79) has actually decreased from 0.0387 to 0.0164. One of the reasons for fitting a multilevel model is that single-level models tend to underestimate the standard errors in the fixed part, so what is the cause of this counter-intuitive result?

Results Table

Copy

	Trend 1-level	S.E.	Trend 2-level	S.E.
Response	smr		smr	
Fixed Part				
cons	125.6769	0.2962	125.6986	0.5439
(year-79)	-1.9822	0.0387	-1.9845	0.0164
Random Part				
Level: cons				
Level: id				
Var(cons)	137.2831	2.5854	24.4935	0.4807
Level: district				
Var(cons)			112.8966	8.0625

To understand this apparent anomaly, it is necessary to consider the confidence that we have in any predicted value $\widehat{y}_{ij} = \widehat{\beta}_0 + \widehat{\beta}_1 x_{1ij}$. The variance of our predicted value $\widehat{y}_{ij}$ is given by

$$\text{var}(\hat{y}_{ij}) = \text{var}\left(\hat{\beta}_0\right) + x_{1ij}^2\text{var}\left(\hat{\beta}_1\right) + 2x_{1ij}\text{cov}\left(\hat{\beta}_0, \hat{\beta}_1\right)$$

From the current (2-level) model, we have estimates of $\text{var}\left(\hat{\beta}_0\right)$ and $\text{var}\left(\hat{\beta}_1\right)$ as $(0.5439)^2$ and $(0.0164)^2$, respectively. However, there is no estimate of the covariance in the **Equations** window. This parameter is stored by MLwiN, but we will have to find it.

Columns C1096–C1099 are used by MLwiN to store, respectively, the random parameter estimates, their estimated covariance matrix, the fixed parameters and their estimated covariance matrix. Both covariance matrices are stored in lower diagonal form. Take a look at these four columns in the **Data** window.

Go to **Data Manipulation** menu
Select **View or edit data**
Click on the **view** button
Scroll down and highlight C1096, C1097, C1098 and C1099
Click the **OK** button and resize the window if necessary

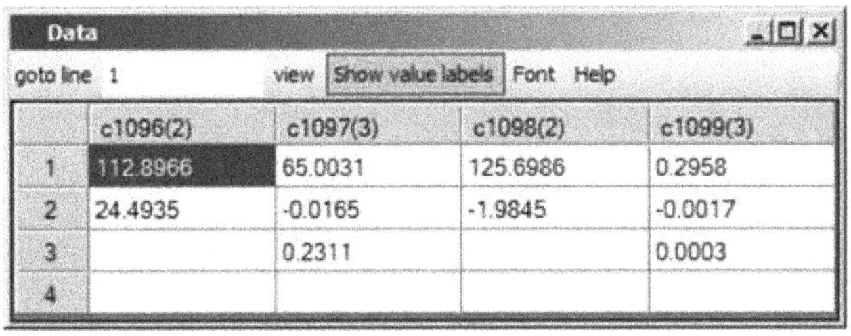

	c1096(2)	c1097(3)	c1098(2)	c1099(3)
1	112.8966	65.0031	125.6986	0.2958
2	24.4935	-0.0165	-1.9845	-0.0017
3		0.2311		0.0003
4				

Looking at columns C1098 and C1099 we find the estimated distribution of the fixed parameters to be

$$\begin{bmatrix} \hat{\beta}_0 \\ \hat{\beta}_1 \end{bmatrix} \sim N\left(\begin{bmatrix} 125.6982 \\ -1.9845 \end{bmatrix}, \begin{bmatrix} 0.2958 & \\ -0.0017 & 0.0003 \end{bmatrix} \right)$$

Our estimates of the two parameters are therefore not independent; we find a negative correlation of about -0.2 between the intercept and the slope. We can use the **Predictions** window to plot the predicted line and a 95% confidence envelope. First save the data so that we can return to the current model when we have finished our exploration.

Go to **File** menu
Select **Save worksheet as...**
Type **lmdpapp1.ws** as the new filename
Click the **Save** button

The Predictions window is described in more detail when it is used later in this tutorial. At this stage we will do little more than detail the commands. To start with we will obtain the predicted values of the SMR for each COUNTY, DISTRICT and YEAR based on the fixed part of the model alone, together with 1.96 times the standard error of these estimates. (A 95% confidence interval can be constructed as the estimate ± 1.96 standard errors.) At the moment, the fixed part of the model just contains the intercept and the time trend YEAR79.

Go to **Model** menu
Select **Predictions**
Click on β_0 and β_1
In the drop-down list by **Output from prediction to** select C12
Edit the multiplier of **S.E.** to 1.96
In the drop-down list by **S.E. of** select **Fixed**
In the drop-down list by **Standard Error output to** select C13
Click on **Calc**

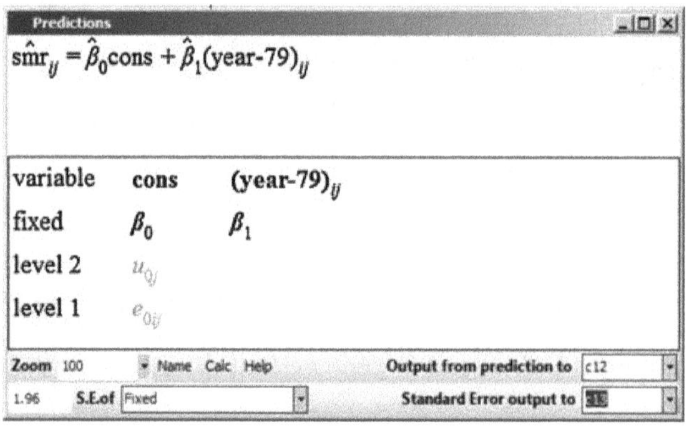

C12 now contains our predicted regression line and C13 contains 1.96 times the standard error of the fixed parameters. We can plot these using the **Customised Graph** window, plotting the predicted values against YEAR as a line graph.

Go to the **Graphs** menu
Select **Customised Graph(s)**
Select the second dataset, **D2**, from the pull-down list at the top left of the window
From the drop-down list by **y** select C12
From the drop-down list by **x** select YEAR
Change the **plot type** to **line**
Click the **Apply** button

This produces a line graph of the predicted mean SMR. We can add confidence intervals around this line using the **y errors** feature on the **error bars** tab:

In the **Customised Graph** window, click on the **error bars** tab
Select C13 to be the **y errors +** and the **y errors –**
Change the **y error type** to **lines**
Click on **Apply**

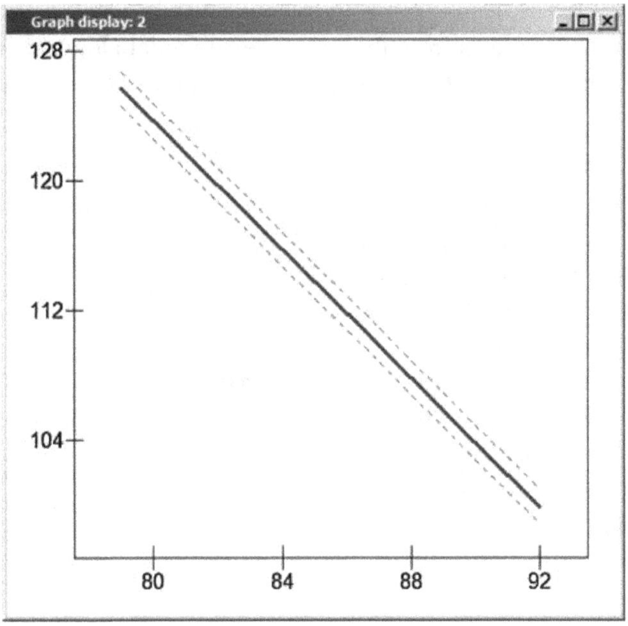

This is the predicted regression line together with 95% confidence intervals. We will now compare this with the single-level model. We start by removing CONS from the random part of the model at level 2 and then we re-estimate the model.

In the **Equations** window, click on u_{0j}
Remove the tick by **j(district)**
Click on **Done**
Click on **More**

This returns us to the single-level model that we had fitted previously. We can now use the **Predictions** window again to obtain the predicted values of the SMR based on the fixed part of the model, together with appropriate multiples of the standard errors of these estimates.

In the **Predictions** window, ensure that both fixed terms are included but not the random terms
In the drop-down list by **Output from prediction to** select C14
Edit the multiplier of **S.E.** to 1.96
In the drop-down list by **S.E. of** select **Fixed**
In the drop-down list by **Standard Error output to** select C15
Click on **Calc**

We can plot the estimates from this single-level model alongside those from the 2-level model using the **position** feature of the **Customised Graph** window.

In the **Customised Graph** window, click on row **2** under **ds #**
From the drop-down list by **y** select C14
From the drop-down list by **x** select YEAR
Change the **plot type** to **line**
Click on the **error bars** tab
Select C15 to be the **y errors +** and the **y errors –**
Change the **y error type** to **lines**
Click on the **position** tab
Click in the box on row **1**, column **2**
Click on **Apply**

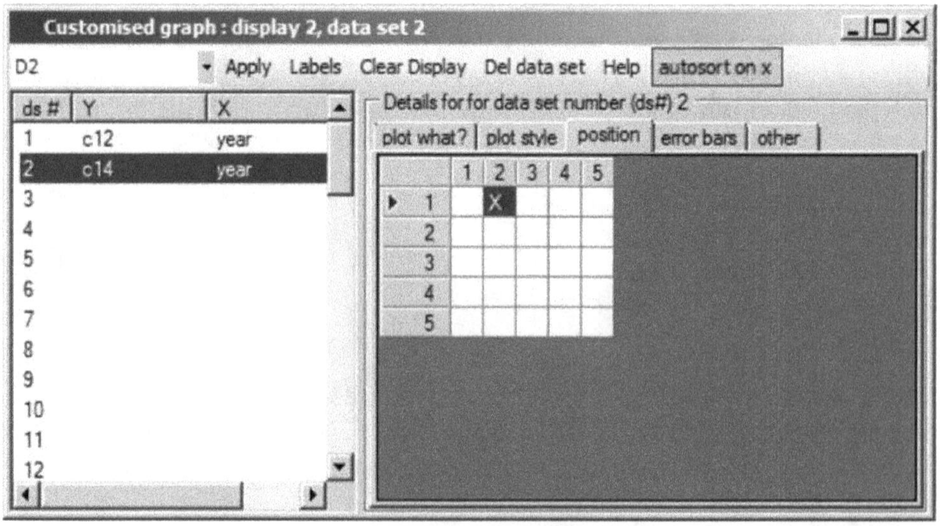

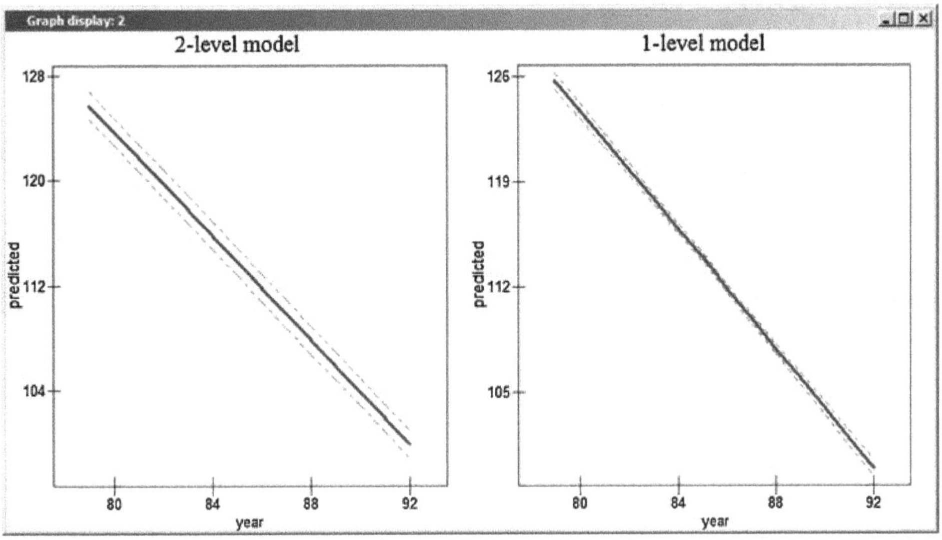

(Note: the above graphs have added titles.) We can see that the confidence envelope around the predicted mean is much tighter under the 1-level model than the 2-level model. We can confirm this by looking at the variables C12–C15 in the **Names** window:

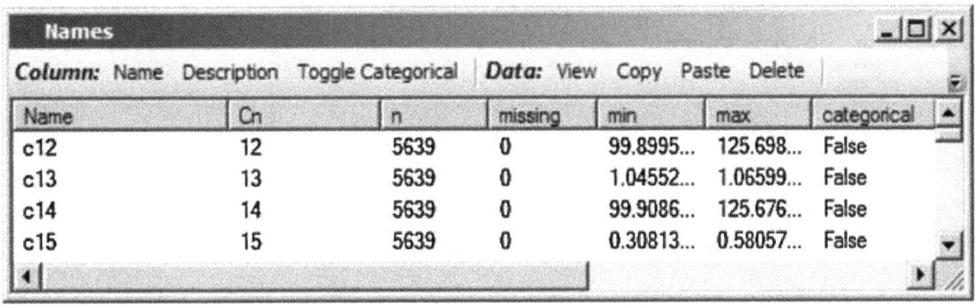

Name	Cn	n	missing	min	max	categorical
c12	12	5639	0	99.8995...	125.698...	False
c13	13	5639	0	1.04552...	1.06599...	False
c14	14	5639	0	99.9086...	125.676...	False
c15	15	5639	0	0.30813...	0.58057...	False

C13, 1.96 times the standard error under the 2-level model, varies between 1.046 and 1.066; C15, 1.96 times the standard error under the single-level model, takes values ranging between 0.308 and 0.581. The single-level estimates show signs of 'misestimated precision'—ignoring the data hierarchy leads to a confidence envelope that is too tight.

Retrieve the saved worksheet before returning to the section on the hierarchy viewer:

Go to **File** menu
Select **Open** worksheet
Choose **lmdpappl.ws** as the filename
Click the **Open** button

References

Gelman A, Hill J (2007) Data analysis using regression and multilevel/hierarchical models. Cambridge University Press, Cambridge

Leyland AH (2004) Increasing inequalities in premature mortality in Great Britain. J Epidemiol Commun Health 58:296–302

Leyland AH, McLeod A (2000) Mortality in England and Wales, 1979-1992. An introduction to multilevel modelling using MLwiN. MRC Social and Public Health Sciences Unit occasional paper no. 1. MRC Social and Public Health Sciences Unit, Glasgow

Snijders TAB, Bosker RJ (2012) Multilevel analysis: an introduction to basic and advanced multilevel modeling. Sage, Los Angeles

12

Multilevel Logistic Regression through a Specialist Multilevel Modeling Software

Abstract This chapter contains a tutorial for analysing a dichotomous response variable in multilevel analysis using multilevel logistic regression.

After introducing the multilevel logistic regression model, we move on to the example data set that will be used. This concerns variation in referral rates of general practitioners (GPs) to physiotherapists. The outcome or dependent variable is whether or not a patient was referred to a physiotherapist, something that may be influenced by characteristics of both patient and GP. We briefly discuss the theoretical model that the authors of this study applied to formulate hypotheses to explain the apparent variation in referrals.

The data were collected in the late 1980s in the Netherlands. The structure of the data was that consultations for problems with the locomotive system (the main reason for referral to physiotherapists) were nested within GPs.

In the chapter we describe the analysis of these data using MLwiN.

Keywords Tutorial · Multilevel analysis · Logistic regression · Physiotherapy · Referral

Many research problems involve a response variable which is dichotomous; for example, a patient has a good or a poor outcome following surgical intervention. Such data are often assumed to arise from a binomial distribution and may be modelled using logistic regression. More generally, data may be in the form of a proportion (such as the proportion of GP consultations resulting in a referral to physiotherapy) and may be modelled in a similar manner. This chapter shows how a multilevel logistic regression model is formulated for binomial data clustered within higher-level units. We then introduce the example and the data set used. This is followed by an application within MLwiN. Further details on multilevel modelling and MLwiN are available from the Centre for Multilevel Modelling http://www.bristol.ac.uk/cmm/. The materials have been written for MLwiN v3.01. The teaching version of the software is available from https://www.bristol.ac.uk/cmm/software/mlwin/download/.

Multilevel Logistic Regression Model

Let y_{ij} denote a binary response (0 or 1) for the *i*th individual in the *j*th unit, and let π_{ij} denote the probability of a 'success' (i.e. $y_{ij} = 1$). The binomial distribution is characterised by two parameters: the probability of success π_{ij} and the number of 'trials' n. So if the outcome were the proportion of GP consultations that resulted in physiotherapy, the denominator n would be the total number of relevant consultations. For a logistic regression model, when each data item refers to an individual response with a dichotomous outcome rather than a proportion, the denominator is always equal to one. This means that we have

$$y_{ij} \sim \text{Binomial}(1, \pi_{ij})$$

In a random intercept multilevel logistic regression model, we then model the transformed probability π_{ij} as a linear combination of a series of covariates or explanatory variables x_{pij} together with a random effect for each higher-level unit u_{0j} so that we can write

$$\text{logit}(\pi_{ij}) = \log\left(\frac{\pi_{ij}}{1 - \pi_{ij}}\right) = \beta_0 + \beta_1 x_{1ij} + \cdots + u_{0j}$$

As for the multilevel linear regression model, we make an assumption about the distribution of the higher-level residuals u_{0j}

$$u_{0j} \sim N(0, \sigma^2_{u0})$$

Alternative *link functions* to the logit link can be employed for dichotomous outcomes; common alternatives are the probit and complementary log-log links. The logit link has the advantage that the parameter estimates β_p can be interpreted as log odds ratios (and so, when exponentiated, they can be interpreted as odds ratios). For further details of link functions, the reader is referred to general works such as that by McCullagh and Nelder (1989).

Example: Variation in the GP Referral Rate to Physiotherapy

Until recently, patients in the Netherlands (from where the data used in this example are drawn) had to be referred by a GP before they could visit a physiotherapist. GPs are still the major source of referrals to physiotherapists in primary healthcare. Patients are predominantly referred to physiotherapists when they have complaints relating to the locomotive system. Of all patients that present their problem to their

GP, a varying proportion is referred to a physiotherapist. The aim of the original study was to explain the variation between GPs in physiotherapy referrals (Uunk et al. 1992).

The authors followed the logic that was explained in Chap. 2. The average referral rate of the GPs in their sample for patients with complaints related to the locomotive system was 24%. This percentage varied between GPs from a low of 11% to a high of 45%. So some GPs referred only one out of ten patients with problems in the locomotive system to a physiotherapist, whilst at the other end of the scale almost half of another GP's patients were referred. The authors constructed an explanatory model based on social production function (SPF) theory (again see Chap. 2; Lindenberg 1996).

The GPs could either treat the patients themselves, including the use of a 'wait and see' policy, or they could refer patients to a physiotherapist. The dependent variable is therefore dichotomous. Following SPF theory it was assumed that GPs have two goals: improving their patients' health and increasing their own well-being. It was further assumed that both GPs and patients had resources that they could use to reach their goals. The theoretical model is given in Fig. 12.1.

Starting from the right-hand side of Fig. 12.1, the dependent variable is whether a patient is referred to physiotherapy or not. Preceding this are two boundary conditions: firstly, patients have to visit their GP with health complaints for which referral to a physiotherapist is a relevant alternative. The authors restricted the data to patients with complaints of the locomotive system. Hence this condition was fulfilled. The separate diagnoses were used in the analysis to take the case-mix of different GPs into account. The second condition is that there are physiotherapists to whom patients can be referred. That condition is always fulfilled globally, but there

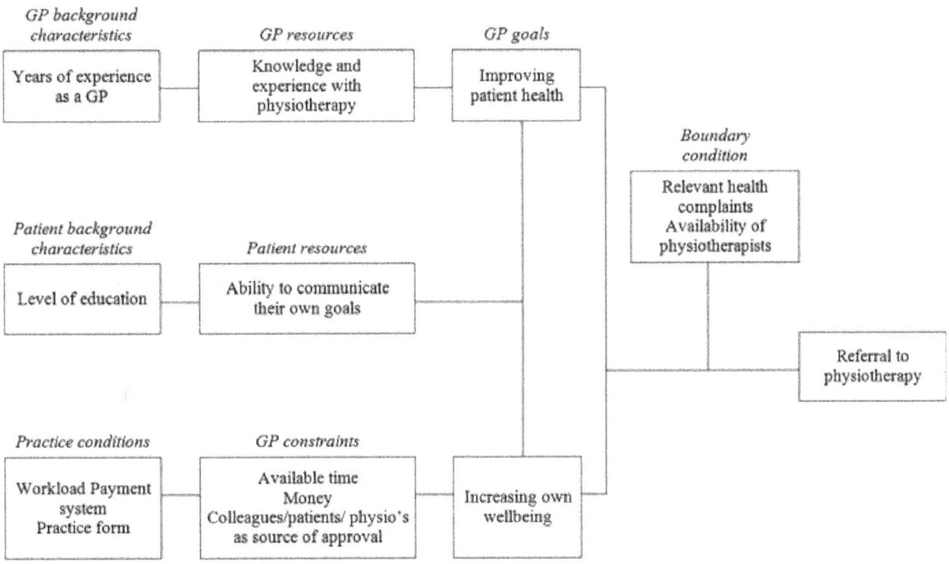

Fig. 12.1 Theoretical model to explain variation in referrals to physiotherapy

is variation in the local availability of physiotherapists within the practice area of the GPs. This variable was therefore used as a control variable.

The assumption was that GPs want to improve their patients' health. Whether they can realise this goal by referring a patient to physiotherapy might depend on their knowledge of and experience with physiotherapy. As the authors did not have a direct measure of this, they used the number of years of experience that each GP had working as a GP. It is also assumed that GPs want to achieve personal goals: well-being and social approval (from patients, colleagues and physiotherapists). Their workload and the way they were paid (depending on whether a patient was publicly or privately insured) were both assumed to influence well-being. The type of practice was considered a potential influence of sources of social approval: in single-handed practices, GPs depend more on their patients for social approval. The authors had information on whether GPs had physiotherapists in their social network. They interpreted this information in two ways: either this might influence the possibility of acquiring social approval through the referral of patients to physiotherapists, or it might relate to their knowledge of physiotherapy. Finally, it was assumed that patients themselves might want to visit a physiotherapist and that those patients who had achieved a higher educational level would be better able to put their point forward when discussing this issue with their GP. Patient characteristics such as age and sex were used as control variables. In the example dataset, we will use a less extensive set of variables for the sake of simplicity. However, you will still be able to explore the data and test your own ideas.

The data were collected in 1987 as part of a large national survey of general practice (Van der Velden 1999). The starting point was a sample of 100 GP practices in the Netherlands. The following data are relevant to this example:

- GPs in these practices recorded all contacts with their patients over a period of 3 months, including the diagnosis and whether a patient was referred to a physiotherapist.
- GPs filled in a questionnaire.
- All patients on the list of each practice were sent a short questionnaire to collect social and demographic background variables.

The contacts of the same patients for the same health problem were combined into care episodes. This is especially relevant in the case of referrals where patients might first have a consultation, presenting their problem, and their GP might advise them to wait for a couple of weeks and come back if their complaints did not disappear. If we calculated the referral rate using separate contacts instead of the care episodes, we would therefore tend to find much lower referral rates. Consequently, the data have five levels: the practice, the GPs, the patients, the episodes and the contacts. In this example, we only use two levels: GPs and episodes (most GPs were single-handed at that time and the majority of patients only had one episode during the 3-month period). The data therefore form a two-level strict hierarchy of episodes nested within GPs. Patient characteristics, such as age, are simply distributed over episodes. The outcome of interest is a binary indicator of whether the patient was referred to a physiotherapist or not.

The Data

The data are contained in the MLwiN worksheet ‘fysio.wsz’. When you open the worksheet, you will see the **Names** window providing an overview of all of the variables. Patients (as previously mentioned, these are not strictly speaking patients but episodes) are identified by PATID and GPs by GPID. Columns 3–8 contain data information relating to the patient. PATAGE is the patient’s age in years, ranging from 18 to 98. This variable is subsequently categorised in PAGEGRP. This variable has been declared as a categorical variable; click on the variable name PAGEGRP in the **Names** window and then on the **View** button in the **Categories** section at the top of the **Names** window to display the category names. The categories used are 18–34, 35–44, 45–54, 55–64, 65–74, 75–84 and 85–98. PATSEX is also a categorical variable denoting the patient’s sex—1 for male and 2 for female. Similarly, PATINSUR takes the value 1 if the patient is publicly insured and 0 if they are privately insured. The extent of the patient’s education is contained in the variable PATEDU; this variable has four levels (1 for no formal education, 2 for those with only primary education, 3 for secondary and lower/middle vocational education and 4 for higher vocational and university education).

Names

Column: Name Description Toggle Categorical *Data:* View Copy Paste Delete

Name	Cn	n	missing	min	max	categorical
gpid	1	16700	0	500	844	False
patid	2	16700	0	1	16700	False
patage	3	16700	0	18	98	False
pagegrp	4	16700	0	1	7	True
patsex	5	16700	0	0	1	True
patinsur	6	16700	0	0	1	True
patedu	7	16700	0	1	4	True
diag	8	16700	0	1	13	True
gpexper	9	16700	0	0	3.29999...	False
gpworkload	10	16700	0	0.27700...	4.64900...	False
practype	11	16700	0	1	4	True
location	12	16700	0	1	4	True
gpphysifr	13	16700	0	0	1	True
referral	14	16700	0	0	1	False
cons	15	16700	0	1	1	False
c16	16	0	0	0	0	False

The variable DIAG contains the primary diagnosis resulting from the care episodes. These diagnoses are in 13 mutually exclusive categories:

- diag_1: symptoms/complaints neck
- diag_2: symptoms/complaints back
- diag_3: myalgia/fibrositis
- diag_4: symptoms of multiple muscles
- diag_5: disabilities related to the locomotive system
- diag_6: impediments of the cervical spine
- diag_7: arthrosis cervical spine
- diag_8: lumbago
- diag_9: ischialgia
- diag_10: hernia nuclei pulposi
- diag_11: impediments of the shoulder
- diag_12: epicondylitis lateralis
- diag_13: tendinitis/synovitis

The variables in columns 9–13 relate to the GP. Their experience was measured by the number of years they had worked as a GP; we have rescaled this by dividing by 10 so that GPEXPER, a continuous variable, ranges from 0 to 3.3 indicating that the range of experience was from 0 to 33 years. Also at the level of GP we have workload (GPWORKLOAD), a continuous variable, containing the total number of contacts in the 3-month registration period, measured in thousands of patients, and ranging from 0.277 to 4.649 (i.e. from 277 to 4649 patients). The type of practice, PRACTYPE, is a categorical variable distinguishing between single-handed practices, partnership practices, group practices and health centres. The variable LOCATION differentiates between four categories of practice location: rural, suburban, urban and big city. Finally, the variable GPPHYSIFR indicates whether the GPs have physiotherapists in their social network (taking the value 1 for yes, 0 for no).

REFERRAL is the response variable with 0 indicating that the patient was not referred to a physiotherapist and 1 indicating that they were. (Note the use of 0 and 1 for the responses, not the 1 and 2 used by convention in some other software packages.) Finally, CONS is a column of 1s used to model the intercept in the fixed part of the model; for a random intercept model, this variable will also model the random variation across GPs.

Model Set-Up

Open the **Equations** window and the default unspecified model should appear. Declare REFERRAL to be the response, specify a two-level model and set the level 1 and 2 identifiers to be PATID and GPID, respectively. Next click on the **N** corresponding to the default (normal) distribution for the response and change this to binomial. Accept the default suggestion of a logit link to fit a logistic regression. The window should appear as follows:

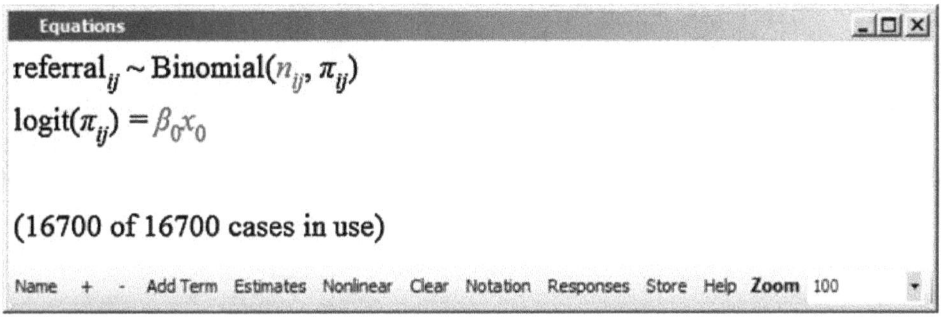

In addition to asking for the model specification—the red $\beta_0 x_0$ term—MLwiN requests the denominator n_{ij}. We can use the binomial distribution to model proportions in which case n_{ij} would be the number of 'attempts'. Since our data refer to individuals, and the response is whether or not an individual patient is referred to physiotherapy, the n_{ij} that we require is just another column of 1s. Click on the n_{ij}, select CONS from the drop-down list and click on **Done**.

Now we can specify the fixed part of the model and the level-2 variance component. It is sensible to start with a mean model to estimate the probability of being referred and see how this varies between GPs. Add CONS as an explanatory variable to estimate the mean probability and let this mean vary across GPs at level 2. The window should now appear as follows (you may need to press the + button at the bottom of the **Equations** window to expand the model that is shown).

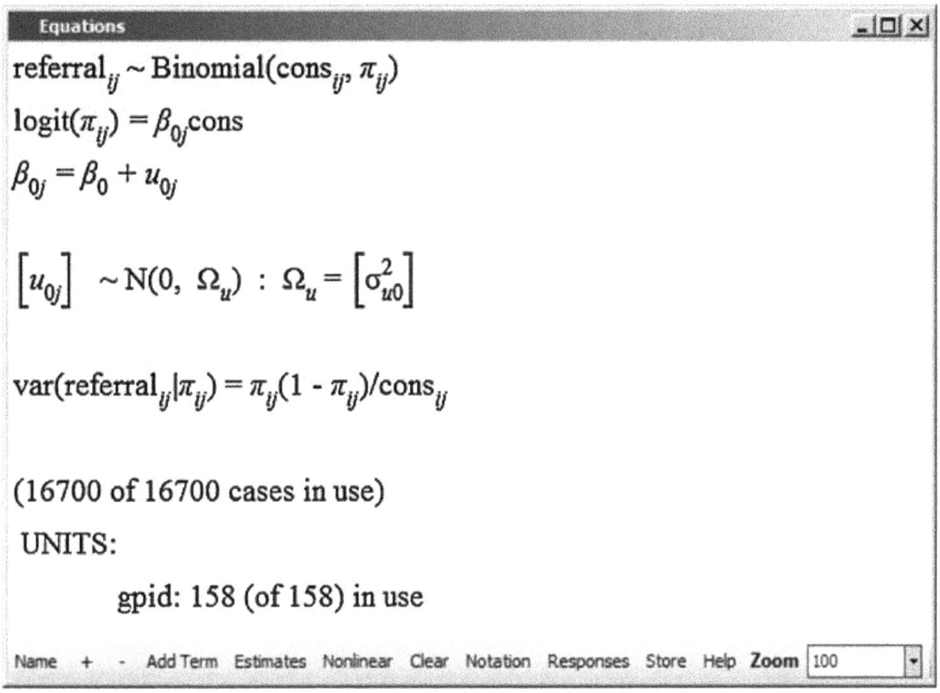

The constant β_0 will estimate the log odds of referral by the average GP and the GP residuals u_{0j}, which are assumed to be normally distributed, will estimate the GP deviations from the mean log odds. The lowest level variance is a function of π_{ij}, the probability of individual i being referred to a physiotherapist by GP j; this is determined by the fact that we are assuming a binomial distribution and we do not estimate this variance explicitly.

Non-linear Settings

Before estimating the model, we need to specify the settings for non-linear estimation. There are three options that can be set, and this is done by clicking on the **Nonlinear** button at the bottom of the **Equations** window. The first option covers the distributional assumption and this relates to whether we wish to assume the variation at level 1 is binomial. For binary data we should assume that this is true rather than testing for over- or under-dispersion (Skrondal and Rabe-Hesketh 2007). The second and third options relate to the estimation procedure used by MLwiN. The estimation procedure is iterative and involves transforming the data and fitting a linear model. The *linearisation* option relates to the Taylor series expansion, which approximates a linear form for the model, and the options are either a first or second order expansion. The linearising expansion uses predicted values from one iteration to estimate the parameters at the next iteration, and *estimation type* relates to whether these predicted values are calculated from the fixed part of the model only (MQL) or from both the fixed and random parts of the model (PQL). The simplest estimation procedure (first order MQL) tends to under-estimate the random parameters (variances), although it is computationally more robust than second order PQL estimation (Goldstein and Rasbash 1996; Rodríguez and Goldman 1995). A rule of thumb is to start with the simpler estimation procedure and, once a model of interest has been established, switch to second order PQL. To start with we shall use the default settings: a binomial distribution with a first order MQL estimation procedure. This can be selected by clicking on **Use Defaults** and then **Done**.

Once these options have been selected, we can estimate the model by clicking on the **Start** button at the top of the MLwiN window.

Model Interpretation and Model Building

The mean model should appear as follows:

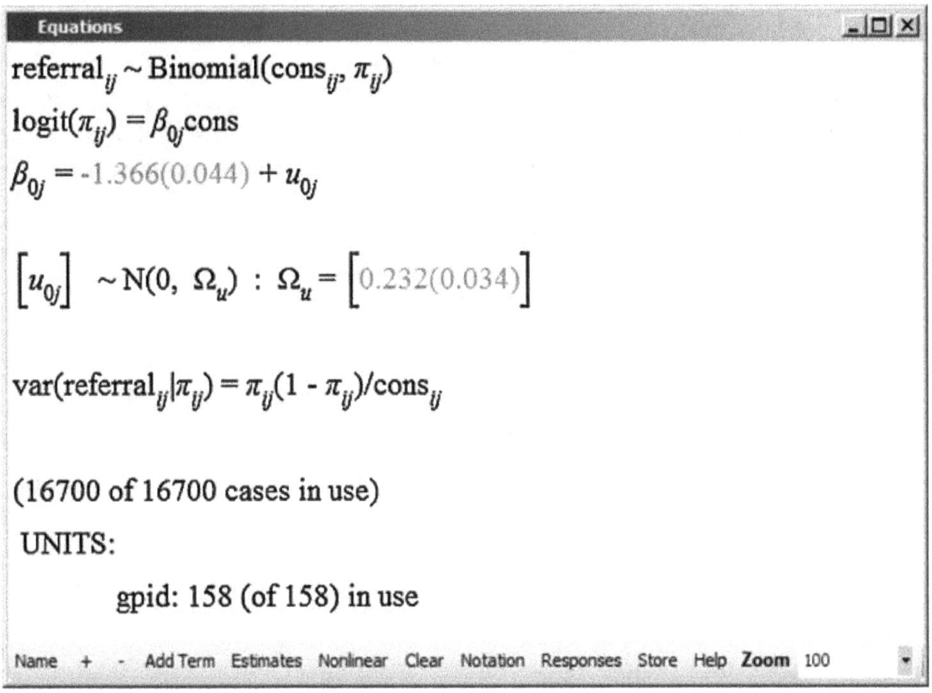

Taking the antilogit function of the intercept (i.e. $\exp(\beta_0)/[1 + \exp(\beta_0)]$) gives the probability of being referred by the average GP to be 0.203. There is a great deal of variation between GPs and we can use this estimate to calculate a 95% confidence interval for the proportion of patients receiving a referral from their GP, again using the antilogit function. Thus, in 95% of GPs the probability of referral is between antilogit $\left(-1.366 - 1.96\sqrt{0.232}, -1.366 + 1.96\sqrt{0.232}\right) = (0.090, 0.396)$.

In Chap. 6, we considered ways of examining the magnitude of the variance for multilevel logistic regression models. Firstly, the intraclass correlation coefficient can be approximated as

$$\rho_{\mathrm{I}} = \frac{\sigma_{u0}^2}{\sigma_{u0}^2 + 3.29}$$

suggesting that 6.6% of the variability in whether a patient is referred to a physiotherapist can be attributed to differences between GPs. Secondly, we can calculate a median odds ratio (MOR) as

$$\text{MOR} = \exp\left(0.954\sqrt{\sigma_{u0}^2}\right)$$

This suggests that the median of all pairwise comparisons between GPs gives an odds ratio of 1.58. There is therefore considerable variation between GPs and we can go on to see how much of this variation can be explained by differences in patient populations. Firstly, add the two control variables, age and sex, as explanatory variables to the current model: PAGEGRP and PATSEX. As reference categories use women in the youngest age group. Then add the diagnoses contained in the variable DIAG, with the first category (symptoms or complaints of the neck) as the reference category. Now estimate this new model to obtain:

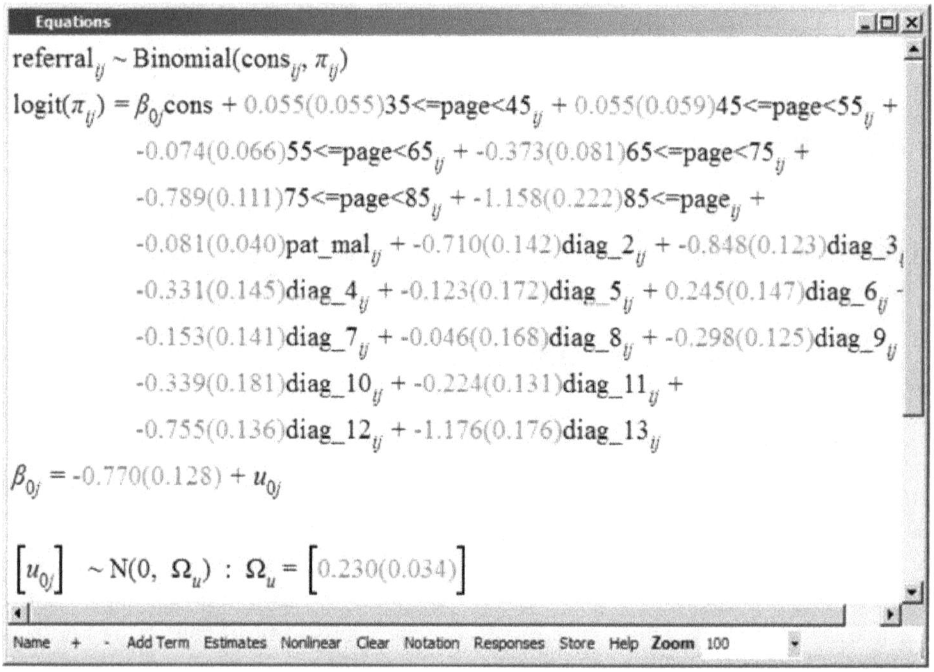

Note that MLwiN does not provide an estimate of $-2*loglikelihood$ for logistic regression models. This is because the estimation procedure used is not maximum likelihood but pseudo-likelihood. There has been a change in the estimate associated with the intercept β_0. This is now an estimate of the log odds of referral by the average GP for a patient with the baseline characteristics, in this case a female aged 18–34. All of the covariate estimates are on the log odds scale and thus represent the change in log odds associated with a unit increase in each explanatory variable. By taking the exponential of these estimates, we can obtain estimates of the odds ratio (OR) of referral relative to an appropriate baseline group. The OR for referral for patients aged 35–44, relative to those aged 18–34, is exp(0.055) or 1.06; 95% confidence intervals are given by $\exp(0.055 \pm 1.96 \times 0.055)$ or (0.95, 1.18). The 95% confidence interval contains 1 suggesting that the odds of referral to a physiotherapist are not significantly different between the 18–34 and 35–44 age groups. The parameter estimates suggest a non-linear relationship with age and, relative to the younger patients, older patients (those aged 65 and over) are less likely to be referred to a physiotherapist. Relative to the youngest group, the OR of referral is 0.69 (0.59, 0.81) for those aged 65–74, 0.45 (0.37, 0.56) for those aged 75–84 and 0.31 (0.20, 0.49) for those aged 85 and over. Men are less likely to be referred than women, although this is of borderline significance (OR = 0.92; 95% C.I. 0.85, 1.00).

After taking account of differences in patient populations and diagnoses, we see that the between GP variation has remained virtually unchanged. This is quite uncommon, as often a large part of the apparent variation between high level units is due to differences between individuals. It is, however, also possible for the variance between higher-level units to increase in multilevel models following the addition of variables at the lower (in this case patient) level. Snijders and Bosker (2012) provide an explanation as to why this is likely to happen in multilevel logistic regression models. In essence, since the variance in a binary outcome y_{ij} is constrained to be equal to $\pi_{ij}(1 - \pi_{ij})$ (see Chap. 6), the addition of a level 1 variable will tend to result in an increase in the level 2 variance so that the *proportion* of unexplained variation at level 1 will decrease.

We can now check for the effect of the other patient variables; add both PATEDU and PATINSUR to the current model, using the lowest educated and those with private insurance as the reference categories.

Equations

$$\text{referral}_{ij} \sim \text{Binomial}(\text{cons}_{ij}, \pi_{ij})$$

$$\begin{aligned}\text{logit}(\pi_{ij}) = {} & \beta_{0j}\text{cons} + 0.094(0.056)\text{35<=page<45}_{ij} + 0.140(0.061)\text{45<=page<55}_{ij} + \\ & 0.044(0.070)\text{55<=page<65}_{ij} + -0.243(0.085)\text{65<=page<75}_{ij} + \\ & -0.639(0.115)\text{75<=page<85}_{ij} + -1.012(0.224)\text{85<=page}_{ij} + \\ & -0.091(0.040)\text{pat\_mal}_{ij} + -0.700(0.142)\text{diag\_2}_{ij} + -0.833(0.123)\text{diag\_3}_{ij} \\ & -0.321(0.145)\text{diag\_4}_{ij} + -0.111(0.173)\text{diag\_5}_{ij} + 0.263(0.148)\text{diag\_6}_{ij} + \\ & -0.135(0.142)\text{diag\_7}_{ij} + -0.037(0.168)\text{diag\_8}_{ij} + -0.288(0.125)\text{diag\_9}_{ij} \\ & -0.351(0.181)\text{diag\_10}_{ij} + -0.217(0.131)\text{diag\_11}_{ij} + \\ & -0.759(0.136)\text{diag\_12}_{ij} + -1.168(0.177)\text{diag\_13}_{ij} + \\ & 0.364(0.184)\text{edu\_primary}_{ij} + 0.585(0.183)\text{edu\_secondary}_{ij} + \\ & 0.851(0.198)\text{edu\_higher}_{ij} + 0.081(0.050)\text{publicins}_{ij}\end{aligned}$$

$$\beta_{0j} = -1.423(0.228) + u_{0j}$$

$$\left[u_{0j}\right] \sim \text{N}(0, \Omega_u) : \Omega_u = \left[0.230(0.034)\right]$$

Name + - Add Term Estimates Nonlinear Clear Notation Responses Store Help Zoom 100

These two new covariates offer further insight into the pattern of referrals: there is a steady increase in the probability of referral with increasing educational level of those patients who present with complaints of the locomotive system. Relative to those with no education, those with higher education have more than twice the odds of being referred for physiotherapy (OR = 2.34; 95% C.I. 1.59, 3.45). The type of insurance (and thus the way GPs are remunerated) does not significantly affect the chance of being referred; those with public insurance show a small and insignificant increase in the odds of referral (OR = 1.08; 95% C.I. 0.98, 1.19). Once again, the addition of these patient characteristics makes no difference to the variance between GPs.

Finally we add the five GP-level variables: GPEXPER, GPWORKLOAD, PRACTYPE (reference: single-handed practices), LOCATION (reference: rural) and GPPHYSIFR (reference: those GPs who do not have friends who are physiotherapists).

Equations

$$
\begin{aligned}
\text{logit}(\pi_{ij}) = \beta_{0j}\text{cons} &+ 0.096(0.057)\text{35<=page<45}_{ij} + 0.145(0.062)\text{45<=page<55}_{ij} + \\
&0.048(0.071)\text{55<=page<65}_{ij} + -0.243(0.086)\text{65<=page<75}_{ij} + \\
&-0.643(0.115)\text{75<=page<85}_{ij} + -1.006(0.226)\text{85<=page}_{ij} + \\
&-0.091(0.041)\text{pat\_mal}_{ij} + -0.703(0.144)\text{diag\_2}_{ij} + -0.846(0.125)\text{diag\_3} \\
&-0.319(0.147)\text{diag\_4}_{ij} + -0.112(0.174)\text{diag\_5}_{ij} + 0.259(0.149)\text{diag\_6}_{ij} - \\
&-0.136(0.143)\text{diag\_7}_{ij} + -0.044(0.169)\text{diag\_8}_{ij} + -0.293(0.127)\text{diag\_9}_{ij} \\
&-0.352(0.183)\text{diag\_10}_{ij} + -0.222(0.132)\text{diag\_11}_{ij} + \\
&-0.770(0.138)\text{diag\_12}_{ij} + -1.178(0.178)\text{diag\_13}_{ij} + \\
&0.367(0.185)\text{edu\_primary}_{ij} + 0.587(0.184)\text{edu\_secondary}_{ij} + \\
&0.842(0.199)\text{edu\_higher}_{ij} + 0.076(0.050)\text{publicins}_{ij} + \\
&-0.009(0.061)\text{gpexper}_{j} + 0.029(0.056)\text{gpworkload}_{j} + \\
&0.235(0.113)\text{prac\_duo}_{j} + 0.158(0.131)\text{prac\_group}_{j} + \\
&0.353(0.157)\text{healthcentre}_{j} + 0.002(0.099)\text{suburb}_{j} + 0.205(0.122)\text{urban}_{j} \\
&0.613(0.205)\text{bigcity}_{j} + 0.221(0.094)\text{gpphysifr\_y}_{j}
\end{aligned}
$$

$$\beta_{0j} = -1.846(0.296) + u_{0j}$$

$$\left[u_{0j}\right] \sim \text{N}(0,\ \Omega_u) : \Omega_u = \left[0.196(0.030)\right]$$

Name + - Add Term Estimates Nonlinear Clear Notation Responses Store Help Zoom 100

We have now built our final model. GPs working in joint practice and those in health centres (which usually include physiotherapists) refer slightly more patients than those in solo practice. The odds of referral are increased among GPs working in one of the big cities (OR = 1.85; 95% C.I. 1.23, 2.76) and GPs who have physiotherapists as friends or acquaintances are also more likely to refer patients (OR = 1.25; 95% C.I. 1.04, 1.50). Neither the experience of the GP nor their workload appears to influence the likelihood of referring patients to physiotherapy.

Altogether the GP characteristics have reduced the variation between GPs from 0.230 in the previous model to 0.196 (a reduction of about 15%). Although we would expect the introduction of variables at the GP level to decrease the variance between GPs, calculation of the intraclass correlation coefficient shows that 5.6% of the unexplained variation in patient referrals is attributable to differences between GPs. The median odds ratio for this model is 1.52.

A Note on Estimation

The current estimation procedure, first order MQL, is known to produce biased estimates (Goldstein and Rasbash 1996; Rodríguez and Goldman 1995) although it is a reasonable tool for model building. In practice, we recommend that you obtain the final results that you wish to report using second order PQL estimation. (There are alternative methods of estimation available in MLwiN including the parametric bootstrap and Markov chain Monte Carlo or MCMC. Some other packages also include the option of maximum likelihood estimates obtained using numerical integration.) The screenshot below replicates our final model using second order PQL.

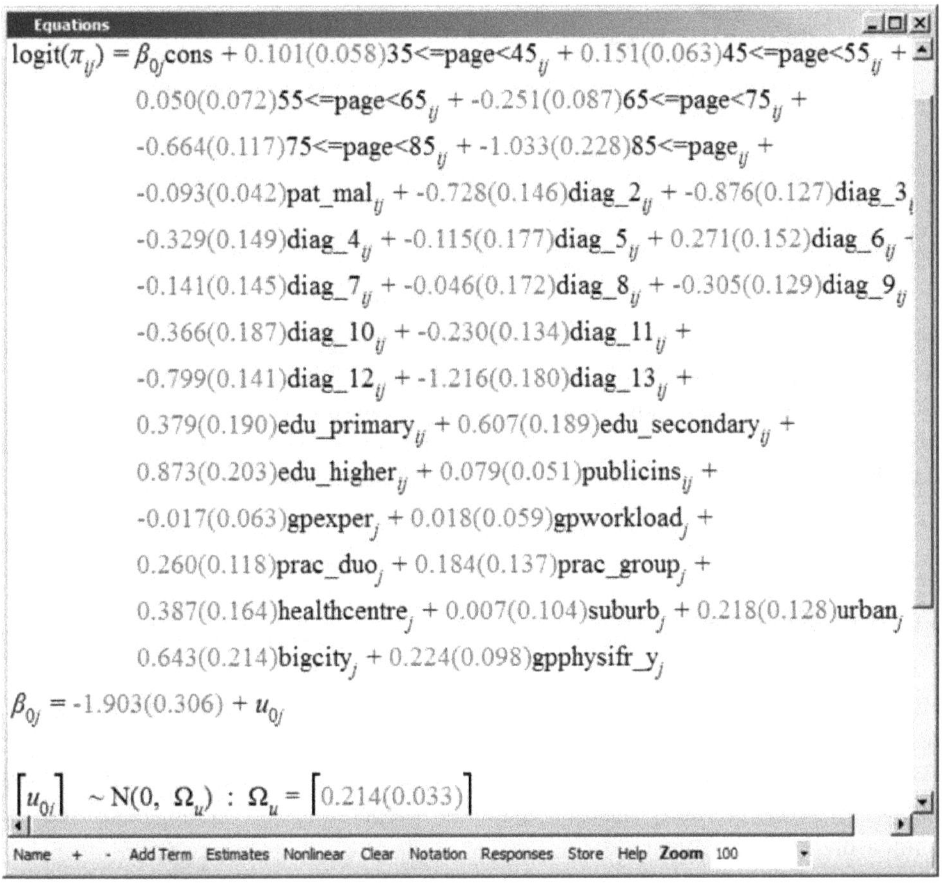

These estimates differ markedly from those obtained using first order MQL. The level 2 variance estimated using second order PQL is considerably larger giving an intraclass correlation coefficient of 0.061 and a median odds ratio of 1.56. There are also changes in the fixed part of the model; for example, the estimate of the odds ratio associated with the practice being located in a big city (compared to rural practices) has increased to 1.90 (95% C.I. 1.25, 2.90).

As for a linear multilevel model, we can calculate residuals for multilevel logistic regression models. The residuals from our final model are shown below for the 158 GPs.

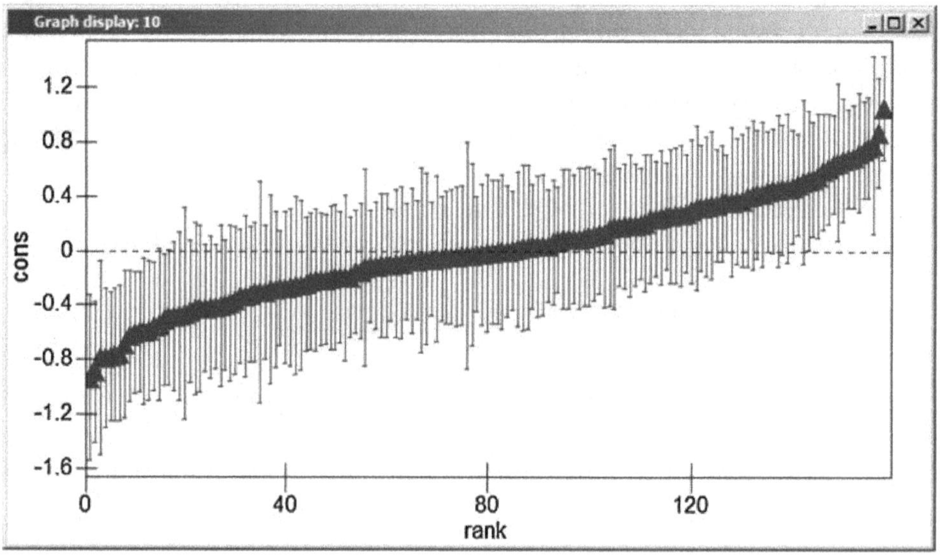

These residuals are now on a log odds scale; patients attending the GP with the largest residual (1.046) have an odds ratio of 2.85 (95% C.I. 1.94, 4.17) of being referred to chemotherapy relative to the average GP after taking patient and GP characteristics into account. Note the varying magnitude of the 95% confidence intervals around the GP residuals; those GPs about whom we have more data (i.e. those with more patients) have smaller confidence intervals.

Further Exercises

Explore the random slope variance for variables such as the insurance status of the patients. It was expected that privately insured patients would be referred less often. We did not find such an effect, but it might still be the case that *some* GPs are less likely to refer privately insured patients (depending on some measured or unmeasured GP variables).

Look at the GP residuals to check for outliers and explore the effects any outliers may have on the current model.

References

Goldstein H, Rasbash J (1996) Improved approximations for multilevel models with binary responses. J R Stat Soc Ser A 159:505–513
Lindenberg S (1996) Continuities in the theory of social production functions. In: Ganzeboom H, Lindenberg S (eds) Verklarende sociologie: opstellen voor Reinhard Wippler. Thesis Publishers, Amsterdam
McCullagh P, Nelder JA (1989) Generalized linear models, 2nd edn. Chapman & Hall/CRC, Boca Raton
Rodríguez G, Goldman N (1995) An assessment of estimation procedures for multilevel models with binary responses. J R Stat Soc Ser A 158:73–89
Skrondal A, Rabe-Hesketh S (2007) Redundant overdispersion parameters in multilevel models for categorical responses. J Educ Behav Stat 32:419–430
Snijders TAB, Bosker RJ (2012) Multilevel analysis: an introduction to basic and advanced multilevel modeling. Sage, Los Angeles
Uunk WJG, Groenewegen PP, Dekker J (1992) Verwijzingen van huisartsen naar fysiotherapeuten: een verklaring en analyse van verschillen tussen huisartsen. Mens en Maatschappij 67:389–411
Van der Velden K (1999) General practice at work: its contribution to epidemiology and health policy. NIVEL, PhD thesis Erasmus University, Utrecht

13

Untangling Contextual and Compositional Effects

Abstract This chapter contains a tutorial that helps to untangle contextual and compositional effects. We start from a typical, empty table and then proceed to fill this table. The example data set concerns patterns of incidence of cardiovascular disease in small areas in Scotland. The outcome or dependent variable is whether or not a survey respondent had self-reported doctor-diagnosed cardiovascular disease. The first step in the analysis is to estimate a null model. We then estimate the fixed effects of two individual-level variables, social class and smoking status, one by one. The final model looks at the fixed effects of all three variables. With these steps the empty table can be filled and we can interpret the results in terms of context and composition.

In this chapter, we describe the analysis of these data using MLwiN.

Keywords Tutorial · Multilevel analysis · Compositional effect · Contextual effects · Cardiovascular disease

As we pointed out in Chap. 7, there is frequent debate in the literature over the relative contributions of composition and context in the statistical explanation of individual-level outcomes, such as self-reported health and the incidence and prevalence of disease or mortality. This tutorial provides an application of the insights from Chap. 7. In this tutorial we will be looking at the patterning of the prevalence of cardiovascular diseases in Scotland. In particular, we consider whether the prevalence of disease is related to an individual social determinant (occupational social class), an individual biological determinant (current smoking status) or an area-based social determinant. As an area-based social determinant we used area deprivation measured by the Carstairs score, a Census-based variable derived from the social class of the heads of households, male unemployment, lack of car ownership and overcrowding (Carstairs 1995; Carstairs and Morris 1990). As with the previous two chapters, the software used in this chapter is MLwiN. Further details on multilevel modelling and MLwiN are available from the Centre for Multilevel Modelling http://www.bristol.ac.uk/cmm/. The materials have been written for MLwiN v3.01. The teaching version of the software is available from https://www.bristol.ac.uk/cmm/software/mlwin/download/.

The Data

The data are contained in the worksheet 'CVD-data.wsz' and are taken from the 1998 Scottish Health Survey, and the analysis is related to a published paper (Leyland 2005). The data refer to 8804 respondents aged between 18 and 64. The outcome considered is a self-report of a doctor-diagnosed cardiovascular disease (CVD) condition (angina, diabetes, hypertension, acute myocardial infarction, etc.). This is a binary response, whether (1) or not (0) respondents have CVD condition.

Names

Column: Name Description Toggle Categorical **Data:** View Copy Paste Delete

Name	Cn	n	missing	min	max	categorical
age	1	8804	0	18	74	False
sex	2	8804	0	1	2	True
sc	3	8804	0	1	3	True
cvddef	4	8804	0	0	1	False
carstair	5	8804	0	-6.2300...	12.5299...	False
smoke	6	8804	0	1	5	True
id	7	8804	0	1	8842	False
area	8	8804	0	1	312	False
cons	9	8804	0	1	1	False
age3	10	8804	0	5832	405224	False
age3*ln(age)	11	8804	0	16856.6...	174411...	False
f.age3	12	8804	0	0	405224	False
f.age3*ln(age)	13	8804	0	0	174411...	False
f	14	8804	0	0	1	False
bcons.1	15	8804	0	1	1	False
denom	16	8804	0	1	1	False
c17	17	0	0	0	0	False

The independent variables at individual level on which we focus in the tutorial are social class and smoking status. Occupational social class is used in three categories: high social class (1 and 2: professional and managerial), intermediate (3: skilled workers), and low (4 and 5 and missing: semiskilled and unskilled manual workers and those for whom social class was missing). Smoking has been categorised as never smoked, light smokers (<10 cigarettes per day), moderate (10–19) and heavy (20+) smokers as well as former smokers. Age and sex are used as control variables in all analyses. At the area level the Carstairs index is used as a continuous variable.

The survey was cluster-sampled, with respondents clustered within 312 small areas (postcode sector, average population about 5500).

Structure of the Analysis

As a first exploratory step in the analysis, examine the mean Carstairs score by social class and current smoking, and also smoking patterns by social class, to see the dependency between the variables.

After that, we are going to examine a series of models with a view to determining the relationship between the prevalence of CVD diseases and individual social class, current smoking and area deprivation. We will conduct these analyses with a table in mind, filling in the table as we progress (see Table 13.1).

Estimating the Null Model

The first model to fit is a null model. We will adjust all of the models we fit for age and sex, but we are not going to report the estimates associated with these factors; these are 'nuisance variables' and we are going to control for differences between areas in their age and sex composition.

We then set up a two-level model with the response variable CVDDEF and with levels defined by AREA and ID. This is a binomial response with a logit link function and with the denominator given by the constant CONS. We will add CONS to the fixed part of the model and allow for random intercepts across areas by letting the coefficient of CONS vary at random at level 2 (i.e. across areas). It is important that we have a well-fitting model at individual level, otherwise unmeasured individual effects might appear as contextual effects. We have used fractional polynomials in age (Royston et al. 1999) together with interactions with sex to find a parsimonious model that adequately controls for age and sex; these are already included in the model that can be found in the **Equations** window. We can start off by fitting this model using the first order MQL approximation but then move on to the second order PQL approximation. This is then the null model on which we base subsequent analyses.

Table 13.1 Outline of a table to report the analysis to untangle context and composition

		Null		Social class		Smoking		Deprivation		Social class + deprivation		Smoking + deprivation	
Variable		OR	CI	OR	CI	OR	CI	OR	CI	OR	CI	OR	CI
	Fixed part												
Social class													
	1&2			Baseline						Baseline			
	3												
	4&5												
	p												
Smoking													
	<10												
	10 < 20												
	20+												
	Ex-smoker												
	Never smoked					Baseline						Baseline	
	p												
Area deprivation													
	p												
	Random part												
Area variance													
Individual variance		[a]		[a]		[a]		[a]		[a]		[a]	
ICC													
R^2													

[a]Individual variance for multilevel logistic regression models approximated by $\pi^2/3$ (Snijders and Bosker 2012)

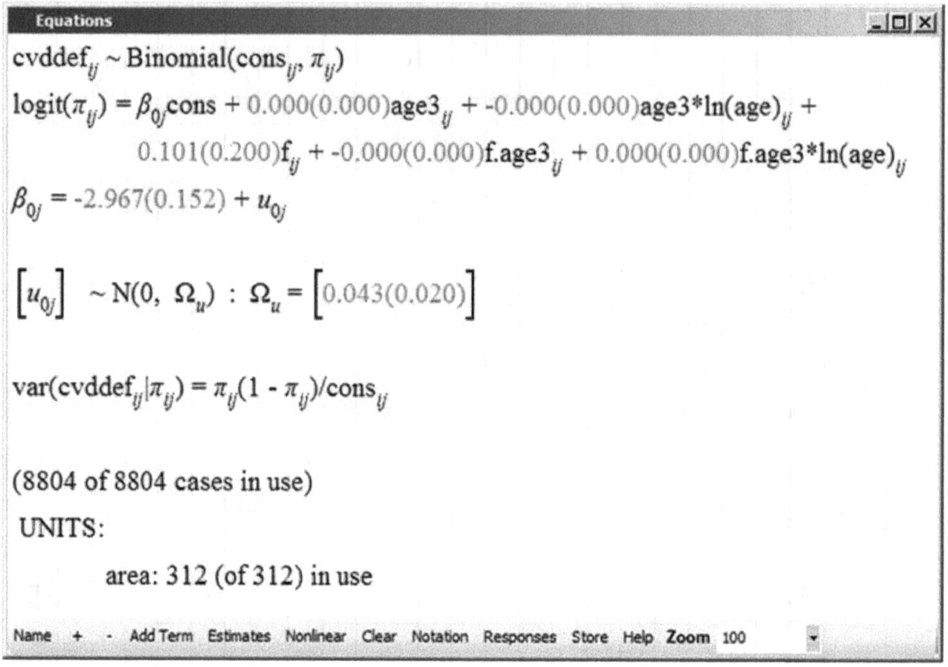

We can estimate the ICC from this model using the approximation that the individual-level variance is given by $\pi^2/3$ (= 3.290). So a level 2 variance of 0.043 gives an ICC of 0.013; just over 1% of the variation in the prevalence of CVD diseases is attributable to differences between areas.

A useful diagnostic measure is the R-squared which indicates how much of the total variation has been explained by the fixed part of the model. For multilevel logistic regression, we approximate the explained variation by the variance of the linear predictor (that is, the variance of the fixed part of the model which is on a log odds scale) and get the total variance by adding the variance of the linear predictor to the variance at the higher levels plus our estimate of the variance at the individual level. In other words,

$$R^2 = \mathrm{VLP}/\left(\mathrm{VLP} + \sigma_{u0}^2 + \pi^2/3\right)$$

where VLP is the variance of the linear predictor. We can calculate the linear predictor using the Predictions window and including all variables in the fixed part (but not the random part).

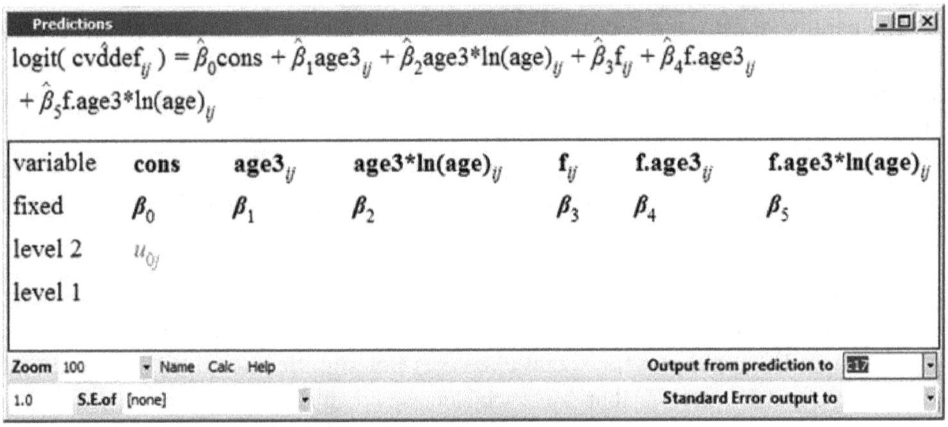

We can use the **Averages and correlations** window to estimate the standard deviation of this prediction as 0.921. The variance is the square of the standard deviation; this gives VLP = 0.848 and so R-squared = 20.3%.

The values of the ICC, VLP and R-squared can be obtained for any two-level multilevel logistic regression model by running the macro 'modeldiag.txt'. (To run the macro make sure that the output window of the **Command interface** is open, then open the macro using the **File** menu and click **Execute**.)

Fixed Effects

The first model that we want to fit is the model containing individual social class (variable SC). There are three categories of social class; we will fit two dummy variables keeping social class 1 and 2 as the reference category.

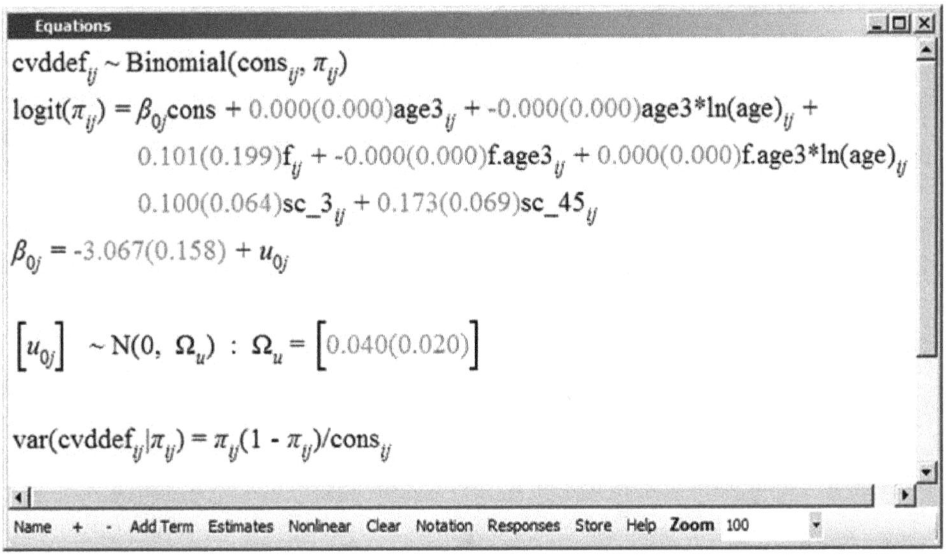

The parameter estimate for social class 3 is a log odds ratio; we can convert this to an odds ratio by exponentiating: $\exp\{0.100\} = 1.105$, so the odds of CVD diseases are 10.5% higher in social class 3 than in social classes 1 and 2. Similarly we can obtain 95% confidence intervals as $\exp\{0.100 \pm 1.96 \times 0.064\} = (0.975, 1.253)$. Since the 95% confidence interval for this odds ratio includes 1, it suggests that the odds ratio for social class 3 is not significantly different from that for social classes 1 and 2.

Odds ratios and 95% confidence intervals can be obtained for all parameter estimates from any logistic regression model by running the macro 'or.txt'.

Although the odds ratio for social class 3 is not significantly different from that for social classes 1 and 2, that for social classes 4 and 5 is significant (the 95% confidence intervals do not include 1). Since we would expect the social class effect to increase across social class categories—CVD prevalence is likely to be higher in social class 3 than in social classes 1 and 2, and higher still among social classes 4 and 5 than in social class 3—we test for a linear trend in the social class variable. We do this by removing the categorical social class variable from the model, fitting social class using a continuous variable created for this purpose (i.e. with values 1, 2 and 3) and testing for the significance of this single variable. This can be done using the **Intervals and tests** window from the **Model** menu.

We can now continue by fitting models containing just smoking and just deprivation (again including age and sex as these were contained in the null model). (Click on a variable in the **Equations** window and choose **Delete term** to remove it from the current model.)

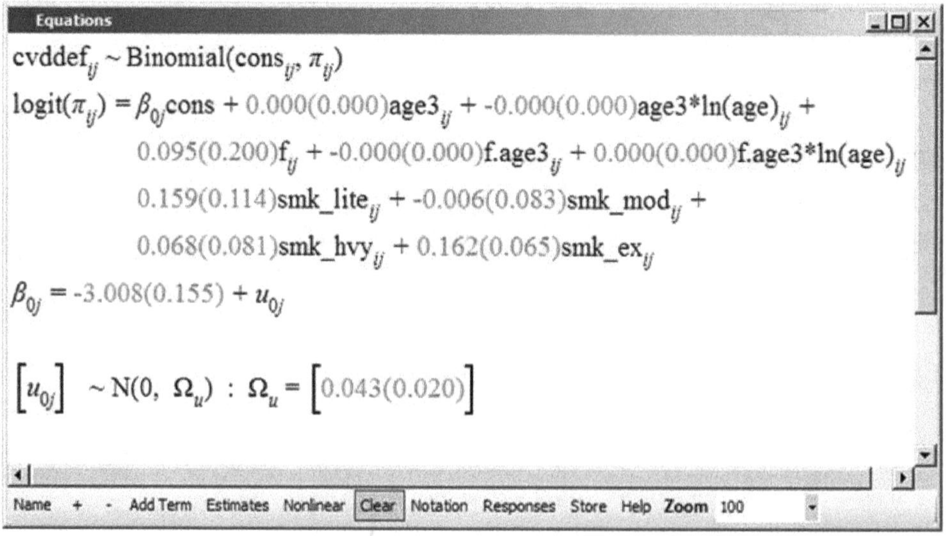

Compared to the reference group of never smokers, the prevalence of CVD diseases is no higher in any of the smoking categories but is significantly higher among the ex-smokers. As a prevalence study this may reflect an increased likelihood of giving up smoking once a respondent has been told by a doctor that they have a cardiovascular disease. The categories of smoking are not ordered and so testing the significance of this variable involves testing the significance of differences between categories rather than a test for trend.

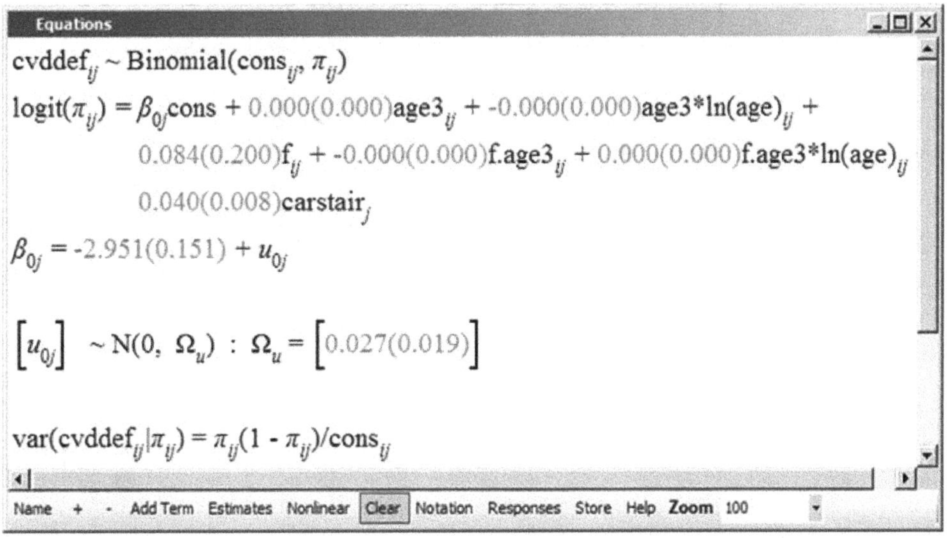

Area deprivation is coded with positive values indicating areas of higher deprivation and negative values indicating areas of lower deprivation. The effect of deprivation is clearly significant; we can consider whether the effects of social class and smoking are significant after controlling for area deprivation. At the same time we will see whether the effect of area deprivation remains significant once individual factors are taken into account. The significant effect of individual social class is attenuated and becomes non-significant when area deprivation is taken into account whilst area deprivation remains significantly related to the prevalence of CVD diseases. The effect of individual smoking status remains insignificant following adjustment for area deprivation.

Basically, with these models we can complete Table 13.1 such that it becomes Table 13.2. This presents a neat summary of the fixed and random parts of the models that we have fitted. The strong influence of the context can be seen through the persistent significance of the area deprivation score even after adjustment for individual factors.

Table 13.2 Estimates from model

		Null		Social class		Smoking		Deprivation		Social class + deprivation		Smoking + deprivation	
Variable		OR	CI	OR	CI	OR	CI	OR	CI	OR	CI	OR	CI
	Fixed part												
Social class													
	1&2			Baseline						Baseline			
	3			1.11	(0.97, 1.25)					1.07	(0.94, 1.21)		
	4&5			1.19	(1.04, 1.36)					1.12	(0.97, 1.28)		
	p			0.012						0.123			
Smoking													
	<10					1.17	(0.94, 1.47)					1.15	(0.92, 1.43)
	10 < 20					0.99	(0.84, 1.17)					0.95	(0.80, 1.12)
	20+					1.07	(0.91, 1.26)					1.01	(0.86, 1.19)
	Ex-smoker					1.18	(1.03, 1.34)					1.18	(1.03, 1.34)
	Never smoked					Baseline						Baseline	
	p					0.093						0.053	
Area deprivation													
								1.04	(1.02, 1.06)	1.04	(1.02, 1.06)	1.04	(1.03, 1.06)
	p							0.000		0.000		0.000	
	Random part												
Area variance		0.043		0.040		0.043		0.027		0.026		0.026	
Individual variance		[a]		[a]		[a]		[a]		[a]		[a]	
ICC		0.013		0.012		0.013		0.008		0.008		0.008	
R^2		0.203		0.203		0.204		0.207		0.207		0.208	

[a]Individual variance for multilevel logistic regression models approximated by $\pi^2/3$ (Snijders and Bosker 2012)

Additional Models

There are a variety of other models that we may wish to fit. One of the reasons for the closer relationship between the Carstairs score and the prevalence of CVD diseases may be because the Carstairs score is a continuous variable—indicating a broad range of deprivation—whilst our measure of occupational social class is categorical with just three categories. To satisfy our curiosity that this is not just a measurement issue, we can categorise the deprivation measure into three approximately equal groups and fit some of these models again.

As we discussed in Chap. 3, contextual variables may be direct observations made on areas detailing, for example, the provision of services. They may be derived from alternative data sources (as in this case: the Carstairs score is based on Census variables). Another possibility is to create contextual variables through the aggregation of individual variables collected in the study. Think about creating a contextual variable describing the social class of the neighbourhood. A simple example would be the proportion of the survey respondents in each area who were in social classes 4 and 5; an alternative might be the difference between the proportion in social classes 4 and 5 and the proportion in social classes 1 and 2. Such variables can be created using the **Multilevel data manipulations** window found under the **Data manipulation** menu. These variables permit further examination of the relative importance of composition versus context, given that both descriptors are derived from the same source, but also illustrate how an important contextual descriptor can be created within the data set in the absence of an externally validated measure such as the Carstairs score.

The aggregation of an individual variable to an area level can change its interpretation. We can construct an area-based smoking score to illustrate this. If an individual is given a score of 3 for a heavy smoker, 2 for a moderate smoker, 1 for a light smoker and 0 for an ex-smoker or a non-smoker, then the average of this score at an area level provides information about current smoking behaviour in an area in terms both of smoking prevalence and dose. The relationship of such a variable to the prevalence of CVD diseases is different to the relationship between individual smoking behaviour and CVD disease prevalence; the area smoking score—just like the area social class score—acts as a marker of area deprivation.

References

Carstairs V (1995) Deprivation indices: their interpretation and use in relation to health. J Epidemiol Community Health 49(Suppl 2):S3–S8

Carstairs V, Morris R (1990) Deprivation and health in Scotland. Health Bull 48:162–175

Leyland AH (2005) Socioeconomic gradients in the prevalence of cardiovascular disease in Scotland: the roles of composition and context. J Epidemiol Community Health 59:799–803

Royston P, Ambler G, Sauerbrei W (1999) The use of fractional polynomials to model continuous risk variables in epidemiology. Int J Epidemiol 28:964–974

Snijders TAB, Bosker RJ (2012) Multilevel analysis: an introduction to basic and advanced multilevel modeling. Sage, Los Angeles

Permissions

All chapters in this book were first published by Springer by Alastair H. Leyland & Peter P. Groenewegen; hereby published with permission under the Creative Commons Attribution License or equivalent. Every chapter published in this book has been scrutinized by our experts. Their significance has been extensively debated. The topics covered herein carry significant information for a comprehensive understanding. They may even be implemented as practical applications or may be referred to as a beginning point for further studies.

We would like to thank the editorial team for lending their expertise to make the book truly unique. They have played a crucial role in the development of this book. Without their invaluable contributions this book wouldn't have been possible. They have made vital efforts to compile up to date information on the varied aspects of this subject to make this book a valuable addition to the collection of many professionals and students.

This book was conceptualized with the vision of imparting up-to-date and integrated information in this field. To ensure the same, a matchless editorial board was set up. Every individual on the board went through rigorous rounds of assessment to prove their worth. After which they invested a large part of their time researching and compiling the most relevant data for our readers.

The editorial board has been involved in producing this book since its inception. They have spent rigorous hours researching and exploring the diverse topics which have resulted in the successful publishing of this book. They have passed on their knowledge of decades through this book. To expedite this challenging task, the publisher supported the team at every step. A small team of assistant editors was also appointed to further simplify the editing procedure and attain best results for the readers.

Apart from the editorial board, the designing team has also invested a significant amount of their time in understanding the subject and creating the most relevant covers. They scrutinized every image to scout for the most suitable representation of the subject and create an appropriate cover for the book.

The publishing team has been an ardent support to the editorial, designing and production team. Their endless efforts to recruit the best for this project, has resulted in the accomplishment of this book. They are a veteran in the field of academics and their pool of knowledge is as vast as their experience in printing. Their expertise and guidance has proved useful at every step. Their uncompromising quality standards have made this book an exceptional effort. Their encouragement from time to time has been an inspiration for everyone.

The publisher and the editorial board hope that this book will prove to be a valuable piece of knowledge for students, practitioners and scholars across the globe.

Index

Printed in the USA
CPSIA information can be obtained
at www.ICGtesting.com
JSHW051352091023
49903JS00006B/125

9 781646 475896